Substance and Non-Substance Related Addictions

Evaristo Akerele
Editor

Substance and Non-Substance Related Addictions

A Global Approach

Springer

Editor
Evaristo Akerele
Department of Psychiatry
New Jersey Medical School
Rutgers University
Newark, NJ, USA

ISBN 978-3-030-84833-0 ISBN 978-3-030-84834-7 (eBook)
https://doi.org/10.1007/978-3-030-84834-7

This Springer imprint is published by the registered company Springer Nature Switzerland AG
The registered company address is: Gewerbestrasse 11, 6330 Cham, Switzerland

I dedicate this book to my mother Elizabeth Folashade Akerele (nee Daniel), SRN, SCM

Foreword

I was so happy to be asked by Dr. Akerele to write the foreword for this very important book. The recognition and treatment of substance use disorders (SUD) has never been more important. So many major developments are underway that it is impossible to include mention of them all.

With regard to the opioid crisis, we are still losing the battle with more than 93,000 drug overdoses in 2020, the highest number ever reported in US history. The isolation and economic pressures of the COVID-19 pandemic are certainly contributing to the increased numbers of not only opioid use but also alcohol, tobacco, cocaine, and methamphetamine. Prescription opioid misuse is still a major problem, in addition to the increased availability of fentanyl and its derivatives in the illicit drug supply.

On other fronts, cannabis use is also climbing, with more daily users and individuals with cannabis use disorder, as a result. Changing attitudes about drug policy and legalization are creating a seismic shift in the culture and resulting in new conversations about substance use and substance use disorders. While some of this is undoubtably good and will help reduce stigma as well as racial bias and decriminalization, changes are coming so fast that one wonders how much the public really comprehends in these complex debates. The rising use of psychostimulants, both recreationally and as possible therapeutic agents, is another rapidly developing area with many unknowns. Medical decision-making by state ballot initiative is generally not prudent and, in many cases, overreaches available evidence. Legalization and federal drug classification are being considered seriously for the first time, and the USA can look to its global partners for some implementation models.

Juxtaposed with these changing public attitudes and increased drug use patterns is a dearth of education in substance use disorders, especially for healthcare providers. Current training of physicians in the recognition and treatment of SUD is felt by many to be inadequate to meet the needs of such a diverse and growing population of patients. The scope of training on SUDs is disproportionate to the population health need to address these problems, and many with SUDs go undiagnosed and untreated. Despite marked advances in the science of addiction, which includes an expanding range of evidence-based pharmacologic and behavioral treatments, the educational requirements in psychiatry and other medical training specialties have not shifted, leaving many ill prepared to manage SUDs in practice. This book can help to fill the gap by providing current evidence that is accessible to many types of audiences.

In addition, too often materials are limited to only a US or Western perspective. Consideration of the global impact of substance abuse disorders is a major achievement of this book. In addition to the designated chapters, a global perspective is integrated throughout, with regard to regional, epidemiological, cultural, and treatment issues, making this a unique and timely resource.

The addition of a whole new set of behavioral addictions warrants additional attention as well. In addition to gambling, new neuroscience has brought greater understanding and insights into how we view other compulsive behaviors including sex and food addiction. All clinicians need to recognize Internet addiction and consider the influence of technology and social media on clients they serve.

This book provides many clinical pearls and gives perspectives on an ever-changing human problem of addiction. The experts who have contributed are well regarded as thought leaders in the field. I hope you will find it as a great resource as I have.

Jill M. Williams, MD
Professor of Psychiatry and Director of the Division of Addiction Psychiatry
Rutgers University-Robert Wood Johnson Medical School
New Brunswick, NJ, USA

Preface

Substance use disorder is a significant public health issue. As a physician, I have had the opportunity to work with individuals struggling with this disease. In this brief introduction, I highlight the social issues, my experience in the field, and the global relevance of this disease.

The social, economic, and financial impact on lives of both patients and their families have become evident to me. In most cases, substance use culminates in loss of home, job, and relationships as well as significant medical issues. Family members such as children and spouses are secondary victims with significant trauma sequelae. In addition to these Herculean challenges, individuals with substance use disorder have to confront the immense societal stigma associated with drug use. The stigma exists in multiple strata which include but are not limited to the general public and medical field and individuals with substance disorders. The public generally see individuals with substance use disorders as being responsible for their own plight; therefore, they have less empathy for such individuals. In the medical field, substance use, until quite recently, was significantly marginalized. In psychiatry, treatment and training in substance use disorders was not a top priority.

As a result, access to care is often much more challenging for individuals with substance use disorders. Furthermore, social stigma is further aggravated by the pecking order that exists among individuals with substance use disorder. Individuals with alcohol use disorder are at the very top of the totem pole. The situation has gradually improved in recent years.

I have been fortunate to work with this population from a variety of perspectives. Initially as a clinician, then as a researcher at Columbia University working on pharmacological treatments for substance use. Later on, I continued to work with this patient population from various positions of leadership, which included Vice President and Chair of Psychiatry and Behavioral Health, Vice President of Medical Affairs at Phoenix House, United Nations Consultant, and several national positions in the American Psychiatric Association.

As professionals, we have focused on substance use disorders as they affect primarily the United States of America. During my service as a consultant for the United Nations, I became painfully aware of the global impact of substance use disorders. Often these global perspectives are not shared with our students, residents, and fellows. I felt a need to change this narrative. In addition to the glaring absence of global substance use disorder, I became aware that there is a dearth of literature on the identification and treatment of behavioral disorders such compulsive sexual behavior (sex addiction), gambling, and food and Internet addiction. As a researcher and educator, I realized the need to fill this gap and provide a truly comprehensive education on addiction to the next generation of leaders in this field.

In this book I have tried to address all the issues elucidated above. I have brought non-substance behavioral disorders out of the shadows to be placed vis-a-vis substance use disorders. I have attempted to introduce the concept of substance use disorders as a global challenge. Finally, I have included both established leaders and emerging future leaders of our field.

I wish to acknowledge all the contributors to this book for their time-consuming effort and dedication. Special thanks to my past and present colleagues at Columbia, Rutgers, Interfaith, Harlem, and Mount Sinai, without whom this book would not have been possible. There is an old African proverb that states, "it takes a village to raise a child." I would go one step further by saying it takes the world to successfully address this public health challenge. Finally I want to thank my children, Andreea, Christa and Anna.

Newark, NJ, USA Evaristo Olanrewaju Akerele

Contents

Contributors

Evaristo Akerele, MD, MPH, DFAPA Department of Psychiatry, New Jersey Medical School, Rutgers University, Newark, NJ, USA

Tiffany Christian Mount Sinai Morningside Hospital, New York, NY, USA

Eric D. Collins, MD Columbia University Vagelos College of Physicians & Surgeons, New York, NY, USA

Naomi Dambreville, MA The City College of New York, New York, NY, USA

CUNY Graduate Center, New York, NY, USA

Ralph Fader The Mount Sinai Hospital, New York, NY, USA

Michael Ferguson Department of Psychiatry and Behavioral Medicine, Virginia Tech Carilion School of Medicine, St. Roanoke, VA, USA

Tiesha T. Gregory Department of Psychology, Columbia University, New York, NY, USA

Diego Garces Grosse, MD Rutgers New Jersey Medical School, Newark, NJ, USA

Marc Grifell Guàrdia Department of Psychology, Columbia University, New York, NY, USA

Department of Psychiatry and Legal Medicine, Universitat Autònoma de Barcelona, Cerdanyola del Vallés and IMIM (Hospital del Mar Medical Research Institute), Bellaterra, Spain

Sasidhar Gunturu, MD BronxCare Health System, Icahn School of Medicine, New York, NY, USA

Columbia University, New York, NY, USA

Carl L. Hart, PhD Department of Psychology, Columbia University, New York, NY, USA

Division on Substance Abuse, New York State Psychiatric Institute and Department of Psychiatry, Columbia University Irving Medical Center, Vagelos College of Physicians and Surgeons, New York, NY, USA

Mariely Hernandez, MA The City College of New York, New York, NY, USA

CUNY Graduate Center, New York, NY, USA

Oluwole Jegede, MD, MPH Department of Psychiatry and Behavioral Sciences, Yale University, New Haven, Connecticut, USA

Panagiota Korenis, MD BronxCare Health System, Icahn School of Medicine, New York, NY, USA

Albert Einstein College of Medicine, St. George's University School of Medicine, West Indies, Grenada

Frances Rudnick Levin, MD Columbia University Medical Center, New York, NY, USA

New York State Psychiatric Institute, New York, NY, USA

Christopher Medina-Kirchner Department of Psychology, Columbia University, New York, NY, USA

Paroma Mitra, MD, MPH Bellevue Hospital Center, New York University Grossman School of Medicine, New York, NY, USA

Nidal Moukaddam, MD, PhD Menninger Department of Psychiatry & Behavioral Sciences, Baylor College of Medicine, Houston, TX, USA

Mohammad Naqvi, MD Department of Investigational Cancer Therapeutics, The University of Texas MD Anderson Cancer Center, Houston, TX, USA

Olawale Ojo, MD, MSc Interfaith Medical Center, Brooklyn, NY, USA

Olaniyi Olayinka, MD, MPH Department of Psychiatry and Behavioral Sciences, Interfaith Medical Center, Brooklyn, NY, USA

Tolulope Olupona, MD Psychiatry Residency Training Program, Interfaith Medical Center, Brooklyn, NY, USA

Tolu Olupona Department of Psychiatry and Behavioral Sciences, Interfaith Medical Center, Brooklyn, NY, USA

Kate O'Malley Department of Psychological Sciences, Swinburne University, Hawthorn, VIC, Australia

Biren Patel, MD Behavioral Health, Kelsey-Seybold Clinics, Houston, TX, USA

Neelambika Revadigar, MD Columbia University, New York, NY, USA

Isabelle Silverstone-Simard, MD, FRCPC McGill University, Montreal, QC, Canada

Maria A. Sullivan Department of Psychiatry, Columbia University College of Physicians and Surgeons, New York State Psychiatric Institute, New York, NY, USA

Samantha Swetter Dartmouth's Geisel School of Medicine, Hanover, NH, USA

Brentt Swetter, MS, MEd Tarrytown, NY, USA

Geoffrey Talis, MD, MS Rutgers NJMS University Hospital, Newark, NJ, USA

Anil A. Thomas, MD Department of Psychiatry, NYU Grossman School of Medicine, New York, NY, USA

Khai Tran, MD BronxCare Health System, Icahn School of Medicine, New York, NY, USA

Jeffery J. Wilson, MD, DFAACAP Department of Psychiatry and Behavioral Medicine, Virginia Tech Carilion School of Medicine, St. Roanoke, VA, USA

Ching Tary Yu, MD, FRCPC Columbia University, New York, NY, USA

Part I

Comorbid and Age Related Drug Use

1 Drug Use and Mental Health: Comorbidity between Substance Use and Psychiatric Disorders

Maria A. Sullivan

Introduction

The co-occurrence of substance use disorders (SUDs) and non-substance use psychiatric disorders is commonly referred to as dual diagnosis. This comorbidity is most common for mood disorders, especially depression. Along with environmental risks, a genetic predisposition is believed to underlie the development of comorbid disorders [46]. Dual diagnosis is of great concern because it is often associated with higher disease severity, poor physical and social functioning, increased rates of psychiatric hospitalization including emergency admissions, self-harm, and suicide [39, 81, 83, 98]. In addition, comorbid drug users have an increased rate of high-risk behaviors and sexually transmitted infections (e.g., HIV), as well as more psychosocial impairments such as unemployment and homelessness, and high rates of violent and criminal behavior [98].

Clinical management of individuals with dual diagnosis can pose unique challenges In a large US national sample, Krawczyk et al. [50] found that 28% of patients discharged from substance treatment facilities had psychiatric comorbidity and 38% did not complete treatment. Clients with psychiatric comorbidity had higher odds of not completing either alcohol or substance treatment, as well as an earlier time to attrition, relative to those without comorbidity. Individuals with psychiatric comorbidities seeking or receiving treatment for substance use disorders face particular challenges that affect their ability to complete treatment. And conversely, the presence of a comorbid substance use disorder is associated with a poor response to treatment for many psychiatric disorders. In this chapter, we describe evidence for the prevalence of co-occurring psychiatric disorders and substance use disorders and the effects of this comorbidity on treatment course. We suggest that these findings call for further efforts to integrate treatment for psychiatric comorbidities in substance use treatment settings.

Epidemiology: Prevalence of Psychiatric and Substance Use Disorder Comorbidity

Comorbidity of Substance Use Disorder (SUD) and Anxiety Disorders

Numerous studies with different methods have shown a significant association between anxiety disorders and alcohol use disorders [77]. Recent epidemiological studies have reported lifetime prevalence rates of 23.5% alcohol dependence and 20.4% alcohol misuse in patients with social

M. A. Sullivan (✉)
Department of Psychiatry, Columbia University College of Physicians and Surgeons, New York State Psychiatric Institute, New York, NY, USA
e-mail: mas23@cumc.columbia.edu

E. Akerele (ed.), *Substance and Non-Substance Related Addictions*,
https://doi.org/10.1007/978-3-030-84834-7_1

phobia [27]. Conversely, the lifetime prevalence of social anxiety disorder among patients with alcohol dependence is about 11% [70]. Anxiety symptoms are associated with a worse course of alcohol use disorder, marked by early relapse following detoxification [88].

Using data from the 2001–2002 National Epidemiologic Survey on Alcohol and Related Conditions (N = 43,093) and the Alcohol Use Disorder and Associated Disabilities Interview Schedule-DSM-IV Version as the diagnostic instrument, Alegria et al. [2] determined that GAD-SUD (2.04%) constitutes half of the lifetime prevalence of GAD (4.14%) in the US adult population. With respect to lifetime risk factors, individuals with GAD-SUD were more likely than those with GAD-NSUD to have had a vulnerable family environment, a family history of antisocial behavior, and a family history of AUD/SUD. The onset of SUD preceded the onset of GAD among those with GAD-SUD, suggesting that SUD, at least in some cases, may facilitate the initiation of GAD. Furthermore, GAD-SUD is associated with high overall vulnerability for additional psychopathology, particularly in the externalizing spectrum, as well as higher disability. Individuals with GAD-SUD also had significantly higher rates of use of alcohol and drugs to relieve symptoms of anxiety among those with GAD-NSUD; this behavior may provide temporary relief from the anxiety symptoms, but may increase symptoms in the long term. Taken together, these findings suggest a stronger predisposition for psychopathology among individuals with GAD-SUD that is further exacerbated by the use of substances [2].

A complex comorbidity exists between alcohol use disorder (AUD) and post-traumatic stress disorder. Because of the associations between at-risk drinking, violence, and accidents, individuals with AUD are frequently exposed to extreme stress and the subsequent development of PTSD [13, 58]. The externalizing disorders common in AUD (e.g., attention-deficit/hyperactivity disorder, conduct disorder, and antisocial personality disorder) are also associated with impulsive and risk-taking behaviors leading to trauma [16].

Post-traumatic stress disorder (PTSD) also conveys an increased risk for the development of substance use disorders (SUD). In patients diagnosed with PTSD, the prevalence of comorbid substance use ranges from 19% to 35% and comorbid alcohol abuse ranges from 36% to 52% [82, 84]. Among patients with PTSD, opioid use disorder is a less common but increasing comorbidity. In a large patient population of veterans who initiated PTSD treatment in the Department of Veterans Affairs (VA) between 2004 and 2013 ($N = 731{,}520$), comorbid opioid use disorder diagnoses increased from 2.5% in 2004 to 3.4% in 2013. Patients with comorbid opioid use disorder used more health services and had more comorbidities than other patients with PTSD [91].

Emotional processing theory posits that PTSD symptoms are maintained, in part, by negative trauma-related cognitions about the world as entirely dangerous and the self as entirely incompetent [25]. Recovery from PTSD therefore involves modifying these cognitions; this is the mechanism by which negative cognitions mediate change in PTSD symptoms during exposure therapy [63]. PTSD often precedes SUD, and a recent analysis revealed that frequency and intensity of negative alterations in cognition and mood predicted alcohol use disorder (AUD), but re-experiencing symptoms, hyperarousal, and avoidance did not [11]. These findings suggest that those who experience negative alterations in cognition and mood may be at increased risk of developing AUD, and that we may be able to predict which individuals in clinical settings will be strong candidates for new combined PTSD/SUD treatments. For instance, prolonged exposure therapy and oral naltrexone for reducing alcohol use among those with comorbid PTSD/AD exert a combined effect through reduction in both PTSD symptoms and craving (McLean et al. 2015).

Comorbid PTSD/SUD is associated with a more complex and costly clinical course when compared with either disorder alone, including increased chronic physical health problems, poorer social functioning, higher rates of suicide attempts, more legal problems, increased risk of violence, worse treatment adherence, and less improvement during treatment [57]. In the treatment of comorbid PTSD/SUD, pharmacotherapy should not replace trauma-specific psychotherapy [77], and psychosocial interventions are the preferred treatment model.

Comorbidity of SUD and Mood Disorders

In the United States, the lifetime prevalence of illicit drug abuse is estimated at 19.4% in mood disorders [47] and 24% in major depressive disorder [104]. The presence of drug abuse has been shown to increase the risk for depression fivefold [81, 83]. Using the 2001–2 National Epidemiologic Survey on Alcohol and Related Conditions (NESARC) as a representative sample of the US adult population (N = 43,093), Blanco et al. [10] found that the lifetime prevalence of major depressive disorder without SUD (MDD-NSUD) was 7.41%, whereas that of MDD-SUD was 5.82% and the prevalence of substance-induced mood disorder was quite low, at 0.26%. The researchers noted that a family history of psychopathology and most childhood and adulthood risk factors were more common in MDD-SUD than in MDD-NSUD. Similarly, Sher et al. [90] reported that individuals with MDD and alcohol use disorder (AUD) were more likely to have a family history of AUD and abuse during childhood than those with MDD and no AUD comorbidity. The results by Blanco et al. [10] suggest that SUD is a marker for greater severity in individuals with MDD; MDD-SUD is characterized by earlier age at MDD onset, higher number of MDD criteria met, higher number of depressive episodes, and higher rates of psychiatric comorbidity, compared to MDD-NSUD. Further, some risk factors – such as a family history of psychopathology -- may not be disorder-specific but, instead, shared between MDD and SUD [60].

Compared to other psychiatric disorders, the rates of comorbidity with alcohol use disorder are highest in bipolar disorder. In the Epidemiological Catchment Area (ECA) Study [81, 83], frequencies of 46.2 and 39.2%, respectively, for bipolar I and II were reported. Recent epidemiologic studies (NESARC; [8]) found frequencies of 54.6% and 51.8% for bipolar I and bipolar II disorders. Among bipolar patients, male gender, history of higher number of manic episodes, and previous history of suicidality are associated with higher susceptibility to substance use disorder (SUD). Thus, in individuals with bipolar disorder at increased risk of drug abuse, more intensive therapeutic interventions should be considered to prevent development of SUD [61]. Further, bipolar disorder is associated with an increased risk of behavioral addictions; pathological gambling and kleptomania are the most prevalent conditions, followed by compulsive buying, compulsive sexual behavior, and internet addiction [103].

A recent study examined co-occurrence of tobacco use, substance use, and mental health problems, and its moderation by gender, among 32,202 US adults from Wave 1 (2013–2014) of the nationally representative longitudinal Population Assessment of Tobacco and Health (PATH) Study. In this nationally representative sample of US adults, Conway et al. (2017) demonstrated that female tobacco users are at increased risk for substance use and mental health problems.

There has also been recent research examining depressive traits that appear to be prevalent in opioid use disorder. In a large (N = 1195) study of Italian heroin addicts, Maremmani et al. [59] identified five personality dimensions: “worthlessness and being trapped,” “somatic symptoms,” “sensitivity-psychoticism,” “panic-anxiety,” and “violence-suicide.” These clusters of traits – which were independent of demographic or clinical characteristics, as well as other substances used -- discriminated patients affected by substance use disorders from those affected by non-substance psychiatric disorders. The researchers concluded that these findings suggest that the SUDs result in a trait-dependent, rather than state-dependent, psychopathology. Similarly, there is evidence that certain personality disorders (i.e., antisocial and schizotypal) are particularly linked with chronicity in substance use disorders [7]. Even though the types of personality disorders seen in individuals with drug and alcohol use disorder are similar, the prevalence of any personality disorder is higher among patients with drug use disorder than alcohol use disorder [73].

Comorbidity of SUD and Schizophrenia

The schizophrenic psychoses have high comorbidity with both alcohol and substance use disorders. The lifetime prevalence of alcohol-related disorders with psychosis rose from 29% in the 1990s to 51% in 2019 [76]. Individuals with schizophrenia are also more likely than those without the disorder to smoke cigarettes, heavily use alcohol, heavily use cannabis, and use recreational drugs; these factors contribute to the premature mortality and increased disability observed in patients with schizophrenia [35]. Emerging data have revealed that individuals who smoke tobacco also have a two-fold increased risk of onset of schizophrenia spectrum disorders [89]. It appears that the smoking of tobacco may play a role in early information processing deficits observed in schizophrenia [79].

A recent meta-analysis of SUDs in epidemiological and treatment-seeking patients diagnosed with schizophrenia or first episode psychosis [41] found that the prevalence of any substance use disorder (SUD) was 41.7%, followed by illicit drugs (27.5%), cannabis (26.2%), alcohol (24.3%), and stimulant use (7.3%). Patients with SUD had an earlier age of onset of schizophrenia. A meta-regression showed that prevalence increased over time for illicit drugs but not for other substances, including alcohol. Further, a meta-analysis revealed that SUD in schizophrenia is highly prevalent, and rates have not changed over time. This finding indicates substance use disorders are difficult to treat in this patient population and more studies are needed to help develop better prevention, detection, and treatment of SUDs in persons with schizophrenia and comorbid disorders.

In an analysis of studies including individuals with psychosis who had a history of substance use, misuse, and dependency related to alcohol, cannabis, and cocaine, Donoghue et al. [22] analyzed how varying levels of use of each particular substance affected cognitive functioning. In contrast to what was expected, they found that individuals who used certain drugs performed better on some cognitive tests than those who did not use drugs. Specifically, cocaine users had better psychomotor processing speed and attention than non-users, but had deficits in memory and verbal ability. Individuals with psychosis who used cannabis had better overall functioning than those who did not use cannabis. The authors recommended caution in interpreting these findings, as individuals able to seek out and acquire drugs, despite the limitations of their psychosis, may be higher functioning and have more neurological capacity than their non-using peers. They noted that longitudinal studies are needed to enable an in-depth assessment of the extent of impairment resulting from long-term substance misuse.

Four theories have been advanced to explain the pathogenesis of the comorbidity between schizophrenia and SUD: (1) the self-medication hypothesis suggests that the use of substances ameliorates some symptoms of schizophrenia [48, 92], (2) schizophrenia and SUD share a common genetic mechanism involving dysregulation in the dopamine-regulated reward circuitry [14, 31, 85]; (3) diathesis-neural stress model: genetic predisposition, combined with the environmental stressor of chronic substance use, results in the onset of schizophrenia [26, 105]; and (4) impaired social and occupational function, together with a limited social environment, together increase the risk of substance use [75]. Co-occurring SUD is present in half of patients with schizophrenia, which is a 3–four-fold higher prevalence than in the general population [35]. Comorbid substance use disorder has a negative impact on clinical outcomes in patients with schizophrenia, including more severe symptoms, less treatment compliance, increased hospitalizations and medical comorbidities [18, 72, 94].

Comorbidity of SUD and Attention-Deficit/Hyperactivity Disorder

Attention-deficit/hyperactivity disorder (ADHD) is associated with an increased risk of developing SUD later in life [15]. Using the largest available meta-analyses of genome-wide association studies (GWAS) of ADHD ($n = 53, 293$) and lifetime cannabis use ($n = 32,330$) to examine their causal relationship, Soler Artigas et al. [93] found that the data supported that ADHD is causal for lifetime cannabis use, with an odds ratio of 7.9 for cannabis use in individuals with ADHD in comparison to individuals without ADHD (95% CI (3.72, 15.51), $P = 5.88 \text{ X } 10^{-5}$). These results highlight the clinical importance of assessing for substance misuse in the context of clinical interventions for ADHD.

Patients with ADHD-SUD comorbidity typically have an early onset of substance use disorder and a faster transition from less severe to more serious SUD [24]. In an analysis of Waves 1 and 2 of the NESARC data, [4] found that each additional ADHD symptom was generally associated with a proportional increase in odds of substance dependence. Individuals with persistent ADHD, compared to those with remittent ADHD or healthy controls, are at significantly higher risk of developing an SUD. ADHD persisters have also been found to have higher prevalence rates of nicotine dependence (24.2%) than ADHD remitters (16.7%) and healthy controls (4.3%) [42]. With respect to the impact of ADHD on the course of specific substance use disorder, Estevez-Lamorte et al. [23] analyzed a large ($N = 4975$) sample of Swiss men and found that men with ADHD were more likely to exhibit persistent and risky alcohol and nicotine use, and to mature out of risky cannabis use. Further, they identified that early age of alcohol initiation distinguished between persistence and maturing out of AUD, while the course of nicotine use disorder and cannabis use disorder was related to ADHD symptoms and SUD severity at baseline. These findings suggest that among those with ADHD, substance-specific prevention strategies, particularly if implemented before early adulthood, may represent a critical intervention for reducing the persistence of substance use disorders [23].

ADHD-SUD comorbidity is highly prevalent in addiction treatment settings; in a meta-analysis of 29 studies, 23.1% of patients with SUD also had adult ADHD [102]. Despite seeking treatment more frequently than those without SUD, adults with ADHD-SUD comorbidity have more difficulty remaining abstinent [53] and report a reduced quality of life with more professional, social, and personal problems [49].

Racial and Ethnic Disparities in Dual Diagnosis

In a study drawing on data from two waves of the NESARC, Szaflarski et al. [95] documented significant associations between nativity, race-ethnicity, and dual diagnosis in the US adult population. Immigrants and some racial-ethnic groups (e.g., people of African and Mexican descents) were less likely than US-natives and Europeans to have a dual diagnosis versus having no SUD or depressive/anxiety disorder alone. Conversely, immigrants and minorities were more likely than their native and European counterparts to have a depressive/anxiety disorder alone rather than a dual diagnosis. There was no nativity-based difference in having a SUD alone versus dual diagnosis, although people of African and Mexican origins were more likely to have this condition, compared with Europeans.

Within a US sample of African American and Caribbean Black men and women, significant challenges in accessing and receiving substance disorder treatment have been identified [80]. Black Americans delay seeking treatment, have shorter treatment durations, and experience significant social and health-related consequences because of their substance use, compared to White Americans [12, 69]. For many Black adults, these consequences include poverty, unemployment, lack of a high school diploma or GED, health ailments, and drug-related legal problems [29, 52]. Redmond et al. [80] found that, among those who sought help, African

Americans most commonly sought help from "other health professionals" (81%), and from self-help groups or other informal sources of care (75.9%). Caribbean Blacks also sought help more often from "other health professionals" (86.7%), followed by mental health professionals (62.2%). African American (32.3%) and Caribbean Black (33.3%) respondents were least likely to seek help from a psychiatrist. These findings suggest that individuals with substance and psychiatric comorbidity may be especially unlikely to receive effective care. Preventive psychoeducation on the value of treatment is needed, as many African American and Caribbean Black individuals may not be aware that avoiding or delaying treatment is associated with a lengthier duration of substance disorder problems, which can have associated health and social consequences [80].

Neurobiology of Comorbid Substance Use Disorders and Psychiatric Disorders

Preclinical work has investigated whether depression-like states increase vulnerability to drug-taking behaviors in animals. It has long been recognized that psychosocial stressors produce depression-like phenotypes in animals. But recent research has demonstrated that post-weaning isolation stress and repeated social defeat generally increases initial drug intake and makes animals more sensitive to the rewarding effects of drugs of abuse, as shown by increased drug self-administration. This increased drug acquisition following post-weaning social isolation may be mediated through changes in protein expression that support potentiated dopamine release in the nucleus accumbens. It is of note that these chronic psychosocial stress paradigms both consistently produce depression-like behaviors in animals and also exert an impact on drug-taking behaviors [64].

The genetic underpinnings for the high comorbidity between psychiatric disorders and substance use disorders have not been fully elucidated. Common genetic factors influencing the co-occurrence of anxiety disorders and SUD, as well as mood disorders and SUD, have been sought through genome-wide association studies (GWAS). Genome-wide linkage scans have revealed significant quantitative trait loci for drug dependence (14q13.2-q21.2, LOD = 3.322) and a broad anxiety phenotype (12q24.32-q24.33, LOD = 2.918). Significant positive genetic correlations were observed between anxiety and each of three addiction subtypes: lifetime history of alcohol dependence, drug dependence, or chronic smoking ($\rho g = 0.550–0.655$) [40]. A linkage signal for anxiety recently identified on 12q24 spans the location of TMEM132D, an emerging gene of interest from previous genome-wide association studies of anxiety traits [40]. Likewise, in analyses adjusted for MDD status in three alcohol dependence GWAS data sets, Andersen et al. [5] observed significant evidence for an association between the MDD polygenic risk score and alcohol dependence (best $P = 0.007$).

In a genome-wide association study of genetic susceptibility to substance use disorders (SUDs) and other psychiatric disorders, significant associations with SUDs were detected for schizophrenia, using polygenic scores [34]. This finding indicates that SUDs share genetic susceptibility with SCZ to a greater extent than with other psychiatric disorders, including externalizing disorders such as attention-deficit/hyperactivity disorder. These researchers noted that women have a lower probability to develop substance abuse/dependence than men at similar polygenic scores, probably because of a higher social pressure against excessive drug use in women. A genetic risk for schizophrenia has also been linked to prospective cannabis use patterns during adolescence [37]. There are indications that increased risk for substance and nicotine use, found for certain dopaminergic polymorphisms (e.g., DRD4–7 for frequent cannabis use or DRD2 A1-allele for alcohol use), is under the influence of environmental factors such as low parental monitoring or childhood trauma [32]. In addition, life-course effects on alcohol consumption have been reported for dopaminergic genes [33].

Diagnostic Considerations and Therapeutic Approaches

There are two separate types of substance disorders described in DSM-5. There are those that are conditions of use (substance use disorders) and those that are induced by the misuse of substances (e.g., psychosis, withdrawal, anxiety, and dysfunction). Substance-induced mood disorders represent a separate diagnostic. According to DSM-5, independent depression that develops outside the context of drug use cannot be entirely causally attributed to substance use and persists even when abstinence is sustained. By contrast, substance-induced depression, while warranting clinical attention, occurs only within the context of substance use and is expected to resolve with abstinence [3]. When assessing for the presence of psychiatric disorders comorbid with substance use disorders, it is essential to take a careful history and apply DSM-5 criteria for primary vs. substance-induced mood disorder, anxiety disorder, or psychotic disorder. A recent investigation has found that 10% of individuals presenting for substance abuse treatment had possible schizophrenia or psychotic illness; these results support the need for routine screening for psychiatric issues, including schizophrenia/psychosis-like symptoms, in adults entering substance use disorder treatment settings [100]. Although the distinction between substance and non-substance (psychiatric) disorders has important prognostic and therapeutic implications, in clinical practice it can often be difficult to differentiate between these two conditions, as they rely upon chronological and symptom severity criteria that patients may be unable to provide with precision [19]. Overall, DSM categories are broadly defined, and their application relies considerably on clinical judgment.

In a review of the evidence of diagnostic accuracy for screening and diagnostic tests to be used in populations with SUD and severe mental illness (SMI) conditions, Larun et al. [51] identify two screening tests for SUD in patients with SMI: (1) the CAGE (Chemical Use, Abuse, and Dependence Scale) to identify alcohol use disorder, both current and lifetime; and (2) the AUDIT (Alcohol Use Disorders Identification Test). The authors noted one screening tests for SMI in patients with SUD which has the strongest evidence base: the PDSQ (Psychiatric Diagnostic Screening Questionnaire). Among the available validated diagnostic tests, Larun et al. [51] determined that the PRISM (Psychiatric Research Interview for Substance and Mental Disorders) showed good concordance (kappa 0.63–0.90) when compared to a reference standard (e.g., clinical interview or Structured Clinical Interview for DSM-5, SCID).

It is recommended that co-occurring independent depression be addressed immediately with antidepressants or psychotherapy, while substance-induced depression is best managed by careful observation of its course while focusing primarily on the treatment of the substance use disorder (Nunes et al. 2009). Two meta-analyses have validated the efficacy of antidepressant medication for comorbid depression and alcohol use disorder, with studies showing the strongest effects when patients are required to be abstinent before depression was diagnosed [66]. With respect to other substance use disorders comorbid with depression, Dakwar et al. [19] found that cannabis dependence was highly associated with independent depression ($p < 0.001$), while cocaine dependence was highly associated with substance-induced depression ($p < 0.05$) in a sample ($N = 242$) of cocaine, cannabis, and/or opioid-dependent, treatment-seeking individuals. Independent depression was found to be significantly associated with female gender, higher Hamilton-D score, and post-traumatic stress disorder (PTSD). The finding of a strong association between cannabis dependence and independent depression is consistent with research implicating the endocannabinoid system in mood regulation [38]. Future studies should seek to further elucidate the effect of depression category on the prognosis of SUD, its illness course, and response to treatment. Trials of psychotherapeutic or behavioral treatments may enable the development of treatment algorithms that integrate the skill sets of mental health and substance abuse clinicians [65].

Attention-deficit hyperactivity disorder (ADHD) is also highly prevalent in substance use disorder (SUD). In a group of treatment-seeking high-dose benzodiazepine-dependent patients ($N = 167$), 31.7% of the sample screened positive for adult ADHD. Patients who were ADHD-positive showed a significantly higher prevalence of poly-drug abuse than did those who were ADHD-negative [96]. Guidelines recommend that when ADHD coexists with other psychopathologies in adults, the most impairing condition should generally be treated first [43]. Although the diagnostic assessment of ADHD is usually postponed until after a period of abstinence, this practice delays timely treatment. In a recent study of treatment-seeking adult SUD patients with a comorbid diagnosis of adult ADHD ($N = 127$), the authors found that in 95.3% of SUD patients with ADHD, the diagnosis of ADHD remained stable during abstinence, although the subtype of ADHD was less stable between assessments. These findings suggest that SUD patients can reliably be evaluated for ADHD during active substance use [101].

Co-occurring psychiatric syndromes are likely to be important in the search for a nosology grounded in the pathophysiology of the substance use disorders [68]. The high prevalence of comorbid substance and non-substance use disorders points to a common etiology with shared genetic and neurobiological features. And, from a clinical perspective, diagnostic acumen can lead to early identification of the concurrent conditions, thereby permitting timely interventions in which effective treatment of one disorder can result in an improved prognosis for the other disorder.

Treatment Course: Prognostic Implications

In light of the heightened risk for self-medication in patients with anxiety and mood disorders, clinicians should be particularly vigilant at monitoring for the presence of substance use problems early in the course of psychiatric treatment [7]. The simultaneous treatment of comorbid disorders is commonly referred to as integrated treatment. Integrated treatment of dual disorders often involves an interdisciplinary team, including social workers, psychotherapists, counselors, and case managers [44]. In the case of comorbid conditions for which pharmacologic options are limited (e.g., schizophrenia and cannabis use disorder), the intensity of psychotherapies and behavioral treatments must be increased. One behavioral treatment that has been proven highly effective for the treatment of comorbid substance and psychiatric disorders in an intensive outpatient setting is Contingency Management [45].

Among individuals ($N = 507$) seeking outpatient treatment for substance use disorders, Sanchez et al. [87] found that one fifth (21%; $n = 106$) screened positive for depression. After controlling for anxiety and PTSD symptoms, presence of depressive symptoms remained significantly associated with fewer coping strategies ($P = 0.001$), greater impairment in social adjustment ($P < 0.001$), and poorer health status ($P < 0.001$), but not to days of drug use in the last 90 days ($P = 0.14$). The presence of depressive symptoms was associated with fewer coping strategies and poorer social adjustment. Since coping skills are a significant predictor of addiction outcomes, screening for and enhancing coping among depressed patients may be an important evidence-based intervention to improve global functioning among substance abusers, as an adjunct to usual treatment [87].

A cross-sectional study of individuals seeking SUD treatment ($N = 1276$) found that substance-dependent patients had impaired quality of life, especially in the mental component of the SF-36 (Maigre et al. 2017). Impaired physical quality of life was independently associated with medical condition, age, being female, depressive disorder, and anxiety disorder. Depression disorder, any personality disorder, active consumption last month, attention-deficit hyperactivity disorder, anxiety disorder, and suicide attempt were independently associated with worse mental quality of life. These findings emphasize the significance of dual diagnosis in the impairment of health-related quality of life in substance-dependent patients, particularly with regard to the mental component. In addicted patients with low scores on SF-36, psychiatric comorbidity should be evaluated and treated in an integrated approach.

Recent findings from a register-based cohort-based study in Denmark of people born since 1955 suggest that having any substance use disorder (SUD) is associated with at least a three-fold increased risk of completed suicide, compared to those having no SUD [71]. Alcohol misuse was associated with an increased risk of completed suicide in all populations with hazard ratios (HR) between 1.99 [95% confidence interval (CI) = 1.44–2.74] and 2.70 (95% CI = 2.40–3.04). Other illicit substances were associated with a two- to three-fold risk increase of completed suicide in all populations except bipolar disorder. However, cannabis use disorder was associated with increased risk of attempted suicide only in people with bipolar disorder (HR = 1.86, 95% CI = 1.15–2.99). Alcohol and other illicit substances each displayed strong associations with attempted suicide, HR ranging from 3.11 (95% CI = 2.95–3.27) to 3.38 (95% CI = 3.24–3.53) and 2.13 (95% CI = 2.03–2.24) to 2.27 (95% CI = 2.12–2.43), respectively. Cannabis was associated with suicide attempts only in people with schizophrenia (HR = 1.11, 95% CI = 1.03–1.19) [71].

Blanco et al. [10] found that individuals with MDD-SUD were less likely to receive pharmacologic treatment for depression than those with MDD-NSUD, despite evidence that antidepressants are efficacious for treatment of depressive symptoms and modestly improve SUD (Nunes et al. 2004, [21]). In particular, the use of lithium has been found to result in reduced craving and improved near-term clinical outcomes in patients with comorbid bipolar and substance use disorders [28, 78]. Nonetheless, the finding by Blanco et al. [10] is consistent with the established clinical approach to delay initiating pharmacotherapy in SIDD and encourage abstinence. In this NESARC sample, individuals with SIDD reported greater use of substances to relieve their depressive symptoms, suggesting that in the absence of antidepressant treatment some individuals may resort to self-medication.

By contrast, individuals with generalized anxiety disorder (GAD)-SUD are as likely as those with GAD-NSUD to receive medication for anxiety symptoms [2]. Alegria et al. suggest caution in the use of benzodiazepine in individuals with GAD-SUD due to the increased risk for dependence of prescription drugs among individuals with SUD [9]. Thus, antidepressants (e.g., SSRIs), many of which are effective for GAD, may be preferable as first-line treatment for most individuals with GAD-SUD [67].

It is also important to recognize that while all antipsychotics improve the positive symptoms of schizophrenia, second generations appear most effective in reducing cravings in SUDs. The atypical antipsychotic clozapine has been found to be the most effective medication in reducing alcohol and cannabis use [30, 56, 86], while findings on other medications are equivocal [45]. A systematic review of pharmacological approaches to schizophrenia with comorbid SUD found that the efficacy of clozapine for SUD improvement in schizophrenic patients was superior to that of first-generation antipsychotics in polysubstance users. When compared to second-generation antipsychotics, clozapine was superior to risperidone but equal to olanzapine or ziprasidone in polysubstance and cannabis users [6].

The presence of psychiatric comorbidity exerts a negative influence on SUD prognosis and treatment outcome. Krawczyk et al. [50] found that 28% of patients discharged from substance treatment facilities had psychiatric comorbidity, and 38% did not complete treatment. Clients with psychiatric comorbidity had higher odds of not completing substance treatment relative to those without comorbidity [OR = 1.28 (1.27–1.29)] and an earlier time to attrition [HR = 1.14 (1.13–1.15)]. Psychiatric comorbidity was most strongly associated with treatment non-completion and rate of attrition in those admitted primarily for alcohol [OR = 1.37 (1.34–1.39); HR = 1.19 (1.17–1.21), respectively].

Yet in the population of patients seeking treatment for depression, concurrent SUD does not necessarily predict poor treatment outcome for the mood disorder. In an exploratory analysis of the effect of concurrent substance use disorder on single and combination antidepressants for the treatment of MDD, Davis et al. [20] found no significant differences between the MDD-SUD and MDD-NSUD groups in terms of dose, time in treatment, response to assigned treatment or remission at Week 12 and 28. Thus, patients with MDD and concurrent SUD are as likely to respond and remit to a single or combination antidepressant treatment as those presenting without SUD. And in a 14-week double-blind trial evaluating the combination of sertraline and naltrexone for the treatment of patients with depression and alcohol dependence, patients in the sertraline-naltrexone group combination were more likely than those in the groups that received only naltrexone, only sertraline, or double placebo to achieve abstinence from alcohol (53.7% vs. 21.3–27.5%) and delay relapse to heavy drinking (98 days vs. 23–29 days) and less likely to be depressed by the end of treatment or report a serious adverse event [74].

These findings highlight the need for the concurrent treatment of depressive symptoms and substance use disorder in patients with MDD-SUD and SIDD. Integrating psychotherapy and pharmacotherapy for comorbid substance use and mood disorders should be considered [10], since reduction in depressive symptoms may improve the course of SUD, and decreases in substance use may contribute to improved mood. Since MDD and SUD are highly co-prevalent, and this comorbidity frequently presents with greater psychopathological and medical severity, as well as worse social function, it is important to treat both MDD and SUD simultaneously, rather than to treat both conditions separately [97].

Although treatment rates for substance use disorders are only half that of major depression, SUD increases the likelihood of depression treatment among comorbid cases [36]. More intensive treatment is often required for MDD patients with concomitant SUD, and an integrated treatment model can permit its implementation. Further controlled trials are needed to examine the impact of each condition upon the other, and to identify optimal treatment approaches for this challenging comorbid presentation.

The only evidence-based guideline offering treatment recommendations for AUD and comorbid psychiatric disorders was recently published in Germany, using methodological criteria for the highest quality ("S3-criteria") as defined by the Association of Scientific Medical Societies in Germany (Preuss et al. 2017). Among these recommendations are that patients with psychosis and comorbid alcohol use disorders should receive psychotherapy after adequate stabilization. Similarly, comorbid depression should be treated beginning 3–4 weeks after withdrawal, and cognitive behavioral therapy has been reported as effective for both depression and AUD, in the majority of studies. For bipolar disorder and AUD, integrated therapy with cognitive behavioral therapy is recommended, with the addition of valproic acid if necessary. An integrated psychotherapeutic treatment strategy is recommended for PTSD patients, with stabilizing, trauma-focused therapeutic interventions. These S3 guidelines based on clinical research are intended to facilitate evidence-based decision-making in psycho- and pharmacotherapy to treat comorbid alcohol use and other psychiatric disorders. As the authors note, further research is urgently needed to support evidence-based clinical approaches to other substance and psychiatric comorbidities.

For the treatment of adults with combined ADHD and SUD, studies have suggested that a combination of pharmacotherapy and psychotherapy is most useful [99, 106]. In an international consensus statement, an expert panel offered recommendations on the treatment of comorbid ADHD and SUD [17]. The authors advised that pharmacotherapy should not be avoided; rather, this approach should be critically encouraged in patients with ADHD and SUD -- with a preference for high doses of long-acting stimulants in ADHD patients with stimulant use disorders, or atomoxetine in patients with alcohol use disorder. Treatment of ADHD can be effective in reducing ADHD symptoms without worsening the substance use disorder. Clinicians should consider treating both ADHD and SUD with their own medication simultaneously, that is, for patients with ADHD and an alcohol use disorder, treatment with atomoxetine and with naltrexone, nalmefene, acomprosate, or topiramate [17]. This panel recommended a multimodal integrated approach: combining pharmacotherapy (for ADHD and SUD) with a non-pharmacological intervention that targets both the ADHD and SUD, such as an integrated CBT, while noting that further research is needed. Optimizing treatment for comorbid SUD and ADHD can have a significant effect on public health [55]. A recent large registry-based study suggested that individuals with ADHD who received medications had a significant reduction in criminality compared to those who did not, with a relative risk reduction of32% in men and 41% in women [54].

In sum, the integration of mental health and substance use disorder treatment as well as behavioral treatments such as CBT has demonstrated efficacy [62]. Certain pharmacotherapeutic approaches to the treatment of comorbid psychiatric and substance use disorders have also shown promise. The atypical antipsychotic clozapine has demonstrated preliminary efficacy in the treatment of co-occurring schizophrenia and substance use disorder, as well as naltrexone and disulfiram for comorbid alcohol use disorder, methadone or buprenorphine for opioid use disorder and bupropion and varenicline for tobacco use disorder. Additional research is needed to define optimal pharmacological treatment approaches for these concurrent conditions [1].

Conclusion

Mood, anxiety, and psychotic disorders commonly occur with alcohol and substance use disorders. Exploration of the neurobiology of substance use disorders and mood and anxiety disorders has identified shared neural circuitry in mood, anxiety, and substance use disorders. Genome-wide studies have pointed to, but not fully elucidated, the genetic factors that underlie the high rates of comorbidity between substance use and psychiatric disorders. Environmental factors, such as low parental monitoring and trauma, also play a contributory role in this shared etiology. In light of the extent to which psychiatric and substance use disorders co-occur, careful clinical consideration should be given to assessing for the presence of one category of disorder in patients presenting for treatment of the other.

Diagnosis of co-occurring disorders requires a comprehensive psychiatric and substance use disorder assessment. Empirically validated screening and diagnostic instruments may be helpful in this regard, but the overlap of symptoms between SUD and psychiatric disorders requires clinical skill to review the history of the emergence of each disorder and their temporal relation to each other.

Treatment of co-occurring disorders should include management of diagnoses simultaneously, often with a combination of pharmacotherapy and psychotherapy, to improve symptom management, and treatment adherence. While pharmacotherapies are often more effective in targeting the non-substance-related comorbidity, available pharmacotherapies which specifically target reducing substance use should be used as available and needed, while integrating pharmacotherapy with evidence-based psychotherapies and behavioral therapies should enhance treatment outcomes for patients with substance and psychiatric comorbidities.

References

1. Akerman SC, Brunette MF, Noordsy DL, Green AI. Pharmacotherapy of co-occurring schizophrenia and substance use disorders. Curr Addict Rep. 2014;1(4):251–60.
2. Alegria AA, Hasin DS, Nunes EV, Liu SM, Davies C, Grant BF, Blanco C. Comorbidity of generalized anxiety disorder and substance use disorders: results from the National Epidemiologic Survey on alcohol and related conditions. J Clin Psychiatry. 2010;71(9):1187–95. quiz 1252–1253
3. American Psychiatric Association. Diagnosis and statistical manual of mental disorders (DSM-5). Washington DC; 2013.
4. Ameringer KJ, Leventhal AM. Associations between Attention Deficit Hyperactivity Disorder Symptom Domains and DSM-IV Lifetime Substance Dependence. Am J Addict. 2013;22(1) https://doi.org/10.1111/j.1521-0391.2013.00325.x.
5. Andersen AM, Pietrzak RH, Kranzler HR, Ma L, Zhou H, Liu X, Kramer J, Kuperman S, Edenberg HJ, Nurnberger JI Jr, Rice JP, Tischfield JA, Goate A, Foroud TM, Meyers JL, Porjesz B, Dick

DM, Hesselbrock V, Boerwinkle E, Southwick SM, Krystal JH, Weissman MM, Levinson DF, Potash JB, Gelernter J, Han S. Polygenic Scores for Major Depressive Disorder and Risk of Alcohol Dependence. JAMA Psychiat. 2017;74(11):1153–60.
6. Arranz B, Garriga M, García-Rizo C, San L. Clozapine use in patients with schizophrenia and a comorbid substance use disorder: a systematic review. Eur Neuropsychopharmacol. 2018;28(2):227–42.
7. Baigent M. Managing patients with dual diagnosis in psychiatric practice. Curr Opin Psychiatry. 2012;25(3):201–5.
8. Bega S, Schaffer A, Goldstein B, Levitt A. Differentiating between bipolar disorder types I and II: results from the National Epidemiologic Survey on alcohol and related conditions (NESARC). J Affect Disord. 2012;138:46–53.
9. Blanco C, Alderson D, Ogburn E, et al. Changes in the prevalence of non-medical prescription drug use and drug use disorders in the United States: 1991–1992 and 2001–2002. Drug Alcohol Dep. 2007;90:252–60.
10. Blanco C, Alegría AA, Liu SM, Secades-Villa R, Sugaya L, Davies C, Nunes EV. Differences among major depressive disorder with and without co-occurring substance use disorders and substance-induced depressive disorder: results from the National Epidemiologic Survey on Alcohol and Related Conditions. J Clin Psychiatry. 2012;73(6):865–73.
11. Boland M, Rielage JK, Hoyt T. The power of negative mood in predicting posttraumatic stress disorder and alcohol abuse comorbidity. Psychol Trauma. 2018;10(5):572–5.
12. Breslau J, Kendler KS, Su M, Aguilar-Gaxiola S, Kessler RC. Lifetime risk and persistence of psychiatric disorders across ethnic groups in the United States. Psychol Med. 2005;35:317–27.
13. Brown PJ, Wolfe J. Substance abuse and post-traumatic stress disorder comorbidity. Drug Alcohol Depend. 1994;35(1):51–9.
14. Chambers RA, Krystal JH, Self DW. A neurobiological basis for substance abuse comorbidity in schizophrenia. Biol Psychiatry. 2001;50(2):71–83.
15. Charach A, Yeung E, Climans T, Lillie E. Childhood attention-deficit/hyperactivity disorder and future substance use disorders: comparative meta-analyses. J Am Acad Child Adolesc Psychiatry. 2011;50:9–21.
16. Chilcoat HD, Breslau N. Posttraumatic stress disorder and drug disorders: testing causal pathways. Arch Gen Psychiatry. 1998;55(10):913–7.
17. Crunelle CL, van den Brink W, Moggi F, Konstenius M, Franck J, Levin FR, van de Glind G, Demetrovics Z, Coetzee C, Luderer M, Schellekens A. ICASA consensus group, Matthys F. International Consensus Statement on Screening, Diagnosis and Treatment of Substance Use Disorder Patients with Comorbid Attention Deficit/Hyperactivity Disorder. Eur Addict Res. 2018;24(1):43–51.
18. Crump C, Winkleby MA, Sundquist K, et al. Comorbidities and mortality in persons with schizophrenia: a Swedish national cohort study. A large cohort study demonstrating the premature morbidity and mortality in patients with schizophrenia. Am J Psychiatry. 2013;170(3):324–33.
19. Dakwar E, Nunes EV, Bisaga A, Carpenter KC, Mariani JP, Sullivan MA, Raby WN, Levin FR. A comparison of independent depression and substance-induced depression in cannabis-, cocaine-, and opioid-dependent treatment seekers. Am J Addict. 2011;20(5):441–6.
20. Davis LL, Pilkinton P, Wisniewski SR, Trivedi MH, Gaynes BN, Howland RH, Zisook S, Balasubramani GK, Fava M, Rush AJ. Effect of concurrent substance use disorder on the effectiveness of single and combination antidepressant medications for the treatment of major depression: an exploratory analysis of a single-blind randomized trial. Depress Anxiety. 2012;29(2):111–22.
21. Davis LL, Wisniewski SR, Howland RH, et al. Does comorbid substance use disorder impair recovery from major depression with SSRI treatment? An analysis of the STAR*D level one treatment outcomes. Drug Alcohol Depend. 2010;107(2–3):161–70.
22. Donoghue K, Doody GA. Effect of illegal substance use on cognitive function in individuals with psychotic disorder: a review and meta-analysis. Neuropsychology. 2012;26(6):785–801.
23. Estévez-Lamorte N, Foster S, Eich-Höchli D, Moggi F, Gmel G, Mohler-Kuo M. Adult attention-deficit/hyperactivity disorder, risky substance use and substance use disorders: a follow-up study among young men. Eur Arch Psychiatry Clin Neurosci. 2018 Nov 27; https://doi.org/10.1007/s00406-018-0958-3.
24. Fatséas M, Hurmic H, Serre F, Debrabant R, Daulouède JP, Denis C, Auriacombe M. Addiction severity pattern associated with adult and childhood attention deficit hyperactivity disorder (ADHD) in patients with addictions. Psychiatry Res. 2016;246:656–62.
25. Foa EB, Huppert JD, Cahill SP. Emotional processing theory: an update. In: Rothbaum BO, editor. Emotional processing theory: an update. New York: Emotional Processing Theory; 2006. p. 3–24. An Update.
26. Fowles D. Schizophrenia: diathesis-stress revisited. Annu Rev Psychol. 1992;43(1):303–36.
27. Galbraith T, Heimberg RG, Wang S, Schneier FR, Blanco C. Comorbidity of social anxiety disorder and antisocial personality disorder in the National Epidemiological Survey on alcohol and related conditions (NESARC). J Anxiety Disord. 2014;28:57–66.
28. Geller B, Cooper TB, Sun K, Zimmerman B, Frazier J, Williams M, Heath J. Double-blind and placebo-controlled study of lithium for adolescent bipolar

disorders with secondary substance dependency. J Am Acad Child Adoles Psychiatry. 1998;37:171–8.
29. Godette DC, Headen S, Ford CL. Windows of opportunity: fundamental concepts for understanding alcohol-related disparities experienced by young blacks in the United States. Prev Sci. 2006;7:311–87.
30. Green AI, Burgess ES, Dawson R, Zimmet SV, Strous RD. Alcohol and cannabis use in schizophrenia: effects of clozapine vs. risperidone. Schizophr Res. 2003;60(1):81–5.
31. Green AI, Zimmet SV, Strous RD, et al. Clozapine for comorbid substance use disorder and schizophrenia: do patients with schizophrenia have a reward-deficiency syndrome that can be ameliorated by clozapine? Harv Rev Psychiatry. 1999;6(6):287–96.
32. Groenman AP, Greven CU, van Donkelaar MM, Schellekens A, van Hulzen KJ, Rommelse N, Hartman CA, Hoekstra PJ, Luman M, Franke B, Faraone SV, Oosterlaan J, Buitelaar JK. Dopamine and serotonin genetic risk scores predicting substance and nicotine use in attention deficit/hyperactivity disorder. Addict Biol. 2016;21(4):915–23.
33. Guo G, Wilhelmsen K, Hamilton N. Gene-lifecourse interaction for alcohol consumption in adolescence and young adulthood: five monoamine genes. Am J Med Genet B Neuropsychiatr Genet. 2007;144b:417–23.
34. Gurriarán X, Rodríguez-López J, Flórez G, Pereiro C, Fernández JM, Fariñas E, Estévez V, Arrojo M, Costas J. GenPol study group. Relationships between substance abuse/dependence and psychiatric disorders based on polygenic scores. Genes Brain Behav. 2018;4:e12504.
35. Hartz SM, Pato CN, Medeiros H, et al. Comorbidity of severe psychotic disorders with measures of substance use. JAMA Psychiat. 2014;71(3):248–54.
36. Hasin D, Kilcoyne B. Comorbidity of psychiatric and substance use disorders in the United States: current issues and findings from the NESARC. Curr Opin Psychiatry. 2012;25(3):165–71.
37. Hiemstra M, Nelemans SA, Branje S, van Eijk KR, Hottenga JJ, Vinkers CH, van Lier P, Meeus W, Boks MP. Genetic vulnerability to schizophrenia is associated with cannabis use patterns during adolescence. Drug Alcohol Depend. 2018;190:143–50.
38. Hill MN, Gorzalka BB. The endocannabinoid system and the treatment of mood and anxiety disorders. CNS Neurol Disord Drug Targets. 2009;8(6):451–8.
39. Hirschfield R, Hasin D, Keller M, Endicott J, Wunder J. Depression and alcoholism: comorbidity in a longitudinal survey. In: Maser J, Cloninger C, editors. Comorbidity of mood and anxiety disorders. Washington, DC: American Psychiatric Press; 1990. p. 293–304.
40. Hodgson K, Almasy L, Knowles EE, Kent JW, Curran JE, Dyer TD, Göring HH, Olvera RL, Fox PT, Pearlson GD, Krystal JH, Duggirala R, Blangero J, Glahn DC. Genome-wide significant loci for addiction and anxiety. Eur Psychiatry. 2016;36:47–54.
41. Hunt GE, Large MM, Cleary M, Lai HMX, Saunders JB. Prevalence of comorbid substance use in schizophrenia spectrum disorders in community and clinical settings, 1990-2017: systematic review and meta-analysis. Drug Alcohol Depend. 2018;191:234–58.
42. Ilbegi S, Groenman AP, Schellekens A, Hartman CA, Hoekstra PJ, Franke B, Faraone SV, Rommelse NNJ, Buitelaar JK. Substance use and nicotine dependence in persistent, remittent, and late-onset ADHD: a 10-year longitudinal study from childhood to young adulthood. J Neurodev Disord. 2018;10(1):42.
43. Katzman MA, Bilkey TS, Chokka PR, Fallu A, Klassen LJ. Adult ADHD and comorbid disorders: clinical implications of a dimensional approach. BMC Psychiatry. 2017;17(1):302.
44. Kelly TM, Daley DC. Integrated treatment of substance use and psychiatric disorders. Soc Work Public Health. 2013;28(3–4):388–406.
45. Kelly TM, Daley DC, Douaihy A. Treatment of substance abusing patients with comorbid psychiatric disorders. Addict Behav. 2012;37(1):11–24.
46. Kessler RC. The epidemiology of dual diagnosis. Biol Psychiatry. 2004;56:730–7.
47. Kessler RC, Berglund P, Demler O, Jin R, Koretz D, Merikangas KR. National Comorbidity Survey R the epidemiology of major depressive disorder: results from the National Comorbidity Survey Replication (NCS-R). JAMA. 2003;289(23):3095–105.
48. Khantzian EJ. The self-medication hypothesis of substance use disorders: a reconsideration and recent applications. Harv Rev Psychiatry. 1997;4(5):231–44.
49. Kronenberg LM, Goossens PJ, van Etten DM, van Achterberg T, van den Brink W. Need for care and life satisfaction in adult substance use disorder patients with and without attention deficit hyperactivity disorder (ADHD) or autism spectrum disorder (ASD). Perspect Psychiatr Care. 2015;51:4–15.
50. Krawczyk N, Feder KA, Saloner B, Crum RM, Kealhofer M, Mojtabai R. The association of psychiatric comorbidity with treatment completion among clients admitted to substance use treatment programs in a U.S. national sample. Drug Alcohol Depend. 2017;1(175):157–63.
51. Larun L, Helseth V, Bramness JG, Haugurud H, Hoie B, Grawe RW, Kornor H, Landhein A, Lossius K, Hammerstrom KT, Waal H. Dual diagnoses – substance use disorder and severe mental illness: Part I – accuracy of screening and diagnostic instruments. Oslo, Norway: Knowledge Centre for the Health Services at The Norwegian Institute of Public Health (NIPH); 2007 Dec. Report from Norwegian Knowledge Centre for the Health Services (NOKC) No. 21–2007.
52. Lee JA, Mavis BE, Stoffelmayr BE. A comparison of problems of life for blacks and whites entering

substance use programs. J Psychoactive Drugs. 1991;23(3):233–9.
53. Levin FR, Evans SM, Vosburg SK, Horton T, Brooks D, Ng J. Impact of attention-deficit hyperactivity disorder and other psychopathology on treatment retention among cocaine abusers in a therapeutic community. Addict Behav. 2004;29:1875–82.
54. Lichtenstein P, Halldner L, Zetterqvist J, Sjolander A, Serlachius E, Fazel S, et al. Medication for attention deficit-hyperactivity disorder and criminality. N Engl J Med. 2012;367:2006–14.
55. Luo S, Levin FR. Towards Precision Addiction Treatment: New Findings in Co-morbid Substance Use and Attention-Deficit Hyperactivity Disorders. Curr Psychiatry Rep. 2017;19(3):14.
56. Lybrand J, Caroff S. Management of schizophrenia with substance use disorders. Psychiatr Clin N Am. 2009;32(4):821–33.
57. McCauley JL, Killeen T, Gros DF, Brady KT, Back SE. Posttraumatic Stress Disorder and Co-Occurring Substance Use Disorders: Advances in Assessment and Treatment. Clin Psychol (New York). 2012;19(3):1.
58. McFarlane AC. Epidemiological evidence about the relationship between ptsd and alcohol abuse: the nature of the association. Addict Behav. 1998;23(6):813–25.
59. Maremmani AGI, Pani PP, Rovai L, Bacciardi S, Maremmani I. Toward the identification of a specific psychopathology of substance use disorders. Front Psychiatry. 2017:27;8:68.
60. Merikangas KR, Risch NJ, Weissman MM. Comorbidity and co-transmission of alcoholism, anxiety and depression. Psychol Med. 1994;24(1):69–80.
61. Messer T, Lammers G, Müller-Siecheneder F, Schmidt RF, Latifi S. Substance abuse in patients with bipolar disorder: A systematic review and meta-analysis. Psychiatry Res. 2017;253:338–50.
62. Mueser KT, Gingerich S. Treatment of co-occurring psychotic and substance use disorders. Soc Work Pub Health. 2013;28(3–4):424–39.
63. Mueser KT, Rosenberg SD, Xie H, Jankowski MK, Bolton EE, Lu W, et al. Wolfe R. a randomized controlled trial of cognitive-behavioral treatment for posttraumatic stress disorder in severe mental illness. J Consult Clin Psychol. 2008;76:259–71.
64. Ng E, Browne CJ, Samsom JN, Wong AHC. Depression and substance use comorbidity: what we have learned from animal studies. Am J Drug Alcohol Abuse. 2017;43(4):456–74.
65. Nunes EV, Levin FR. Treating depression in substance abusers. Curr Psychiatry Rep. 2006;8(5):363–70.
66. Nunes EV, Levin FR. Treatment of depression in patients with alcohol or other drug dependence: a meta-analysis. JAMA. 2004;291(15):1887–96.
67. Nunes EV, McGrath PJ, Quitkin FM. Treating anxiety in patients with alcoholism. J Clin Psychiatry. 1995;56:3–9.
68. Nunes EV, Rounsaville BJ. Comorbidity of substance use with depression and other mental disorders: from Diagnostic and Statistical Manual of Mental Disorders, fourth edition (DSM-IV) to DSM-V. Addiction. 2006;101(Suppl. 1):89–96.
69. Ojeda VD, McGuire TG. Gender and racial/ethnic differences in use of outpatient mental health and substance use services by depressed adults. Psychiatry Q. 2006;77(3):211–22.
70. Oliveira LM, Bermudez MB, Macedo MJA, Passos IC. Comorbid social anxiety disorder in patients with alcohol use disorder: a systematic review. J Psychiatr Res. 2018;106:8–14.
71. Østergaard MLD, Nordentoft M, Hjorthøj C. Associations between substance use disorders and suicide or suicide attempts in people with mental illness: a Danish nation-wide, prospective, register-based study of patients diagnosed with schizophrenia, bipolar disorder, unipolar depression or personality disorder. Addiction. 2017;112(7):1250–9.
72. Owen RR, Fischer EP, Booth BM, et al. Medication noncompliance and substance abuse among patients with schizophrenia. Psychiatr Serv. 1996;47(8):853–8.
73. Parmar A, Kaloiya G. Comorbidity of personality disorder among substance use disorder patients: A narrative review. Indian J Psychol Med. 2018;40(6):517–27.
74. Pettinati HM, Oslin DW, Kampman KM, et al. A double-blind, placebo-controlled trial combining sertraline and naltrexone for treating co-occurring depression and alcohol dependence. Am J Psychiatry. 2010;167(6):668–75.
75. Polimanti R, Agrawal A, Gelernter J. Schizophrenia and substance use comorbidity: a genome-wide perspective. Genome Med. 2017;9(1):25.
76. Preuss UW (2008) Abhängigkeitserkrankungen und Psychosen: Erkenntnisse und Kontroversen in Vorbereitung auf neue Klassifikationssysteme. Die Psychiatrie 2:61–68. Cited in Preuss et al. 2018.
77. Preuss UW, Gouzoulis-Mayfrank E, Havemann-Reinecke U, Schafer I, Beutel M, Hoch E, Mann KF. Psychiatric comorbidity in alcohol use disorders: results from the German S3 guidelines. Eur Arch Psychiatry Clin Neurosci. 2018;268(3):219–29.
78. Prisciandaro JJ, Brown DG, Brady KT, Tolliver BK. Comorbid anxiety disorders and baseline medication regimens predict clinical outcomes in individuals with co-occurring bipolar disorder and alcohol dependence: Results of a randomized controlled trial. Psychiatry Res. 2011;188(3):361–5.
79. Quednow BB, Brinkmeyer J, Mobascher A, Nothnagel M, Musso F, Grunder G, et al. Schizophrenia risk polymorphisms in the TCF4 gene interact with smoking in the modulation of auditory sensory gating. Proc Natl Acad Sci U S A. 2012;109:6271–6.
80. Redmond ML, Watkins DC, Broman CL, Abelson JM, Neighbors HW. Ethnic and gender differences

in help seeking for substance disorders among black Americans. J Racial Ethn Health Disparities. 2017;4(2):308–16.
81. Regier DA, Farmer ME, Rae DS. Comorbidity of mental disorders with alcohol and other drug abuse. Results from the Epidemiologic Catchment Area (ECA) Study JAMA. 1990a;264:2511–8.
82. Roberts NP, Roberts PA, Jones N, Bisson JI. Psychological therapies for post-traumatic stress disorder and comorbid substance use disorder. Cochrane Database Syst Rev. 2016a;4:CD010204.
83. Regier DA, Farmer ME, Rae DS, Locke BZ, Keith SJ, Judd LL, Goodwin FK. Comorbidity of mental disorders with alcohol and other drug abuse. Results from the epidemiologic catchment area (ECA) study. JAMA. 1990b;264(19):2511–8.
84. Roberts NP, Roberts PA, Jones N, Bisson JI. Psychological therapies for post-traumatic stress disorder and comorbid substance use disorder. Cochrane Database Syst Rev. 2016b;4(4):CD010204.
85. Roth RM, Brunette MF, Green AI. Treatment of substance use disorders in schizophrenia: a unifying neurobiological mechanism? Curr Psychiatry Rep. 2005;7(4):283–91.
86. San L, Arranz B, Martinez-Raga J. Antipsychotic drug treatment of schizophrenic patients with substance abuse disorders. Eur Addict Res. 2007;13:230–43.
87. Sanchez K, Walker R, Campbell AN, Greer TL, Hu MC, Grannemann BD, Nunes EV, Trivedi MH. Depressive Symptoms and Associated Clinical Characteristics in Outpatients Seeking Community-Based Treatment for Alcohol and Drug Problems. Subst Abus. 2015;36(3):297–303.
88. Schellekens AF, de Jong CA, Buitelaar JK, Verkes RJ. Co-morbid anxiety disorders predict early relapse after inpatient alcohol treatment. Eur Psychiatry. 2015;30(1):128–36.
89. Scott JG, Matuschka L, Niemelä S, Miettunen J, Emmerson B, Mustonen A. Evidence of a causal relationship between smoking tobacco and schizophrenia spectrum disorders. Front Psych. 2018;9:607. https://doi.org/10.3389/fpsyt.2018.00607.
90. Sher L, Stanley BH, Harkavy-Friedman JM, et al. Depressed patients with co-occurring alcohol use disorders: a unique patient population. J Clin Psychiatry. 2008;69(6):907–15.
91. Shiner B, Leonard Westgate C, Bernardy NC, Schnurr PP, Watts BV. Trends in Opioid Use Disorder Diagnoses and Medication Treatment Among Veterans With Posttraumatic Stress Disorder. J Dual Diagn. 2017;13(3):201–12.
92. Siris SG. Pharmacological treatment of substance-abusing schizophrenic patients. Schizophr Bull. 1990;16(1):111–22.
93. Soler Artigas M, Sánchez-Mora C, Rovira P, Richarte V, Garcia-Martínez I, Pagerols M, Demontis D, Stringer S; ADHD Group of the Psychiatric Genomics Consortium, International Cannabis Consortium, Vink JM, Børglum AD, Neale BM, Franke B1, Faraone SV, Casas M, Ramos-Quiroga JA, Ribasés M. Attention-deficit/hyperactivity disorder and lifetime cannabis use: genetic overlap and causality. Mol Psychiatry. 2019; https://doi.org/10.1038/s41380-018-0339-3.
94. Swartz MS, Wagner HR, Swanson JW, et al. Substance use in persons with schizophrenia: baseline prevalence and correlates from the NIMH CATIE study. J Nerv Ment Dis. 2006;194(3):164–72.
95. Szaflarski M, Bauldry S, Cubbins LA, Meganathan K. Nativity, Race-Ethnicity, and Dual Diagnosis among US Adults. Res Sociol Health Care. 2017;35:171–91.
96. Tamburin S, Federico A, Morbioli L, Faccini M, Casari R, Zamboni L, Briguglio G, Lugoboni F. Screening for adult attention deficit/hyperactivity disorder in high-dose benzodiazepine dependent patients. Am J Addict. 2017;26(6):610–4.
97. Tirado Muñoz J, Farré A, Mestre-Pintó J, Szerman N, Torrens M. Dual diagnosis in Depression: treatment recommendations. Adicciones. 2018;30(1):66–76.
98. Torrens M, Martin-Santos R, Samet S. Importance of clinical diagnoses for comorbidity studies in substance use disorders. Neurotox Res. 2006;10(3–4):253–61.
99. Torrens M, Rossi PC, Martinez-Riera R, Martinez-Sanvisens D, Bulbena A. Psychiatric co-morbidity and substance use disorders: treatment in parallel systems or in one integrated system? Subst Use Misuse. 2012;47(8–9):1005–14.
100. Trudeau KJ, Burtner J, Villapiano AJ, Jones M, Butler SF, Joshi K. Burden of schizophrenia or psychosis-related symptoms in adults undergoing substance abuse evaluation. J Nerv Ment Dis. 2018;206(7):528–36.
101. van Emmerik-van Oortmerssen K, Vedel E, Kramer FJ, Koeter MW, Schoevers RA, van den Brink W. Diagnosing ADHD during active substance use: feasible or flawed? Drug Alcohol Depend. 2017;180:371–5.
102. van Emmerik-van Oortmerssen K, van de Glind G, van den Brink W, Smit F, Crunelle CL, Swets M, Schoevers RA. Prevalence of attention-deficit hyperactivity disorder in substance use disorder patients: a meta-analysis and meta-regression analysis. Drug Alcohol Depend. 2012;122:11–9.
103. Varo C, Murru A, Salagre E, Jiménez E, Solé B, Montejo L, Carvalho AF, Stubbs B, Grande I, Martínez-Arán A, Vieta E, Reinares M. Behavioral addictions in bipolar disorders: a systematic review. Eur Neuropsychopharmacol. 2018:S0924-977X(18)30847-2.
104. Volkow ND. The reality of comorbidity: depression and drug abuse. Biol Psychiatry. 2004;56(10):714–7.
105. Walker EF, Diforio D. Schizophrenia: a neural diathesis-stress model. Psychol Rev. 1997;104(4):667.
106. Zulauf CA, Sprich SE, Safren SA, Wilens TE. The complicated relationship between attention deficit/hyperactivity disorder and substance use disorders. Curr Psychiatry Rep. 2014;16:436.

ADHD and Co-Occurring Substance Use Disorders

2

Mariely Hernandez, Naomi Dambreville, and Frances Rudnick Levin

Abbreviations

ADHD	Attention-Deficit/Hyperactivity Disorder
AMP	Amphetamine
ASD	Autism Spectrum Disorder
ASRS	Adult ADHD Self-Report Scale
ASU	Adolescent Substance Use
ATX	Atomoxetine
AUD	Alcohol Use Disorder
CD	Conduct Disorder
DBD	Disruptive Behavior Disorders
DLPFC	Dorsolateral Prefrontal Cortex
DMN	Default Mode Network
DSM-5	Diagnostic and Statistical Manual of Mental Disorders, 5th Edition
DSM-IV	Diagnostic and Statistical Manual of Mental Disorders, IV Edition
DUD	Drug Use Disorder
EF	Executive Function
fMRI	functional Magnetic Resonance Imaging
IFC	Inferior Frontal Cortex
LDX	Lisdexamfetamine
MDD	Major Depressive Disorder
MPH	Methylphenidate
MTS	Transdermal methylphenidate system
OFC	Orbitofrontal cortex
OROS-MPH	Osmotic-Release Oral Systems Methylphenidate
PET	Positron Emission Tomography
PFC	Prefrontal Cortex
Proband	Person serving as the starting point of a genetic or family study
PSU	Psychoactive substance use, includes alcohol, nicotine, and illicit drugs
PSUD	Psychoactive substance use disorder, includes alcohol, nicotine, and illicit drugs
RCT	Randomized control trial
SUD	Substance Use Disorder
VMPFC	Ventromedial Prefrontal Cortex

M. Hernandez (✉) · N. Dambreville
The City College of New York, New York, NY, USA

CUNY Graduate Center, New York, NY, USA
e-mail: Mhernandez1@gradcenter.cuny.edu

F. R. Levin
Columbia University Medical Center, New York, NY, USA

New York State Psychiatric Institute, New York, NY, USA
e-mail: frl2@cumc.columbia.edu

Epidemiology, Comorbidity, and Risk

Attention-deficit/hyperactivity disorder (ADHD) is a neurodevelopmental disorder characterized by impairing symptoms of inattention, hyperactivity, and impulsivity across multiple settings,

E. Akerele (ed.), *Substance and Non-Substance Related Addictions*,
https://doi.org/10.1007/978-3-030-84834-7_2

according to the *Diagnostic and Statistical Manual of Disorders* – fifth edition (DSM-5) [3]. The estimated worldwide prevalence of childhood and adolescent ADHD is 5.29% [123, 124]. Although ADHD is typically diagnosed in childhood and can remit over time, symptoms of ADHD can persist into adulthood for up to 65% of affected individuals [43]. The estimated prevalence of adult ADHD ranges from 2.5–4.4% in the United States (US) [75] and 3.4% worldwide [50].

There is ample evidence that childhood onset of ADHD is associated with an increased risk of adverse clinical, functional, and health outcomes in adolescence and adulthood. Research findings consistently indicate that ADHD confers a significant risk for developing an alcohol use disorder (AUD) and/or substance use disorder (SUD) [18, 21, 36, 79], due to shared genetic and phenotypic vulnerabilities and/or psychosocial challenges which increase the likelihood of deviant behavior in adolescence [108].

Prevalence estimates of ADHD among substance use populations vary widely by country and treatment setting, with rates of DSM-5 adult ADHD ranging from 7.6% (Hungary) to 32.6% (Norway), and higher rates of ADHD observed in inpatient facilities for treatment-seeking SUD patients compared to those in outpatient settings [80, 114, 133, 154]. ADHD appears to be over-represented in both treatment and non-treatment-seeking SUD populations. A recent meta-analysis of ADHD in adolescent and adult SUD samples reported an estimated overall prevalence of 25.3% (C.I. 20.0–31.4%, $I^2 = 93.2\%$) in adolescents and 21.0% (C.I. 15.9–27.2%, $I^2 = 91.3\%$) in adults [155]. However, this meta-analysis excluded studies on participants with primary nicotine dependence, treatment studies of patients with a psychiatric disorder and comorbid SUD, and studies reporting on juvenile offenders. Lastly, the inconsistent diagnostic methods of assessing ADHD across the different studies analyzed may limit the conclusions that can be drawn from these findings.

Beyond prevalence rates, numerous studies show that individuals with ADHD initiate psychoactive substance use (PSU) at an earlier age, are more likely to engage in polysubstance use, and escalate their use more rapidly than their non-ADHD peers [49, 58, 87, 109, 110, 162, 165]. Studies of treatment-seeking populations often group participants by the primary substance of use, which can obscure the high incidence of poly-substance use in ADHD and SUD populations, resulting in varying estimates of ADHD in specific SUD populations. The most common addictive substances of abuse are tobacco and alcohol, followed by cannabis [145]. Early initiation of PSU likely begins with nicotine and alcohol due to their legality and widespread availability, and a number of studies have reported that persistent ADHD predicts nicotine use in adolescence as well as drug and alcohol use disorders in adulthood [21, 49, 79, 109, 110].

Adults with ADHD and a co-occurring psychoactive substance use disorder (PSUD) have more severe and complex presentations, as evidenced by the over-representation of ADHD in PSUD treatment-seeking populations compared to general prevalence rates [114, 133, 157]. A recent study on inpatients with AUD reported an estimated ADHD prevalence of 20.5% [87]. Those with ADHD were significantly younger than their non-ADHD counterparts at admission, but reported the same period of alcohol dependence, were more likely to relapse during treatment, and reported a higher rate of co-occurring drug use disorders (DUD), and history of intravenous drug use. Another study in a younger, non-treatment-seeking population of college students with ADHD found that students with ADHD are more likely to report negative consequences of alcohol use despite similar rates and frequencies of alcohol consumption [130].

Outcomes

ADHD, especially when untreated, has been associated with adverse clinical [17, 21], functional [54, 76], and health outcomes [113], including increased mortality [37]. Generally, those with the combined-type presentation are at greater risk for a more severe course and worse outcomes, likely because they have more symptoms than unspecified and predominately inattentive presentations [3]. Individuals with ADHD often present with other co-occurring psychiatric disorders, such as disruptive behavioral disorders (DBD) in childhood (Oppositional Defiant Disorder; Conduct Disorder (CD)) and Antisocial Personality Disorder (ASPD) in adulthood. ADHD and comorbid DBD is believed to be the most predictive of substance use problems, though studies have shown that ADHD confers a risk for SUD, even when controlling for conduct disorder [5, 40, 168]. Individuals with ADHD and comorbid conduct problems likely represent a more severe presentation of ADHD and are thus at an increased risk of substance use problems. A prospective longitudinal study of children with and without ADHD, evaluated from ages 5 to 18, showed that it was growth in ADHD symptoms which led to increases in conduct disorder symptoms and then subsequent substance use in adolescence [138]. Thus, CD mediated the relationship between ADHD and adolescent substance use, but an escalation of ADHD symptoms was driving the risk.

Poor functional outcomes such as academic and occupational underachievement have also been observed in adults with persistent childhood-onset ADHD compared to their non-ADHD peers [76]. A 2012 report analyzing the 33-year follow-up data of a prospective longitudinal study of boys with and without ADHD (mean age: 44 years old) documents significant discrepancies in psychiatric comorbidity, psychosocial functioning, as well as vocational and educational achievement [76]. The ADHD probands had significantly higher rates of ASPD, SUDs, and nicotine dependence, fewer years of education, lower occupational attainment, significantly lower median annual salary (a $40,000 discrepancy), greater lifetime history of incarceration and divorce, and increased mortality, compared to their non-ADHD peers.

In a nationally representative sample, adult ADHD was associated with an increased risk of at least one co-occurring psychiatric disorder, the most common included bipolar disorder, anxiety disorders such as generalized anxiety disorder (GAD), specific phobia, and post-traumatic stress disorder (PTSD), as well as cluster B personality disorders (antisocial, borderline, histrionic, and narcissistic) and schizotypal personality disorder [17]. ADHD in this sample was also associated with an increased risk of functional and occupational problems related to poor planning and deficits in inhibitory control, such as gambling problems, overspending, risky driving behaviors, and abruptly quitting a job. Further, individuals with ADHD also reported a greater number of traumatic events, higher levels of stress, and lower perceived health and social support. Notably, this analysis did not find significant evidence of ADHD as a risk factor for SUD, despite numerous studies demonstrating the opposite [21, 73, 79, 104, 109, 110, 165]. It is likely that the population of adults surveyed were past the vulnerable period of adolescence, when ADHD likely poses greatest risk for substance use initiation and escalation.

Apart from educational and occupational impairment, ADHD is also associated with a number of adverse physical and mental health outcomes, including smoking and substance use, sleep disturbances [146], physical injury [102, 119, 148], motor-vehicle accidents [11, 13], risky sexual behavior [12], obesity [30], and early mortality [113]. Many of these risks are related to ADHD symptoms of inattention and impulsivity, executive functioning deficits in planning and inhibitory control, and sensation-seeking behaviors. However, other risks like early mortality seem to be specific to ADHD in the presence of other comorbid psychiatric conditions such as conduct disorder, substance use problems, and/or depression [22, 76].

Co-Occurring ADHD and SUD

Given that the singular diagnoses of ADHD or SUD, respectively, are associated with a number of adverse outcomes, individuals with co-occurring ADHD and SUD (ADHD+SUD) are at an increased risk for negative outcomes and present an even more difficult population to both diagnose and treat than those with either disorder alone.

Notably, disentangling ADHD from SUD for etiological understanding and diagnostic ability can be difficult given the bidirectional influence of each disorder on the other. Retrospective diagnosis of ADHD in a SUD population can be challenging because of how persistent substance use affects attention and reward pathways to prioritize drug-related cues and promote drug-seeking behaviors [71]. Some of these neurological alterations may persist even after prolonged abstinence from substances, particularly for neurotoxic substances such as alcohol. Further complicating the diagnostic picture is cumulative evidence that childhood ADHD is a risk factor for substance use, and that ADHD youth are more likely to initiate alcohol and substance use earlier than the general population, which can also compromise neurological development [138]. Thus, it is important to identify the presence of symptoms of ADHD in childhood and in the absence of substance use initiation.

Neural Correlates and Genetics

ADHD presents as a phenotypically complex and heterogeneous disorder, which has made it challenging to consistently associate differences in neural structure and neurocognitive functioning with symptoms and functional impairment. Generally, neuropsychological impairments observed in ADHD include problems with executive function (sustained attention, planning, timing, and inhibitory control), processing speed, working memory, and reward processes [9].

These cognitive functions have been associated with specific brain structures and neural pathways via fMRI and PET studies. The prefrontal cortex (PFC) is a primary structure of interest, as it is an advanced cortical region highly involved in the regulation of attention, motivation, and emotion, with different regions of the PFC presumed to mediate specific cognitive functions. Neural pathways associated with different regions of the PFC and cognitive functions have been conceptualized as regions associated with "cool" executive function (EF) and "hot" executive function processes. "Cool" EF pathways involve the dorsolateral prefrontal cortex (DLPFC) and inferior frontal cortex (IFC), which are associated with attention, planning, working memory (DLPFC) as well as inhibitory control and cognitive flexibility (IFC). The "hot" EF pathways are associated with motivation and reward-based cognitive tasks, involving the ventromedial prefrontal cortex (VMPFC) and the orbitofrontal cortex (OFC) [9, 33].

Differing theoretical models conceptualize the cognitive deficits observed in ADHD as either predominately an impairment in functioning of the "cool" EF neural networks regulating inhibitory control, or both the "cool" and "hot" EF network signaling such that high reward salience and sensation seeking dominated by the mesoaccumbens regions overwhelm the underdeveloped pre-frontal regions to impair thoughtful planning and response inhibition [142, 143]. These neural networks are particularly sensitive to changes in chemical compounds involved in signaling, specifically the catecholamines, dopamine, norepinephrine, and epinephrine. These neurotransmitters are crucial to fronto-striatal and mesolimbic circuits regulating attention and motivation, with differences between ADHD groups and controls in dopaminergic activity in these regions [159]. These differences identify important signaling pathways that serve as potential targets for pharmacological intervention.

Structural imaging studies have noted smaller cortical volume in frontal, striatal, and parietal areas as well as subcortical regions in children and adults with ADHD when compared to controls [33]. Functional imaging studies have also reported differences in regional activation between ADHD subjects and controls. Thus, phenotypically observed impairments in cognitive function in the ADHD population have been linked to structural abnormalities and alterations in signaling connectivity between regions. One example is the "default mode" attention network (DMN), which corresponds to several regions along the brain's medial wall [31, 48]. Generally, the DMN is active when individuals are not focused on a cognitive task. The region has been associated with mind wandering, attention to the environment, and one's internal states. During targeted cognitive tasks, however, DMN activation is generally reduced and fronto-striatal activation is increased, thus suppressing environmental intrusion and facilitating goal-oriented cognitive function. In individuals with ADHD, fMRI studies have shown that suppression of the DMN during cognitive tasks is less efficient compared to healthy controls [48]. The inadequate regulation of the brain's DMN in individuals with ADHD is thought to contribute to phenotypically observed difficulties with sustaining attention and distractibility during cognitive tasks. Notably, two different studies have shown that methylphenidate, a psychostimulant, improves regulation of the DMN in ADHD [85, 121].

Conceptualizing the underlying neural basis for cognitive impairments in ADHD permits one to hypothesize the etiology of risk for developing substance use disorders. There is documented evidence that children with ADHD exhibit a slower structural maturation of cortical brain regions involved in the regulation of attentional, motivational, and motor functions [20, 134]. These structural differences are thought to underlie the cognitive deficits observed in adolescents with ADHD, who, with fewer cognitive resources for regulating attention, planning, and anticipating consequences, are more likely to engage in early substance use compared to non-ADHD peers, at an especially vulnerable period in neural development. Recently published data from the Multimodal Treatment Study of Children with ADHD (MTA) showed that the ADHD group initiated the use of alcohol, cigarettes, marijuana, and illicit drugs earlier than the comparison group [109, 110]. The ADHD group also escalated their use of alcohol and non-marijuana illicit drugs faster than the comparison group. Early use, regardless of ADHD status, was predictive of a faster escalation of alcohol, marijuana, cigarette smoking, and illicit drug use by age 21.

Individuals with substance use disorders exhibit similar phenotypic differences as ADHD populations in behavioral tasks compared to controls [118]. In particular, deficits in inhibitory control, delay of gratification, and motivational systems have pointed to a shared profile of impulsivity between ADHD and SUD. A recent familial risk analysis [173] on the heritability of ADHD and SUD confirmed existing evidence that the risk of developing a SUD is highly heritable in families with an affected first-degree relative and that heritability of alcohol and drug use disorders is non-specific, such that the *risk* of developing a psychoactive substance use disorder is familial, and not the specific substance of use. This finding is consistent with some publications [116] but contrary to earlier findings [16, 101]. Interestingly, Yule et al. (2017) also found that ADHD in the proband was predictive of SUDs in relatives, even if the proband did not have a SUD [173]. Lastly, there was evidence of co-segregation of ADHD and *any* SUD, suggesting that risk genes for both disorders are likely inherited together.

Studies on genetic risk of ADHD have not found one specific gene that confers a high risk of developing the disorder, but instead point to a polygenic inheritance [44]. Candidate genes likely associated with the ADHD phenotype include those for dopamine receptors, dopamine transporters, and other proteins involved in cell signaling and gene expression [38]. While candidate gene studies can lend support to observed phenotypic differences between ADHD individuals and healthy controls in the availability of dopamine synaptic markers in specific brain regions [159], more research is needed to bridge the gap between genetic risk and the considerable heterogeneity in the phenotypic expression of ADHD.

Diagnostic Considerations for ADHD

Perhaps to better account for the heterogeneity of ADHD symptom presentation across the lifespan, there were a few changes to ADHD diagnostic criteria in the DSM-5 [3]. These changes are summarized in Table 2.1.

Recently, there has been an emergence or increased awareness of "late-onset" ADHD in adulthood, with some limited support [105, 135]. One possibility is that ADHD symptoms were

Table 2.1 DSM-5 changes to ADHD diagnostic criteria

ADHD Diagnostic Criteria	Changes in DSM-5
Criterion A (symptom clusters of inattention, hyperactivity, and impulsivity)	Symptoms largely unchanged Additional examples of symptom manifestations in adolescence and adulthood provided. Only 5 instead of 6 symptoms required for older adolescents and adults [41].
Criterion B (age of onset)	Changed from symptoms before age 7 to before age 12.
Criterion C	"Evidence of impairment" changed to "evidence of symptoms" in 2 or more settings.
Criterion D	Instead of "clinically significant impairment," individuals should indicate that symptoms have reduced the quality of their psychosocial, academic, and vocational functioning [3, 41].
Criterion E	Autism spectrum disorder (ASD) is no longer exclusionary to an ADHD diagnosis.
Specifiers	Instead of subtypes, specifiers (predominately inattentive, predominately hyperactive, combined, unspecified) are now called "presentations" to reflect how ADHD symptom manifestations may evolve across the lifespan [3, 41].

present earlier during development but did not reach the threshold of impairment due to familial and/or academic support structures. Once these supports were not available and cognitive demands exceeded resources (e.g., in a college setting), pre-existing ADHD symptoms may have then reached a clinical threshold, resulting in functional impairment. Alternatively, a late adolescent or adult-onset ADHD may represent a different disorder outside of the neurodevelopmental conceptualization [105]. A longitudinal study of adult males with adult-onset ADHD did not show the same structural brain abnormalities as individuals with a childhood-onset of symptoms [125, 135].

Lastly, another alternative is that other disorders can "mimic" ADHD symptoms of inattention and distractibility, such as post-traumatic stress disorder (PTSD), depression (MDD), and anxiety disorders [3]. Correctly diagnosing ADHD, particularly in adulthood, is important so that those whose symptoms were previously undetected may receive needed treatment.

Assessment and Diagnosis of Comorbid ADHD and SUD

Evaluating and diagnosing ADHD alone is challenging and is made more complex in individuals with co-occurring SUD. Despite the high prevalence of ADHD in adults with SUD, individuals with SUD often do not report ADHD symptoms without solicitation [32].

Screening instruments are a feasible and reliable method of assessing ADHD in clinical settings. The most commonly used screening measures include the Adult ADHD Self-Report Scale Short Version (ASRS-SV) [74], the Wender Utah Rating Scale (WURS) [160] which assesses childhood ADHD, the Conners' Adult ADHD Rating Scale (CAARS) [28], and the Attention Deficit Scales for Adults (ADSA) [153]. These measures have been used in ADHD+SUD populations with good sensitivity and specificity [32, 84, 97, 161].

Additionally, neuropsychological assessments can help distinguish adults with ADHD from those without [84]. For example, continuous performance tests, which measure sustained attention and inhibitory control, have demonstrated reasonable sensitivity, specificity, and promising positive predictive power, as well as providing clinical information by observation of the patient's behavior during the cognitive task [55, 56, 112]. Screening for substance use in ADHD populations using validated measures and toxicological assessments has also proven beneficial [32]. While these measures are useful for screening patients who may have ADHD, they should always be followed up by an in-depth clinical evaluation or diagnostic interview.

There are several guidelines for evaluating ADHD+SUD [32, 84, 96, 97]. A comprehensive assessment should be completed by a physician or clinical psychologist with training in addiction, differential diagnoses of ADHD, and the specific population (pediatric vs adult). The evaluation should include a standardized diagnostic interview for a thorough clinical history of ADHD symptoms prior to the onset of substance use and during periods of abstinence, as well as an overall history of mental and physical health, and psychosocial functioning. Available diagnostic interviews include the Conners' Adult ADHD Diagnostic Interview for DSM-IV (CAADID) [29], the gold standard for assessing co-occurring ADHD and SUD, the Structured Clinical Interview for DSM-5 (SCID-5) [53], the Psychiatric Research Interview for Substance and Mental Disorders (PRISM) [127], and lastly the Diagnostic Interview for ADHD (DIVA) [128], which has yet to be validated in SUD populations [32, 84].

Clinicians run the risk of both under- and over-diagnosing ADHD in SUD population, a point of concern noted in the literature [32, 84]. Discrepancies exist as to when the diagnostic process should begin. Some researchers suggest starting as soon as possible when there is no serious intoxication and withdrawal symptoms [32]. Others recommend a 2–4 week period of abstinence, while noting that abstinence may be difficult to achieve in outpatient settings [84]. Patients' limited capacity to accurately report their substance use patterns, note periods of abstinence, and recall childhood symptoms of ADHD impacts the ability to distinguish between primary ADHD and substance-induced symptoms [32, 84, 96]. Acute and chronic effects of substance use can present as psychiatric symptoms, such as the changes in attention and psychomotor activity seen in ADHD, intoxication, and recovery, thus leading to misdiagnosis [32, 84, 96].

Accurate attribution of functional impairment to ADHD or SUD symptoms presents an additional challenge, as associated educational and professional consequences of ADHD can also be found in SUD populations. Furthermore, ADHD symptoms have often been mitigated and obscured by compensatory strategies or "environmental scaffolding," employed and strengthened by parental support and/or structured environments [14, 46]. Lastly, some individuals may feign ADHD symptoms to obtain accommodations on exams or prescriptions for stimulants for misuse or diversion, as seen in high school/college athletes seeking performance enhancement [32, 84, 166]. Thus, it is imperative that information is obtained from multiple sources (e.g., partner or parent) and a review of objective data is completed (e.g., school or work evaluations) [32, 84, 96].

Treatment Options for ADHD and Co-Occurring SUD

ADHD is frequently treated with pharmacotherapy, which has proven efficacy in reducing symptoms of inattention and hyperactivity in children and adults [6, 45]. There is ample evidence that psychostimulant treatment of ADHD (e.g., amphetamine and methylphenidate) earlier in childhood can reduce the risk of subsequent substance use compared to those who initiated stimulant treatment for ADHD at a later age [36, 93, 126]. Thus, to prevent adverse outcomes and substance use escalation, early identification and treatment of ADHD in childhood seems to hold the most promise.

Treating adolescent and adult patients with ADHD+ SUD presents additional challenges in SUD treatment settings: they tend to have additional psychiatric comorbidities, more severe SUD, earlier initiation of substance use, and riskier drug use behaviors than their non-ADHD counterparts, likely resulting in poor SUD treatment adherence and increased rates of relapse [149, 152, 163, 172]. Moreover, practitioners may be less willing to prescribe stimulant medication to individuals with ADHD+SUD due to fears of misuse. These concerns can be addressed by long-acting formulations and/or non-stimulant medications in treating ADHD, which are less prone to misuse and diversion.

Evidence-based non-pharmacological interventions for ADHD and/or SUD have been employed in ADHD and co-occurring SUD populations in combination with pharmacotherapy to support, integrate, and optimize long-term treatment outcomes. Psychosocial interventions for adolescents and adults include coaching, behavior modification, and cognitive-behavioral therapies (CBT) for ADHD or SUD that promote psychoeducation, cognitive remediation, and building coping skills [32, 84, 96].

Stimulant Medications

Amphetamine (AMP) is a potent central nervous system stimulant whose primary mechanism of action is to stimulate neurotransmitter release and block the reuptake of dopamine [47, 51, 84, 96]. Amphetamine analogs include methamphetamine, dextroamphetamine, mixed amphetamine salts, and lisdexamfetamine. Methamphetamine is only available in an immediate-release preparation and is rarely prescribed due to concerns of non-medical use and diversion.

Lisdexamfetamine (LDX) is an FDA-approved ADHD treatment for children and adults. LDX remains a therapeutically inactive molecule until after oral ingestion, and is associated with a longer duration of effect and reduced abuse potential [51, 69]. A meta-analysis of five randomized controlled, double-blind studies assessing the efficacy of LDX versus placebo in children and adolescents with ADHD found 30-70 mg per day of LDX to have a greater pooled improvement rate (72% to 21%, respectively) and comparable acceptability and tolerability, indicating it an efficacious treatment for ADHD in this population [91]. In adults with ADHD, the same dosage of LDX was found to be an efficacious alternative stimulant treatment for ADHD that also showed improvement in executive function [90].

Methylphenidate, (MPH) a widely used psychostimulant for the treatment of ADHD, acts therapeutically by blocking dopamine and, to a lesser extent, norepinephrine reuptake in the striatum [47, 51, 84, 96]. The increased dopamine and norepinephrine availability from MPH and AMP have been shown to affect cortical and striatal brain regions related to cognition, executive function, risky decision making, and regulation of reward processes in preclinical and human studies [47]. Produced in multiple formulations, MPH is available in immediate and extended-release preparations. Common side effects of AMP and MPH are mostly related to their stimulant properties and include insomnia, palpitations, increased heart rate and elevated blood pressure, nervousness, emotional lability, and gastrointestinal disturbances such as nausea and vomiting [51, 84, 96]. Rare but serious adverse effects include severe hypertension, seizures, psychosis, and myocardial infarction.

A transdermal methylphenidate system (MTS) ADHD treatment has been FDA approved to deliver once-daily MPH via a drug-in adhesive matrix patch of varying sizes and corresponding dosages worn on the hip over the course of 9 hours [7, 51, 52, 120]. The MTS is a good option for individuals with difficulty swallowing pills, while absorption of MPH is not affected by meals or competitive metabolism of other medications. It has demonstrated safety and efficacy in children and adolescents across multiple settings, is well tolerated after long-term use and after switching from oral MPH medications, and has good quality of life and parental satisfaction with medication responses [52]. Studies have also found MTS to be effective in treating ADHD in adult populations [95, 99]. Adverse reactions to MTS include mild dermal or application site reactions, decreased appetite, and headaches but were otherwise similar to those of other MPH formulations [52].

Lastly, Modafinil is an FDA-approved stimulant drug used to promote wakefulness and treat sleep disorders that has shown to be well tolerated, but exhibits only slight efficacy in treating ADHD in children and adults [8, 57, 70, 86, 147]. Unlike typical stimulants, modafinil acts on histamine and enhances cognitive functions while improving the symptoms of ADHD without resulting in hyperarousal [86]. Modafinil's lack of activation in regions that mediate the reward system and its single route of administration (oral) results in a low abuse potential, allowing it to serve as an alternative, second-line treatment for ADHD, particularly in SUD populations [92, 100].

Non-Stimulant Medications

Non-stimulant medications found effective for use in treating ADHD symptomology include atomoxetine, antidepressants, and alpha-2 agonists. With the exception of atomoxetine, a first-line FDA-approved ADHD medication indicated for use in co-occurring SUD, tic disorders, or cardiovascular disease, non-stimulants are considered off-label, second-line ADHD treatments [51, 84, 96].

Atomoxetine (ATX) is a potent noradrenergic reuptake inhibitor that increases norepinephrine and dopamine in the frontal cortex to effectively treat inattention and impulsivity symptoms in children, adolescents, and adults with ADHD [1, 39, 51, 103, 171]. The therapeutic effects of ATX are produced more gradually than with stimulants, often taking several weeks to manifest. Furthermore, ATX may be used with individuals who are unresponsive to or have difficulty tolerating stimulants [39, 51]. Common side effects of ATX include sedation, appetite suppression, nausea, vomiting, and headache. Rare but serious side effects reported in children and adolescents include increased suicidal ideation and hepatotoxicity. ATX has no known non-medical use potential and is less vulnerable to abuse and diversion, compared to stimulants, so it is an appealing medication option in the treatment of ADHD and co-occurring SUDs. Although published data are limited, the pharmacology of ATX can be associated with improved ADHD symptoms and reduced substance use [171].

Several antidepressants have been considered for off-label treatment of ADHD. Bupropion, a dopaminergic antidepressant, has shown effectiveness in reducing ADHD symptoms, but evidenced no benefit over placebo in SUD patients [27, 81, 164]. Tricyclic antidepressants, which block the reuptake of norepinephrine, show some efficacy in treating ADHD but are less effective than stimulants [170]. Venlafaxine, a norepinephrine-serotonin reuptake inhibitor antidepressant, has limited evidence of efficacy on ADHD in uncontrolled and small placebo-controlled clinical trials [4, 111, 117]. Lastly, monoamine oxidase inhibitors have shown efficacy for ADHD but are contraindicated in SUD populations given the potential for hypertensive crises associated with tyramine-containing foods and medications, limiting their utility [84, 96].

Guanfacine extended release, a norepinephrine alpha-2 agonist, has been shown to improve ADHD symptoms after 1-week of administration and is nearly as effective as stimulants in treating children and adolescents [61, 68, 131, 144], with limited findings in adults [150]. It has also been shown to further reduce ADHD symptoms when co-administered with stimulants among children and adults who have had a limited response to stimulants alone [144]. Common side effects of guanfacine include somnolence, headaches, sedation, and hypotension [26, 131]. Clonidine, molecularly similar to guanfacine, has shown efficacy for the treatment of ADHD although less so than stimulant and other FDA-approved non-stimulant medication [24, 25, 45]. Clonidine extended release also evidenced reduction in ADHD symptoms for those with only a partial response to stimulants [77]. Side effects include sedation, dry mouth, depression, confusion, electrocardiographic changes, and hypertension with abrupt withdrawal.

Pharmacotherapy in Co-occurring ADHD and SUD

Valid concerns have been raised regarding prescribing these medications to patients with addictive disorders, given the potential risk for abuse, difficulties with medication compliance, and the higher tolerance that may require doses higher than those administered in clinical trials [89]. The AAP [60] noted adolescents tend to report misusing stimulants to concentrate, study, and improve grades; "to party" and "get high." While most misuse occurs via oral administration, those who do so via nasal insufflation (i.e., snorting) and to get high are at the greatest risk for a SUD. While longitudinal studies have provided evidence that ADHD medication use prevents adolescent substance use (ASU), results from meta-analyses conclude that medication neither increases nor decreases the risk for ASU

[66, 67, 106, 107]. Thus, drawing conclusions from the literature should be done with caution.

As noted, psychostimulants are the first line of treatment for adults and children with ADHD, yet issues arise when treating adult ADHD in individuals with SUD. Research has shown psychostimulants are safe and effective in treating ADHD symptoms in SUD populations, with low abuse potential, particularly for longer acting formulations [19, 32, 42, 51, 84, 96]. Oral MPH has shown efficacy in treating ADHD symptoms without producing significant effects of euphoria in intravenous cocaine and methylphenidate users [23, 89]. One study of adults with ADHD and a history of illicit stimulant use found MTS to be safe and effective at reducing ADHD symptomology and stimulant use over 8 weeks, thought participants did consume other drugs [99]. Lastly, modafinil has demonstrated reductions in substance use in cocaine [34, 35, 72, 92, 100] and methamphetamine-dependent [136] individuals. In adolescents, psychostimulants are effective in treating ADHD [2, 60] and have not been shown to increase the likelihood of SUD, though it is unknown whether it is protective in preventing later misuse [66].

Noting the long-term changes in ADHD symptomology resulting from medication use that lessen the vulnerability to PSUD is important for future research [67, 108], as well as fully accounting for moderating and mediating clinical factors. For adolescents known to misuse stimulants or suspected of selling or diverting medication, the AAP [60] suggests prescribing a long-acting stimulant, such as OROS-MPH (a long-acting formulation of MPH), or LDX, given its lower abuse potential [69]. Reviews of ASU and co-occurring ADHD provide an overview of pharmacological studies and psychotherapeutic options for this population [66, 174]. Results from two national CTN studies found no differences in subjective levels of euphoria with OROS-MPH, or in patterns of medication misuse in adolescents with and without SUD [169]. A 16-week, multi-site, RCT of OROS-MPH + CBT for ASU versus CBT for ASU + Placebo in adolescents demonstrated overall comparable significant decreases in ADHD symptoms and drug use, but the combined active treatment group had better secondary outcomes, greater drug use reduction, and greater self-reported improvements in problem-solving abilities and focused coping skills [129].

In ADHD+SUD adults, non-stimulant medications have shown efficacy in reducing ADHD symptoms, with mixed results in reducing substance use. An RCT comparing the efficacy of ATX versus placebo in cannabis-dependent individuals found that ATX in combination with Motivational Interviewing (MI) was effective at reducing some ADHD symptoms, but did not significantly reduce substance use [98]. Similar results were seen in an open-label trial of ATX in adults with ADHD and cocaine dependence [82]. Another RCT of ATX versus placebo in ADHD+SUD adolescents found no significant differences between groups on these factors of interest [151].

A recent study investigating the effectiveness of non-stimulant medication treatment in a sample of adults in a correctional facility with ADHD+SUD and other psychiatric disorders showed an improvement in overall clinical severity, a response rate of 64%, and a remission rate of 35% [15]. In an adolescent sample with ADHD+SUD and comorbid mood diagnoses, sustained-release bupropion reduced ADHD symptoms and substance use [141]. These findings support the use of non-traditional and non-stimulant treatment in psychiatrically complex ADHD+ SUD populations and in settings where minimizing the risk for abuse and diversion limits the implementation of first-line ADHD treatments. When both ADHD and PSUD symptoms are treated, SUD patients with more severe ADHD have the potential for greater improvement in ADHD symptomology, thereby increasing the likelihood of improvement in SUD [19, 88, 149].

Luo and Levin (2017) posit that computational modeling can be a tool in using clinical, genetic, and biomarker to support patient-treatment matching and precision addiction medicine, facilitating individually tailored treatment ADHD+SUD patients [89]. Indeed, findings from numerous studies suggest certain treatments are optimal for specific subpopulations: OROS-MPH was found effective at reducing substance use in adolescents with comorbid CD [149] and improved nicotine abstinence in combination with a nicotine patch for adults with more severe ADHD [115], while ATX may be beneficial in ADHD and AUD populations [42, 167].

In non-abstinent ADHD+SUD populations, continued substance use likely impacts the detection of therapeutic effects [59]. A recent systematic review of RCTs for DSM-IV ADHD and comorbid stimulant dependence [171] note that OROS-MPH in higher than usual doses (e.g., up to 180-mg per day) for longer durations can effectively treat ADHD and lessen use in amphetamine users [78]. In cocaine-dependent patients, a three-arm, 14-week RCT of extended-release MAS and CBT/relapse prevention treatment resulted in greater reduction of ADHD symptoms, fewer cocaine positive weeks, a higher proportion of cocaine abstinence, and high treatment retention rates in the active treatment arms [83].

A nationwide study of adult ADHD patients in Sweden treated with MPH found those with comorbid SUD were prescribed 40% higher doses 2 years into treatment than their non-SUD peers [140]. Individuals with diagnoses of stimulant use, comorbid DUD, and AUD had a significant increased risk of exceeding the United States Food and Drug Administration recommended maximum dose of 72 mg per day. Two years into treatment, 37.1% and 6.7% of ADHD+ SUD patients were prescribed 73–180 mg and 181–360 mg of MPH daily, compared to 21.6% and 1.0% of their ADHD-only counterparts, respectively. Together, these findings reflect the need for clinical and dosing guidelines specific to ADHD and SUD populations.

Psychosocial Interventions for ADHD and SUD

While pharmacotherapy is the foundation of ADHD treatment, various psychosocial treatments can be implemented in combination with medication. Psychosocial interventions for ADHD include cognitive behavioral therapy (CBT), psychoeducation, metacognitive training, mindfulness training, coaching and behavioral modification, as well as motivational interviewing (MI). Psychoeducation is an important component of any ADHD intervention, given the pervasive effects of symptoms in multiple areas of functioning and the importance of treatment compliance [96].

Research suggests that a combination of medication and cognitive therapy is more effective than medication alone or medication and psychoeducation [94, 122, 132]. Several of the studies assessing the efficacy of medication also included psychosocial interventions, such as CBT targeting ADHD or SUD symptoms [83, 98, 129]. One RCT assessed the efficacy of CBT or relaxation with educational support in medicated adults with persistent ADHD [132]. Results showed that CBT patients responded well to treatment, their ADHD symptoms were reduced, and they maintained gains over 12 months post-treatment.

Challenges for treatment providers include helping patients distinguish and link the cognitive, behavioral, and physiological symptoms associated with ADHD and those associated with SUD, as seen in a relapse prevention approach [10]. Additionally, ADHD-related impairments in cognitive process can affect gains made in psychosocial treatments. Integrating cognitive enhancement interventions to ADHD+ SUD populations can directly target executive functioning deficits that impede success in skills-based behavioral interventions, particularly for adolescents [66]. Patients' emotional responses to struggling with ADHD+ SUD may lead to inadequate coping skills and further drug use. Results from the first integrated CBT approach for ADHD+SUD adults have recently been published, assessing the efficacy of this treatment compared to standard substance use treatments [156, 158].

Several family-based ADHD interventions for adolescents appear promising for treating ADHD+ SUD in a developmentally appropriate manner. The Medication Integration Protocol (MIP) integrates medication into behavioral treatment planning for adolescents with ADHD and is therefore a useful tool for ADHD+ SUD populations [62–65]. The MIP includes ADHD and medication psychoeducation, reframing patient issues into family problems with potential family solutions, and medication management to enhance adherence. Supporting Teens' Academic Needs Daily (STAND), another psychosocial ADHD treatment that has yet to be used with comorbid ASU but may be applicable in this population, is an 8–10-week protocol integrating behavioral management and academic training to emphasize organization skills, parenting skills, and family problem solving [137, 139].

Conclusion

ADHD confers significant risk for PSUDs and is over-represented in SUD populations. Yet, ADHD+SUD individuals present diagnostic challenges due to shared cognitive and behavioral features of both disorders. Validated screening instruments are useful in identifying probable ADHD, and should be followed by a thorough clinical or diagnostic interview. While stimulant medication is often the most effective treatment for ADHD, clinicians may be reluctant to prescribe them to individuals with co-occurring SUD, due to fears of non-medical use and diversion. Published findings on the efficacy of stimulant, non-stimulant, and psychosocial interventions for ADHD+SUD populations underscore the need for additional research and potential revision of dosing guidelines.

References

1. Adler LA, Spencer TJ, Milton DR, Moore RJ, Michelson D. Long-term, open-label study of the safety and efficacy of atomoxetine in adults with attention-deficit/hyperactivity disorder: an interim analysis. J Clin Psychiatry. 2005;66(3):294–9.
2. American Academy of Pediatrics, Subcommittee on Attention-Deficit/Hyperactivity Disorder, Committee on Quality Improvement. ADHD: clinical practice guideline for the diagnosis, evaluation, and treatment of attention-deficit/hyperactivity disorder in children and adolescents. Pediatr. 2011;128(5):1007–22.
3. American Psychiatric Association. Diagnostic and statistical manual of mental disorders: DSM-5. Arlington, VA: American Psychiatric Association; 2013.
4. Amiri S, Farhang S, Ghoreishizadeh MA, Malek A, Mohammadzadeh S. Double-blind controlled trial of venlafaxine for treatment of adults with attention deficit/hyperactivity disorder. Hum Psychopharmacol Clin Exp. 2012;27(1):76–81.
5. Arias AJ, Gelernter J, Chan G, Weiss RD, Brady KT, Farrer L, et al. Correlates of co-occurring ADHD in drug-dependent subjects: prevalence and features of substance dependence and psychiatric disorders. Addict Behav. 2008;33(9):1199–207.
6. Arnold LE. Methlyphenidate vs amphetamine: comparative review. J Atten Disord. 2000;3(4):200–11.
7. Arnold LE, Lindsay RL, López FA, Jacob SE, Biederman J, Findling RL, Ramadan Y. Treating attention-deficit/hyperactivity disorder with a stimulant transdermal patch: the clinical art. Pediatr. 2007;120(5):1100–6.
8. Arnold VK, Feifel D, Earl CQ, Yang R, Adler LA. A 9-week, randomized, double-blind, placebo-controlled, parallel-group, dose-finding study to evaluate the efficacy and safety of modafinil as treatment for adults with ADHD. J Atten Disord. 2014;18(2):133–44.
9. Arnsten AFT, Rubia K. Neurobiological circuits regulating attention, cognitive control, motivation, and emotion: disruptions in neurodevelopmental psychiatric disorders. J Am Acad Child Adolesc Psychiatry. 2012;51(4):356–67.
10. Aviram RB, Rhum M, Levin FR. Psychotherapy of adults with comorbid attention-deficit/hyperactivity disorder and psychoactive substance use disorder. J Psychother Pract Res. 2001;10(3):179.
11. Barkley RA. Driving impairments in teens and adults with attention-deficit/ hyperactivity disorder. Psychiat Clin North Am. 2004;27:233–60.
12. Barkley RA, Fischer M, Smallish L, Fletcher K. Young adult outcome of hyperactive children: adaptive functioning in major life activities. J Am Acad Child Adolesc Psychiatry. 2006;45:192–202.
13. Barkley RA, Cox D. A review of driving risks and impairments associated with attention-deficit/hyperactivity disorder and the effects of stimulant medication on driving performance. J Saf Res. 2007;38:113–28.
14. Barkley RA, Brown TE. Unrecognized attention-deficit/hyperactivity disorder in adults presenting with other psychiatric disorders. CNS Spectr. 2008;13(11):977–84.
15. Bastiaens L, Scott O, Galus J. Treatment of Adult ADHD without stimulants: effectiveness in a dually diagnosed correctional population. Psychiatry Q. 2018;26:1–6.
16. Bierut L, Dinwiddie S, Begleiter H, Crowe R, Hesselbrock V, Numberger J, et al. Familial transmission of substance dependence: alcohol, mari-

juana, cocaine, and habitual smoking. Arch Gen Psychiatry. 1998;55(11):982–8.

17. Bernardi S, Faraone SV, Cortese S, Kerridge BT, Pallanti S, Wang S, et al. The lifetime impact of attention-deficit hyperactivity disorder: results from the National Epidemiologic Survey on alcohol and related conditions. Psychol Med. 2012;42(4):875–87.
18. Biederman J, Wilens T, Mick E, Milberger S, Spencer TJ, Faraone SV. Psychoactive substance use disorders in adults with attention deficit hyperactivity disorder (ADHD): effects of ADHD and psychiatric comorbidity. Am J Psychiatry. 1995;152:1652–8.
19. Carpentier PJ, Levin FR. Pharmacological treatment of ADHD in addicted patients: what does the literature tell us? Harvard Rev Psychiatry. 2017 Mar;25(2):50.
20. Castellanos FX, Lee PP, Sharp W, Jeffries NO, Greenstein DK, Clasen LS, et al. Developmental trajectories of brain volume abnormalities in children and adolescents with attention deficit/hyperactivity disorder. J Am Med Assoc. 2002;288(14):1740e1748.
21. Charach A, Yeung E, Climans T, Lillie E. Childhood attention-deficit/hyperactivity disorder and future substance use disorders: comparative Meta-analyses. J Am Acad Child Adolesc Psychiatry. 2011;50(1):9–21.
22. Chronis-Tuscano A, Molina BS, Pelham WE, Applegate B, Dahlke A, Overmyer M, et al. Very early predictors of adolescent depression and suicide attempts in children with attention-deficit/hyperactivity disorder. Arch Gen Psychiatry. 2010;67:1044–51.
23. Collins SL, Levin FR, Foltin RW, Kleber HD, Evans SM. Response to cocaine, alone and in combination with methylphenidate, in cocaine abusers with ADHD. Drug Alcohol Depend. 2006;82:158–67.
24. Connor DF, Fletcher KE, Swanson JM. A meta-analysis of clonidine for symptoms of attention-deficit hyperactivity disorder. J Am Acad Child Adolesc Psychiatry. 1999;38(12):1551–9.
25. Connor DF, Barkley RA, Davis HT. A pilot study of methylphenidate, clonidine, or the combination in ADHD comorbid with aggressive oppositional defiant or conduct disorder. Clin Pediatr. 2000;39(1):15–25.
26. Connor DF, Findling RL, Kollins SH, Sallee F, López FA, Lyne A, Tremblay G. Effects of guanfacine extended release on oppositional symptoms in children aged 6–12 years with attention-deficit hyperactivity disorder and oppositional symptoms. CNS Drugs. 2010;24(9):755–68.
27. Conners CK, Casat CD, Gualtieri CT, Weller E, Reader M, Reiss A, Weller RA, Khayrallah M, Ascher J. Bupropion hydrochloride in attention deficit disorder with hyperactivity. J Am Acad Child Adolesc Psychiatry. 1996;35(10):1314–21.
28. Conners CK, Erhardt D, Sparrow EP. Conners' adult ADHD rating scales (CAARS): technical manual. North Tonawanda: MHS; 1999.
29. Conners CK, Epstein J, Johnson DE. Conner's Adult ADHD Diagnostic interview for DSM-IV: CAADID: technical manual. New York, NY: MHS; 2001.
30. Cortese S, Angriman M, Maffeis C, Isnard P, Konofal E, Lecendreux M, et al. Attention-deficit/hyperactivity disorder (ADHD) and obesity: a systematic review of the literature. Crit Rev Food Sci Nutr. 2008;48:524–37.
31. Cortese S, Kelly C, Chabernaud C, Proal E, Di Martino A, Milham MP, et al. Toward systems neuroscience of ADHD: a meta-analysis of 55 fMRI studies. Am J Psychiatry. 2012;169:1038–55.
32. Crunelle CL, van den Brink W, Moggi F, Konstenius M, Franck J, Levin FR, van de Glind G, Demetrovics Z, Coetzee C, Luderer M, Schellekens A. International consensus statement on screening, diagnosis and treatment of substance use disorder patients with comorbid attention deficit/hyperactivity disorder. Eur Addict Res. 2018;24(1):43–51.
33. Cubillo A, Halari R, Smith A, Taylor E, Rubia K. A review of fronto-striatal and fronto-cortical brain abnormalities in children and adults with attention deficit hyperactivity disorder (ADHD) and new evidence for dysfunction in adults with ADHD during motivation and attention. Cortex. 2012;48:194–215.
34. Dackis CA, Lynch KG, Yu E, Samaha FF, Kampman KM, Cornish JW, Rowan A, Poole S, White L, O'Brien CP. Modafinil and cocaine: a double-blind, placebo-controlled drug interaction study. Drug Alcohol Depend. 2003;70(1):29–37.
35. Dackis CA, Kampman KM, Lynch KG, Pettinati HM, O'brien CP. A double-blind, placebo-controlled trial of modafinil for cocaine dependence. Neuropsychopharmacology. 2005;30(1):205.
36. Dalsgaard S, Mortensen PB, Frydenberg M, Thomsen PH. ADHD, stimulant treatment in childhood and subsequent substance abuse in adulthood - a naturalistic long-term follow-up study. Addict Behav. 2014;39:325–8.
37. Dalsgaard S, Ostergaard SD, Leckman JF, Mortensen PB, Pedersen MG. Mortality in children, adolescents, and adults with attention deficit hyperactivity disorder: a nationwide cohort study. Lancet. 2015;385:2190–6.
38. Demontis D, et al. Discovery of the first genome-wide significant risk loci for attention deficit/hyperactivity disorder. Nat Genet. 2018; https://doi.org/10.1038/s41588-018-0269-7.
39. Elbe D. Black TR. Procyshyn RM, editors. Clinical Handbook of Psychotropic Drugs for Children and Adolescents. Hogrefe Verlag: McGrane IR; 2018.
40. Elkins IJ, McGue M, Iacono WG. Prospective effects of attention-deficit/hyperactivity disorder, conduct disorder, and sex on adolescent substance use and abuse. Arch Gen Psychiatry. 2007;64:1145–52. https://doi.org/10.1001/archpsyc.64.10.1145.
41. Epstein JN, Loren REA. Changes in the definition of ADHD in DSM-5: subtle but important. Neuropsychiatry (London). 2013;3(5):455–8.

42. Evren C. Comorbidity of attention deficit-hyperactivity disorder and substance use disorder. J Psychiatry Neurol Sci. 2018;31:115–24.
43. Faraone SV, Biederman J, Mick E. The age-dependent decline of attention deficit hyperactivity disorder: a meta-analysis of follow-up studies. Psychol Med. 2006;36:159–65.
44. Faraone SV, Mick E. Molecular genetics of attention deficit hyperactivity disorder. Psychiatr Clin North Am. 2010a;33(1):159–80.
45. Faraone SV, Glatt SJ. A comparison of the efficacy of medications for adult attention-deficit/hyperactivity disorder using meta-analysis of effect sizes. J Clin Psychiatry. 2010b;71(6):754–63.
46. Faraone SV, Biederman J. Can attention-deficit/hyperactivity disorder onset occur in adulthood? JAMA Psychiat. 2016;73(7):655–6.
47. Faraone SV. The pharmacology of amphetamine and methylphenidate: relevance to the neurobiology of attention-deficit/hyperactivity disorder and other psychiatric comorbidities. Neurosci Biobehav Rev. 2018;87:255–70.
48. Fassbender C, Zhang H, Buzy WM, Cortes CR, Mizuiri D, Beckett L, et al. A lack of default network suppression is linked to increased distractibility in ADHD. Brain Res. 2009;1273:114–28.
49. Fatseas M, Hurmic H, Serre F, Debrabant R, Daulouede JP, Denis C, et al. Addiction severity pattern associated with adult and childhood attention deficit hyperactivity disorder (ADHD) in patients with addictions. Psychiatry Res. 2016;246:656–62.
50. Fayyad J, De Graaf R, Kessler R, et al. Cross-national prevalence and correlates of adult attention-deficit hyperactivity disorder. Br J Psychiatry. 2007;190:402–9.
51. Findling RL. Evolution of the treatment of attention-deficit/hyperactivity disorder in children: a review. Clin Ther. 2008;30(5):942–57.
52. Findling RL, Dinh S. Transdermal therapy for attention-deficit hyperactivity disorder with the methylphenidate patch (MTS). CNS Drugs. 2014;28(3):217–28.
53. First MB, Williams JB, Karg RS, Spitzer RL. User's guide to structured clinical interview for DSM-5 disorders (SCID-5-CV) clinical version. Arlington, VA: American Psychiatric Publishing; 2015.
54. Fredriksen M, Dahl AA, Martinsen EW, Klungsoyr O, Faraone SV, Peleikis DE. Childhood and persistent ADHD symptoms associated with educational failure and long-term occupational disability in adult ADHD. Atten Defic Hyperact Disord. 2014;6:87–99.
55. Gascon GG, Johnson R, Burd L. Central auditory processing and attention deficit disorders. J Child Neurol. 1986;1(1):27–33.
56. Gordon M, Barkley RA, Lovett BJ. Tests and observational measures, in attention-deficit hyperactivity disorder: handbook for diagnosis and treatment. 3rd ed. New York, NY: Guilford Press, Inc.; 2006. p. 69–389.
57. Greenhill LL, Biederman J, Boellner SW, Rugino TA, Sangal RB, Earl CQ, Jiang JG, Swanson JM. A randomized, double-blind, placebo-controlled study of modafinil film-coated tablets in children and adolescents with attention-deficit/hyperactivity disorder. J Am Acad Child Adolesc Psychiatry. 2006;45(5):503–11.
58. Groenman AP, Oosterlaan J, Rommelse N, Franke B, Roeyers H, Oades RD, et al. Substance use disorders in adolescents with attention deficit hyperactivity disorder: a 4-year follow-up study. Addict. 2013;108:1503–11.
59. Halikas JA, Meller J, Morse C, Lyttle MD. Predicting substance abuse in juvenile offenders: attention deficit disorder versus aggressivity. Child Psychiatry Hum Dev. 1990;21(1):49–55.
60. Harstad E, Levy S. Committee on substance abuse. Attention-deficit/hyperactivity disorder and substance abuse. Pediatr. 2014;134(1):e293–301.
61. Hervas A, Huss M, Johnson M, McNicholas F, van Stralen J, Sreckovic S, Lyne A, Bloomfield R, Sikirica V, Robertson B. Efficacy and safety of extended-release guanfacine hydrochloride in children and adolescents with attention-deficit/hyperactivity disorder: a randomized, controlled, phase III trial. Eur Neuropsychopharmacol. 2014;24(12):1861–72.
62. Hogue A, Bobek M, Nager A. Medication integration protocol (MIP): provider manual. The National Center on Addiction and Substance Abuse at Columbia University. 2013.
63. Hogue A, Bobek M, Tau GZ, Levin FR. Clinical strategies for integrating medication interventions into behavioral treatment for adolescent ADHD: the medication integration protocol. Child Fam Behav Ther. 2014;36(4):280–304.
64. Hogue A, Bobek M, Evans SW. Changing academic support in the home for adolescents with attention-deficit/hyperactivity disorder: a family-based clinical protocol for improving school performance. Cogn Behav Pract. 2016;23(1):14–30.
65. Hogue A, Lichvar E, Bobek M. Pilot evaluation of the medication integration protocol for adolescents with ADHD in Behavioral care: treatment Fidelity and medication uptake. J Emot Behav Disord. 2016;24(4):223–34.
66. Hogue A, Evans SW, Levin FR. A Clinician's guide to co-occurring ADHD among adolescent substance users: comorbidity, neurodevelopmental risk, and evidence-based treatment options. J Child Adolesc Subst Abuse. 2017;26(4):277–92.
67. Humphreys KL, Eng T, Lee SS. Stimulant medication and substance use outcomes: a meta-analysis. JAMA Psychiat. 2013;70(7):740–9.
68. Huss M, Dirks B, Gu J, Robertson B, Newcorn JH, Ramos-Quiroga JA. Long-term safety and efficacy of guanfacine extended release in children and adolescents with ADHD. Eur Child Adolesc Psychiat. 2018;27(10):1283–94.
69. Jasinski DR, Krishnan S. Abuse liability and safety of oral lisdexamfetamine dimesylate in individuals

with a history of stimulant abuse. J Psychopharmacol. 2009;23(4):419–27.
70. Kahbazi M, Ghoreishi A, Rahiminejad F, Mohammadi MR, Kamalipour A, Akhondzadeh S. A randomized, double-blind and placebo-controlled trial of modafinil in children and adolescents with attention deficit and hyperactivity disorder. Psychiatry Res. 2009;168(3):234–7.
71. Kalivas PW, Volkow ND. The neural basis of addiction: a pathology of motivation and choice. Am J Psychiatry. 2005;162:1403–13.
72. Kampman KM, Lynch KG, Pettinati HM, Spratt K, Wierzbicki MR, Dackis C, O'Brien CP. A double blind, placebo controlled trial of modafinil for the treatment of cocaine dependence without comorbid alcohol dependence. Drug Alcohol Depend. 2015;155:105–10.
73. Katusic SK, Barbaresi WJ, Colligan RC, Weaver A, Mrazek DA, Jacobsen SJ. Substance abuse among ADHD cases: a population-based birth cohort study. Proceedings of the Pediatric academic society. Seattle (WA); 2003.
74. Kessler RC, Adler L, Ames M, Demler O, Faraone S, Hiripi EV, Howes MJ, Jin R, Secnik K, Spencer T, Ustun TB. The World Health Organization Adult ADHD self-report scale (ASRS): a short screening scale for use in the general population. Psychol Med. 2005;35(2):245–56.
75. Kessler RC, Adler L, Barkley R, et al. The prevalence and correlates of adult ADHD in the United States: results from the National Comorbidity Survey Replication. Am J Psychiatry. 2006;163:716–23.
76. Klein RG, Mannuzza S, Ramos Olazagasti MA, Roizen E, Hutchison JA, Lashua EC, et al. Clinical and functional outcome of childhood attention-deficit/hyperactivity disorder 33 years later. Arch Gen Psychiatry. 2012;69(12):1295–303.
77. Kollins SH, Jain R, Brams M, Segal S, Findling RL, Wigal SB, Khayrallah M. Clonidine extended-release tablets as add-on therapy to psychostimulants in children and adolescents with ADHD. Pediatr. 2011;127(6):e1406–13.
78. Konstenius M, Jayaram-Lindström N, Guterstam J, Beck O, Philips B, Franck J. Methylphenidate for attention deficit hyperactivity disorder and drug relapse in criminal offenders with substance dependence: a 24-week randomized placebo-controlled trial. Addict. 2014;109(3):440–9.
79. Lee SS, Humphreys KL, Flory K, Liu R, Glass K. Prospective association of childhood attention-deficit/hyperactivity disorder (ADHD) and substance use and abuse/dependence: a meta-analytic review. Clin Psychol Rev. 2011;31:328–41.
80. Levin FR, Evans SM, Kleber HD. Prevalence of adult attention-deficit hyperactivity disorder among cocaine abusers seeking treatment. Drug Alcohol Depend. 1998;52:15–25.
81. Levin FR, Evans SM, Brooks DJ, Kalbag AS, Garawi F, Nunes EV. Treatment of methadone-maintained patients with adult ADHD: double-blind comparison of methylphenidate, bupropion and placebo. Drug Alcohol Depend. 2006;81(2):137–48.
82. Levin FR, Mariani JJ, Secora A, Brooks D, Cheng WY, Bisaga A, Nunes E, Aharonovich E, Raby W, Hennessy G. Atomoxetine treatment for cocaine abuse and adult attention deficit/hyperactivity disorder (ADHD): a preliminary open trial. J Dual Diagn. 2009;5(1):41–56.
83. Levin FR, Mariani JJ, Specker S, Mooney M, Mahony A, Brooks DJ, et al. Extended-release mixed amphetamine salts vs placebo for comorbid adult attention-deficit/hyperactivity disorder and cocaine use disorder: a randomized clinical trial. JAMA Psychiat. 2015;72:593–602.
84. Levin FR, Mariani JJ. Co-occurring addictive disorder and attention deficit hyperactivity disorder. In: Miller SC, Fiellin DA, Rosenthal RN, Saitz R, editors. The ASAM principles of addiction medicine. 6th ed. Wolters Kluwer; 2018.
85. Liddle EB, Hollis C, Batty MJ, Groom MJ, Totman JJ, Liotti M, et al. Task-related default mode network modulation and inhibitory control in ADHD: effects of motivation and methylphenidate. J Child Psychol Psychiatry. 2011;52:761–71.
86. Lindsay SE, Gudelsky GA, Heaton PC. Use of modafinil for the treatment of attention deficit/hyperactivity disorder. Ann Pharmacother. 2006;40(10):1829–33.
87. Luderer M, Sick C, Kaplan-Wickel N, Reinhard I, Richter A, Kiefer F, et al. Prevalence estimates of ADHD in a sample of inpatients with alcohol dependence. J Atten Disord. 2018;00(0):1–12.
88. Luo SX, Covey LS, Hu MC, Levin FR, Nunes EV, Winhusen TM. Toward personalized smoking-cessation treatment: using a predictive modeling approach to guide decisions regarding stimulant medication treatment of attention-deficit/hyperactivity disorder (ADHD) in smokers. Am J Addict. 2015;24(4):348–56.
89. Luo SX, Levin FR. Towards precision addiction treatment: new findings in co-morbid substance use and attention-deficit hyperactivity disorders. Curr Psychiatry Rep. 2017;19(3):14.
90. Maneeton N, Maneeton B, Suttajit S, Reungyos J, Srisurapanont M, Martin SD. Exploratory meta-analysis on lisdexamfetamine versus placebo in adult ADHD. Drug Des Dev Ther. 2014;8:1685.
91. Maneeton B, Maneeton N, Likhitsathian S, Suttajit S, Narkpongphun A, Srisurapanont M, Woottiluk P. Comparative efficacy, acceptability, and tolerability of lisdexamfetamine in child and adolescent ADHD: a meta-analysis of randomized, controlled trials. Drug Des Dev Ther. 2015;9:1927.
92. Mann N, Bitsios P. Modafinil treatment of amphetamine abuse in adult ADHD. J Psychopharmacol. 2009;23(4):468–71.
93. Manuzza S, Klein RG, Truong NL, Moulton JL III, Roizen ER, Howell KH, et al. Age of methylphenidate treatment initiation in children with ADHD and

later substance abuse: prospective follow-up into adulthood. Am J Psychiatry. 2008;165:605–9.
94. March JS, Swanson JM, Arnold LE, Hoza B, Conners CK, Hinshaw SP, Hechtman L, Kraemer HC, Greenhill LL, Abikoff HB, Elliott LG. Anxiety as a predictor and outcome variable in the multimodal treatment study of children with ADHD (MTA). J Abnorm Child Psychol. 2000;28(6):527–41.
95. Marchant BK, Reimherr FW, Robison RJ, Olsen JL, Kondo DG. Methylphenidate transdermal system in adult ADHD and impact on emotional and oppositional symptoms. J Atten Disord. 2011;15(4):295–304.
96. Mariani JJ, Levin FR. Treatment strategies for co-occurring ADHD and substance use disorders. Am J Addict. 2007:16(supl):45–56.
97. Matthys F, Stes S, van den Brink W, Joostens P, Möbius D, Tremmery S, et al. Guideline for screening, diagnosis and treatment of ADHD in adults with substance use disorders. Int J Ment Health Addict. 2014;12:629–47. https://doi.org/10.1007/s11469-014-9496-z.
98. McRae-Clark AL, Carter RE, Killeen TK, Carpenter MJ, White KG, Brady KT. A placebo-controlled trial of atomoxetine in marijuana-dependent individuals with attention deficit hyperactivity disorder. Am J Addict. 2010;19(6):481–9.
99. McRae-Clark AL, Brady KT, Hartwell KJ, White K, Carter RE. Methylphenidate transdermal system in adults with past stimulant misuse: an open-label trial. J Atten Disord. 2011;15(7):539–44.
100. Mereu M, Bonci A, Newman AH, Tanda G. The neurobiology of modafinil as an enhancer of cognitive performance and a potential treatment for substance use disorders. Psychopharmacol. 2013;229(3):415–34.
101. Merikangas KR, Stolar M, Stevens DE, Goulet J, Preisig MA, Fenton B, et al. Familial transmission of substance use disorders. Arch Gen Psychiatry. 1998;55(11):973–9.
102. Merrill RM, Lyon JL, Baker RK, Gren LH. Attention deficit hyperactivity disorder and increased risk of injury. Adv Med Sci. 2009;54:20–6.
103. Michelson D, Adler L, Spencer T, Reimherr FW, West SA, Allen AJ, Kelsey D, Wernicke J, Dietrich A, Milton D. Atomoxetine in adults with ADHD: two randomized, placebo-controlled studies. Biol Psychiatry. 2003;53(2):112–20.
104. Milberger S, Biederman J, Faraone S, Wilens T, Chu M. Associations between ADHD and psychoactive substance use disorders: findings from a longitudinal study of high-risk siblings of ADHD children. Am J Addict. 1997;6:318–29.
105. Moffitt TE, Houts R, Asherson P, Belsky DW, Corcoran DL, Hammerle M, et al. Is adult ADHD a childhood-onset neurodevelopmental disorder? Evidence from a four-decade longitudinal cohort study. Am J Psychiatry. 2015;172:967–77.
106. Molina BS, Pelham WE Jr. Childhood predictors of adolescent substance use in a longitudinal study of children with ADHD. J Abnorm Psychol. 2003;112:497–507.
107. Molina BS, Hinshaw SP, Arnold LE, Swanson JM, Pelham WE, Hechtman L, Hoza B, Epstein JN, Wigal T, Abikoff HB, Greenhill LL. Adolescent substance use in the multimodal treatment study of attention-deficit/hyperactivity disorder (ADHD) (MTA) as a function of childhood ADHD, random assignment to childhood treatments, and subsequent medication. J Am Acad Child Adolesc Psychiatry. 2013;52(3):250–63.
108. Molina BS, Pelham WE Jr. Attention-deficit/hyperactivity disorder and risk of substance use disorder: developmental considerations, potential pathways, and opportunities for research. Annu Rev Clin Psychol. 2014;10:607–39.
109. Molina BSG, Howard AL, Swanson JM, Stehli A, Mitchell JT, Kennedy TM, et al. Substance use through adolescence into early adulthood after childhood-diagnosed ADHD: findings from the MTA longitudinal study. J Child Psychol Psychiatr. 2018;59:692–702.
110. Erratum. J Child Psychol Psychiatr. 2018;59:e1–4. https://doi.org/10.1111/jcpp.12970.
111. Motavalli Mukaddes N, Abali O. Venlafaxine in children and adolescents with attention deficit hyperactivity disorder. Psychiatry Clin Neurosci. 2004;58(1):92–5.
112. Murphy KR, Gordon M. Assessment of adults with ADHD. In: Attention-deficit hyperactivity disorder: handbook for diagnosis and treatment. 3rd ed. New York, NY: Guilford Press, Inc.; 2006. p. 425–50.
113. Nigg JT. Attention-deficit/hyperactivity disorder and adverse health outcomes. Clin Psychol Rev. 2013;33:215–28.
114. Notzon DP, Pavlicova M, Glass A, Mariani JJ, Mahony AL, Brooks DJ, Levin FR. ADHD is highly prevalent in patients seeking treatment for cannabis use disorders. J Atten Disord. 2016; https://doi.org/10.1177/1087054716640109.
115. Nunes EV, Covey LS, Brigham G, Hu MC, Levin FR, Somoza E, Winhusen T. Treating nicotine dependence by targeting attention deficit hyperactivity disorder (ADHD): the role of ADHD severity and treatment response in a randomized controlled trial. J Clin Psychiatry. 2013;74(10):983.
116. Nurnberger JI, Wiegand R, Bucholz K, O'Connor S, Meyer ET, Reich T, et al. A family study of alcohol dependence. Arch Gen Psychiatry. 2004;61:1246–56.
117. Olvera RL, Pliszka SR, Luh J, Tatum R. An open trial of venlafaxine in the treatment of attention-deficit/hyperactivity disorder in children and adolescents. J Child Adolesc Psychopharmacol. 1996;6(4):241–50.
118. Ortal S, van de Glind G, Johan F, Itai B, Nir Y, Iliyan I, et al. The role of different aspects of impulsivity as independent risk factors for substance use disorders in patients with ADHD: a review. Curr Drug Abuse Rev. 2015;8(2):119–33.

119. Pastor PN, Reuben CA. Identified attention-deficit/hyperactivity disorder and medically attended, nonfatal injuries: US school-age children, 1997–2002. Ambul Pediatr. 2006;6:38–44.
120. Patrick KS, Straughn AB, Perkins JS, González MA. Evolution of stimulants to treat ADHD: transdermal methylphenidate. Hum Psychopharmacol Clin Exp. 2009;24(1):1–7.
121. Peterson BS, Potenza MN, Wang Z, Zhu H, Martin A, Marsh R, et al. An fMRI study of the effects of psychostimulants on default-mode processing during Stroop task performance in youths with ADHD. Am J Psychiatry. 2009;166:1286–94.
122. Philipsen A. Psychotherapy in adult attention deficit hyperactivity disorder: implications for treatment and research. Expert Rev Neurother. 2012;12(10):1217–25.
123. Polanczyk G, Rohde LA. Epidemiology of attention-deficit/hyperactivity disorder across the lifespan. Curr Opin Psychiatry. 2007;20:386–92.
124. Polanczyk GV, Willcutt EG, Salum GA, Kieling C, Rohde LA. ADHD prevalence estimates across three decades: an updated systematic review and meta-regression analysis. Int J Epidemiol. 2014:434–42.
125. Proal E, Reiss PT, Klein RG, Mannuzza S, Gotimer K, Ramos-Olazagasti MA, et al. Brain gray matter deficits at 33-year follow-up in adults with attention-deficit/hyperactivity disorder established in childhood. Arch Gen Psychiatry. 2011;68(11):1122–34.
126. Quinn PD, Chang Z, Hur K, Gibbons RD, Lahey BB, Rickert ME, et al. ADHD medication and substance-related problems. Am J Psychiatry. 2017;174(9):877–85.
127. Ramos-Quiroga JA, Díaz-Digon L, Comín M, Bosch R, Palomar G, Chalita JP, Roncero C, Nogueira M, Torrens M, Casas M. Criteria and concurrent validity of adult ADHD section of the psychiatry research interview for substance and mental disorders. J Atten Disord. 2015;19(12):999–1006.
128. Ramos-Quiroga JA, Nasillo V, Richarte V, Corrales M, Palma F, Ibáñez P, Michelsen M, Van de Glind G, Casas M, Kooij JS. Criteria and concurrent validity of DIVA 2.0: a semi-structured diagnostic interview for adult ADHD. J Atten Disord. 2016:1087054716646451.
129. Riggs PD, Winhusen T, Davies RD, Leimberger JD, Mikulich-Gilbertson S, Klein C, Macdonald M, Lohman M, Bailey GL, Haynes L, Jaffee WB. Randomized controlled trial of osmotic-release methylphenidate with cognitive-behavioral therapy in adolescents with attention-deficit/hyperactivity disorder and substance use disorders. J Am Acad Child Adolesc Psychiatry. 2011;50(9):903–14.
130. Rooney M, Chronis-Tuscano A, Yoon Y. Substance use in college students with ADHD. J Atten Disord. 2012;16:221–334.
131. Sallee FR, Lyne A, Wigal T, McGough JJ. Long-term safety and efficacy of guanfacine extended release in children and adolescents with attention-deficit/hyperactivity disorder. J Child Adolesc Psychopharmacol. 2009;19(3):215–26.
132. Safren SA, Sprich S, Mimiaga MJ, Surman C, Knouse L, Groves M, Otto MW. Cognitive behavioral therapy vs relaxation with educational support for medication-treated adults with ADHD and persistent symptoms: a randomized controlled trial. J Am Med Assoc. 2010;304(8):875–80.
133. Schubiner H, Tzelepis A, Milberger S, Lockhart N, Kruger M, Kelley BJ, et al. Prevalence of attention-deficit/hyperactivity disorder and conduct disorder among substance abusers. J Clin Psychiatry. 2000;61:244–51.
134. Shaw P, Eckstrand K, Sharp W, Blumenthal J, Lerch JP, Greenstein D, et al. Attention deficit/hyperactivity disorder is characterized by a delay in cortical maturation. Proc Natl Acad Sci U S A. 2007;104(49):19649e19654.
135. Shaw P, Polanczyk GV. Combining epidemiological and neurobiological perspectives to characterize the lifetime trajectories of ADHD. Eur Child Adolesc Psychiatry. 2017;26:139–41.
136. Shearer J, Darke S, Rodgers C, Slade T, Van Beek I, Lewis J, Brady D, McKetin R, Mattick RP, Wodak A. A double-blind, placebo-controlled trial of modafinil (200 mg/day) for methamphetamine dependence. Addict. 2009;104(2):224–33.
137. Sibley MH, Pelham WE, Derefinko KJ, Kuriyan AB, Sanchez F, Graziano PA. A pilot trial of supporting teens' academic needs daily (STAND): a parent-adolescent collaborative intervention for ADHD. J Psychopathol Behav Assess. 2013;35(4):436–49.
138. Sibley MH, Pelham WE Jr, Molina BSG, Coze S, Kipp H, Gnagy EM, et al. The role of early childhood ADHD and subsequent CD in the initiation and escalation of adolescent cigarette, alcohol and marijuana use. J Abnorm Psychol. 2014;123:362–74.
139. Sibley MH, Graziano PA, Kuriyan AB, Coxe S, Pelham WE, Rodriguez L, Sanchez F, Derefinko K, Helseth S, Ward A. Parent–teen behavior therapy+ motivational interviewing for adolescents with ADHD. J Consult Clin Psychol. 2016;84(8):699.
140. Skoglund C, Brandt L, D'Onofrio B, Larsson H, Franck J. Methylphenidate doses in attention deficit/hyperactivity disorder and comorbid substance use disorders. Eur Neuropsychopharmacol. 2017;27(11):1144–52.
141. Solhkhah R, Wilens TE, Daly J, Prince JB, Patten SL, Biederman J. Bupropion SR for the treatment of substance-abusing outpatient adolescents with attention-deficit/hyperactivity disorder and mood disorders. J Child Adolesc Psychopharmacol. 2005;15(5):777–86.
142. Sonuga-Barke EJ. The dual pathway model of AD/HD: an elaboration of neuro-developmental characteristics. Neurosci Biobehav Rev. 2003;27:593–604.
143. Sonuga-Barke EJ. Causal models of attention-deficit/hyperactivity disorder: from common simple deficits to multiple developmental pathways. Biol Psychiatry. 2005;57:1231–8.

144. Spencer TJ, Greenbaum M, Ginsberg LD, Murphy WR. Safety and effectiveness of coadministration of guanfacine extended release and psychostimulants in children and adolescents with attention-deficit/hyperactivity disorder. J Child Adolesc Psychopharmacol. 2009;19(5):501–10.
145. Substance Abuse and Mental Health Services Administration. Key substance use and mental health indicators in the United States: results from the 2017 National Survey on drug use and health (HHS publication no. SMA 18-5068, NSDUH series H-53). Rockville, MD: Center for Behavioral Health Statistics and Quality, Substance Abuse and Mental Health Services Administration; 2018.
146. Surman CB, Adamson JJ, Petty C, Biederman J, Kenealy DC, Levine M, et al. Association between attention-deficit/hyperactivity disorder and sleep impairment in adulthood: evidence from a large controlled study. J Clin Psychiatry. 2009;70:1523–9.
147. Swanson JM, Greenhill LL, Lopez FA, Sedillo A, Earl CQ, Jiang JG, Biederman J. Modafinil film-coated tablets in children and adolescents with attention-deficit/hyperactivity disorder: results of a randomized, double-blind, placebo-controlled, fixed-dose study followed by abrupt discontinuation. J Clin Psychiatry. 2006;67(1):137–47.
148. Swensen A, Birnbaum HG. Ben, Hamadi R, Greenberg P, Cremieux PY, Secnik K. incidence and costs of accidents among attention-deficit/hyperactivity disorder patients. J Adolesc Health. 2004;35:346–9.
149. Tamm L, Trello-Rishel K, Riggs P, Nakonezny PA, Acosta M, Bailey G, Winhusen T. Predictors of treatment response in adolescents with comorbid substance use disorder and attention-deficit/hyperactivity disorder. J Subst Abus Treat. 2013;44(2):224–30.
150. Taylor FB, Russo J. Comparing guanfacine and dextroamphetamine for the treatment of adult attention-deficit/hyperactivity disorder. J Clin Psychopharmacol. 2001;21(2):223–8.
151. Thurstone C, Riggs PD, Salomonsen-Sautel S, Mikulich-Gilbertson SK. Randomized, controlled trial of atomoxetine for attention-deficit/hyperactivity disorder in adolescents with substance use disorder. J Am Acad Child Adolesc Psychiatry. 2010;49(6):573–82.
152. Tiet QQ, Ilgen MA, Byrnes HF, Harris AHS, Finney JW. Treatment setting and baseline substance use severity interact to predict patients' outcomes. Addict. 2007;102:432–40.
153. Triolo SJ, Murphy KR. Attention-deficit scales for adults (ADSA). Brunner/Mazel; 1996.
154. van de Glind G, Konstenius M, Koeter MW, van Emmerik-van Oortmerssen K, Carpentier PJ, Kaye S, et al. Variability in the prevalence of adult ADHD in treatment seeking substance use disorder patients: results from an international multi-center study exploring DSM-IV and DSM-5 criteria. Drug Alcohol Depend. 2014;134:158–66.
155. van Emmerik-van Oortmerssen K, van de Glind G, van den Brink W, Smit F, Crunelle CL, Swets M, et al. Prevalence of attention-deficit hyperactivity disorder in substance use disorder patients: a meta-analysis and meta-regression analysis. Drug Alcohol Depend. 2012;122:11–9.
156. van Emmerik–van Oortmerssen K, Vedel E, Koeter MW, de Bruijn K, Dekker JJ, van den Brink W, Schoevers RA. Investigating the efficacy of integrated cognitive behavioral therapy for adult treatment seeking substance use disorder patients with comorbid ADHD: study protocol of a randomized controlled trial. BMC Psychiatry. 2013;13(1):132.
157. van Emmerik-van Oortmerssen K, van de Glind G, Koeter MW, Allsop S, Auriacombe M, Barta C, et al. Psychiatric comorbidity in treatment-seeking substance use disorder patients with and without attention deficit hyperactivity disorder: results of the IASP study. Addict. 2014;109:262–72.
158. van Emmerik-van Oortmerssen K, Vedel E, Kramer FJ, Blankers M, Dekker JJ, van den Brink W, Schoevers RA. Integrated cognitive behavioral therapy for ADHD in adult substance use disorder patients: results of a randomized clinical trial. Drug Alcohol Depend. 2019:5.
159. Volkow ND, Wang GJ, Kollins SH, Wigal TL, Newcorn JH, Telang F, et al. Evaluating dopamine reward pathway in ADHD: clinical implications. J Am Med Assoc. 2009;302:1084–91.
160. Ward MF, Wender PH, Reimherr FW. The Wender Utah rating scale: an aid in the retrospective diagnosis of childhood attention deficit hyperactivity disorder. Am J Psychiatry. 1993;150(6):885–90.
161. West SL, Mulsow M, Arredondo R. Factor analysis of the attention deficit scales for adults (ADSA) with a clinical sample of outpatient substance abusers. Am J Addict. 2003;12(2):159–65.
162. Wilens TE, Biederman J, Mick E, Faraone SV, Spencer T. Attention-deficit/hyperactivity disorder (ADHD) is associated with early-onset substance use disorders. J Nerv Ment Disord. 1997;185(8):475–82.
163. Wilens TE, Biederman J, Mick E. Does ADHD affect the course of substance abuse? Findings from a sample of adults with and without ADHD. Am J Addict. 1998;7:156–63.
164. Wilens TE, Spencer TJ, Biederman J, Girard K, Doyle R, Prince J, Polisner D, Solhkhah R, Comeau S, Monuteaux MC, Parekh A. A controlled clinical trial of bupropion for attention deficit hyperactivity disorder in adults. Am J Psychiatry. 2001;158(2):282–8.
165. Wilens T. Attention-deficit/hyperactivity disorder and the substance use disorders: the nature of the relationship, subtypes at risk, and treatment issues. Psychiatr Clin North Am. 2004;27(2):283–301.
166. Wilens TE, Adler LA, Adams J, Sgambati S, Rotrosen J, Sawtelle R, Utzinger L, Fusillo S. Misuse and diversion of stimulants prescribed for ADHD: a systematic review of the literature. J Am Acad Child Adolesc Psychiatry. 2008a;47(1):21–31.

167. Wilens TE, Adler LA, Weiss MD, Michelson D, Ramsey JL, Moore RJ, Renard D, Brady KT, Trzepacz PT, Schuh LM, Ahrbecker LM. Atomoxetine treatment of adults with ADHD and comorbid alcohol use disorders. Drug Alcohol Depend. 2008b;96(1–2):145–54.
168. Wilens TE, Martelon M, Joshi G, et al. Does ADHD predict substance-use disorders? A 10-year follow-up study of young adults with ADHD. J Am Acad Child Adolesc Psychiatry. 2011;50:543–53.
169. Winhusen TM, Lewis DF, Riggs PD, Davies RD, Adler LA, Sonne S, et al. Subjective effects, misuse, and adverse effects of osmotic-release methylphenidate treatment in adolescent substance abusers with attention-deficit/hyperactivity disorder. J Child Adolesc Psychopharmacol. 2011;21:455–63.
170. Wolraich ML, Wibbelsman CJ, Brown TE, Evans SW, Gotlieb EM, Knight JR, Ross EC, Shubiner HH, Wender EH, Wilens T. Attention-deficit/hyperactivity disorder among adolescents: a review of the diagnosis, treatment, and clinical implications. Pediatr. 2005;115(6):1734–46.
171. Woon LS, Hazli Z, Gan L. Pharmacotherapy for comorbid Adult attention-deficit hyperactivity disorder and stimulant dependence: a systematic review. Int Med J Malaysia. 2018;1:17(2).
172. Young JT, Carruthers S, Kaye S, Allsop S, Gilsenan J, Degenhardt L, et al. Comorbid attention deficit hyperactivity disorder and substance use disorder complexity and chronicity in treatment-seeking adults. Drug Alcohol Rev. 2015;34:683–93.
173. Yule AM, Martelon M, Faraone SV, Carrellas N, Wilens TE, Biederman J. Examining the association between attention deficit hyperactivity disorder and substance use disorders: a familial risk analysis. J Psychiatr Res. 2017;85:49–55.
174. Zaso MJ, Park A, Antshel KM. Treatments for adolescents with comorbid ADHD and substance use disorder: a systematic review. J Atten Disord. 2015;5:1087054715569280.

3 Substance Use in Older Adults

Paroma Mitra

Introduction

The group of people born after World War Two or people born between 1946 and 1964 are referred to as the baby boomer generation. According to the census report, they began to turn 65 in 2011. By 2029 more than 20% of the population will be over the age of 65 [1].

The baby boomers have had a higher rate of substance use than previous generations and there is a cumulative effect seen presently [2]. The estimate of the number of people using substances will double from 2.8 million (average in 2002–2006) to 5.7 million in 2020 [3].

This group is unique and has needs that need to be addressed. Providers and other professionals need to be familiar with signs and symptoms of substance use in older adults as well as have a cohesive understanding of treatment and needs of this population.

This chapter is further broken down into the four major groups of substance use most common in older adults – each category has epidemiology, screening, impact on the geriatric population (targeting mental and physical health), and treatment considerations for the same.

The tail end of the chapter also speaks to special populations in older adults including but not limited to the LGBTQ community, the incarcerated population, etc.

Alcohol Use

There were surveys done almost 10 years ago that has shown that 40% older adults drink alcohol [2]. The initial thought had been that substance use gradually decreases with age [5], however this thought is being challenged in more recent studies.

In fact, 9% of the older adults that drink have binge drinking and about 2.5% of these can meet the criteria for alcohol use disorder [6].

The general consensus is also that older people may tend to minimize alcohol use and primary care physicians also do not adequately screen for ongoing alcohol use [7]. Some of the risk factors for excess alcohol use include male gender, being Caucasian, and higher socioeconomic class [26].

There is some scientific evidence that moderate drinking (<1 drink/day) [8] may be beneficial to health. There are many physiologic changes that happen in the body – as we age decreased water to fat ratio and decreased metabolization by the liver as well as decreased excretion by the kidney [9]. There are many medical issues that arise with older age alcohol use – prominent

P. Mitra (✉)
Bellevue Hospital Center, New York University Grossman School of Medicine, New York, NY, USA
e-mail: Paroma.Mitra@nyulangone.org

E. Akerele (ed.), *Substance and Non-Substance Related Addictions*,
https://doi.org/10.1007/978-3-030-84834-7_3

issues consist of hemorrhagic stroke, ulcers, cancer of the liver and stomach, hypertension, and arrhythmias [10]. In fact, binge drinking can lead to an increased risk of falls and early cognitive impairment [11]. Also there are moderate to severe interactions with medications [12].

The National Institute on Alcohol Abuse and Alcoholism mandate that there are no more than 3 drinks on any given day and no more than 7 drinks per week [2, 4, 13].

Comorbid alcohol and affective disorders lead to a more complicated course of treatment and more symptoms of isolation and even increased incidence of suicidal ideation [4, 60]. A longitudinal study has shown that new onset affective and anxiety disorders may develop with comorbid alcohol use with people over the age of 50.

All personality and affective disorders were associated with increased chances of both alcohol and tobacco use disorder in older adults; any lifetime mood disorder was associated with increased chances of past-year alcohol use [64].

Diagnosis

Under Diagnostic and Statistical Disorders Manual V, the current version of the DSM, anyone meeting any two of the 11 criteria during the same 12-month period receives a diagnosis of substance use disorder. If one meets two of the criteria then they meet diagnosis for mild, four of the criteria they meet criteria for moderate, and six or more then they meet criteria for severe use [14].

(a) The substance is often taken in larger amounts or over a longer period of time than intended.
(b) There is a persistent desire or unsuccessful effort to cut down or control substance use.
(c) A great deal of time is spent in activities necessary to obtain the substance, use it, or recover from its effects.
(d) Craving, or a strong desire or urge to use the substance.
(e) Recurrent substance use resulting in a failure to fulfill major role obligations at work, school, or home.
(f) Continued substance use despite having persistent or recurrent social or interpersonal problems caused or exacerbated by the effects of alcohol.
(g) Important social, occupational, or recreational activities are given up or reduced because of substance use.
(h) Recurrent substance use in situations where it is physically dangerous.
(i) Substance use is continued despite knowledge of having a persistent or recurrent physical or psychological problem that is likely to have been caused or exacerbated by alcohol.
(j) Tolerance as defined by either of the following: (a) a need for markedly increased amounts of substance to achieve intoxication or desired effect, (b) a markedly diminished effect with continued use of the same amount of substance.
(k) Withdrawal as manifested by either of the following: (a) the characteristic withdrawal syndrome for alcohol like headaches, tremors; (b) alcohol (or a closely related substance, such as a benzodiazepine) is taken to relieve or avoid withdrawal symptoms.

According to DSM-5 these criteria can be modified to the older adult population – for example, criteria a – in older adults, cognitive impairment can be an impediment to monitor substance use. Hence alcohol may be taken for longer periods than intended. Criteria c refers to a long time required to either obtain alcohol or recover from effects – even small amounts may require increased time for recovery. Criteria g looks at role fulfillment in older adults an example of the same may be taking care of younger grandchildren at home if the adult has retired from work. Criteria e looks at social functioning where in older adults this becomes more limited than usual as older adults may not be part of a larger workforce. Criteria j looks at tolerance where tolerance is significantly lowered in older folks. However, in terms of withdrawal, compared to younger adults, this may be subtler or longer drawn out [15].

In older adults, substance use disorder can be a two-tier classification. There is the at-risk population which takes more medication than the desired amount and the population that may misuse or older adults that do not take medication for the intended effect [2, 33].

Screening

As discussed above screening in older adults for alcohol use is limited among primary care staff. Over the past decade, however, there has been more emphasis on addiction and the use of screening language has changed to be less stigmatizing [16]. The use of words like "addict", "criminal", etc., has been highly discouraged by the National Drug Institute. Older adults can be especially sensitive given past experience of legality association with substance use.

There are several screening tools that may be used for alcohol use and the main ones are highlighted below.

The CAGE

The CAGE questionnaire is possibly the most common tool of use in screening for alcohol use. The CAGE questionnaire consists of 4 questions [17]:

- Have you ever felt you should Cut down on your drinking?
- Have people Annoyed you by criticizing your drinking?
- Have you ever felt bad or Guilty about your drinking?
- Have you ever had a drink first thing in the morning to steady your nerves or to get rid of a hangover (Eye opener)?

Unfortunately, the CAGE Questionnaire does not differentiate between lifetime use and current use. Also, sensitivity of the CAGE questionnaire is 86% and specificity is 78% [18]. The CAGE has been expanded to be used in Spanish as well.

The Alcohol Use Disorders Identification Test (AUDIT)

The AUDIT above was developed by the WHO (World Health Organization) and has also been used in older adults [19]. In a sample of almost 200 adults aged 65+ in primary care centers, the AUDIT was found to have a sensitivity of 66.7% and specificity of 95.3% [20]. The AUDIT-C is a shorter form for the AUDIT. The AUDIT-C compromises 10 questions around alcohol consumption, amount, and frequency.

The Michigan Alcohol Screening Test-Geriatric

The MAST was the first test designed for older people [21]. The MAST-G has 24 questions usually presented in the yes/no format with 5 or more positive responses indicating alcohol use that may meet criteria for alcohol use disorder. It focuses on stressors and behavioral indications while using alcohol [22]. The MAST-G has high sensitivity (95%) and specificity (78%) [23].

Short Michigan Alcohol Screening Test-Geriatric [22]

1. When talking with others, do you ever underestimate how much you drink?
2. After a few drinks, have you sometimes not eaten or been able to skip a meal because you didn't feel hungry?
3. Does having a few drinks help decrease your shakiness or tremors?
4. Does alcohol sometimes make it hard for you to remember parts of the day or night?
5. Do you usually take a drink to relax or calm your nerves?
6. Do you drink to take your mind off your problems?
7. Have you ever increased your drinking after experiencing a loss in your life?
8. Has your doctor or nurse ever said they were worried or concerned about your drinking?

9. Have you ever made rules to manage your drinking?
10. When you feel lonely, does having a drink help?

The Comorbidity-Alcohol Risk Evaluation Tool [23, 24]

This Particular Screening tool identifies older adults with specific behaviors that can place them at risk. It is useful in older adults specially with sensitivity of 92% but specificity being somewhat low (51%). The geriatric age group is a particularly high risk given the use of medications as well.

Biological Markers: Laboratory markers like blood alcohol level (acetate metabolite of alcohol can be detected during acute intoxication). Chronic markers of alcohol use include gamma glutyl transferase levels, mean corpuscular volume, HDL level, and carbohydrate-deficient transferrin [36].

Emergency Room visits: There have not been separate studies looking at emergency room visits exclusively due to alcohol use in older adults. However, alcohol in combination with other illicit substances leads to increased visits to emergency rooms in older adults [24].

Treatment in the Elderly

Non-pharmacological

1. Self-help groups: Older adults may also benefit from Alcoholics Anonymous and other supportive community groups. One of the drawbacks of the same however is considering mobility and modes of getting to these and overall preponderance of younger people [25].
2. Brief interventions.

An example of an intervention for at-risk drinking that was done at a primary care center was non-pharmacological. The study had been conducted over 3 months where at-risk drinkers were identified and were randomized. Half the participants received a booklet on alcohol use. The other half received personalized report, booklet on alcohol and aging, drinking diary, advice from the primary care provider, and telephone counseling from a health educator at 2, 4, and 8 weeks [27]. The proportion of at-risk older adults was not reduced but the amount of drinking reduced over a year.

Another example is of the BRITE project [28] (Brief Intervention and Treatment for Elders) which was conducted in the state of Florida. Evidence-based practices such as motivational interviewing techniques were applied at different sites be it homes, primary care settings, or old age facilities. Counselors were trained to do an intervention for 1 to 5 sessions. Some participants also received treatment for 16 sessions using a Cognitive Behavioral Format. Alcohol misuse was identified and reduced. This study has also treated people with other substance use which will be addressed later in the chapter.

Additional studies have shown basic counseling, education by a physician; using care coordinators from a physician's office can be helpful in reducing alcohol use [29].

Pharmacological Treatment

To date, FDA has approved 4 medications for alcohol use disorder namely acamprosate, disulfiram, oral naltrexone, and extended release injectable naltrexone [30, 31].

(a) Acamprosate: This drug increases inhibitory GABA transmission and is given in doses of 666 mg three times a day [30]. In older adults, special consideration must be given to ones with chronic renal disease. It is considered effective but there are no randomized controlled trials for the same.
(b) Disulfiram: This drug is an aldehyde dehydrogenase inhibitor. The dose can range between 250 and 500 mg/da [30]. It is not recommended in older adults because of cardiovascular side effects. It is also not recommended for adults with chronic liver disease [32].

(c) Naltrexone: The maximum is 50 mg/day orally or 380 mg intramuscularly every 4 weeks [30]. Naltrexone is an opioid receptor antagonist. Again special caution must be taken for persons with chronic liver disease. A randomized controlled trial conducted among veterans older than 50 showed that alcohol use is reduced with persons on naltrexone therapy [32, 33, 40]. Also, older adults have been shown as more adherent to medications [39].

Medications like topiramate and gabapentin are being researched for treatment for alcohol use. A word of caution with the use of the medications above is the cognitive effects on older people [34, 35].

During detoxication from acute alcohol intoxication, older adults are more prone to medical symptoms of withdrawal like delirium tremens and seizures [32]. Also short-acting benzodiazepines are preferred for older adults with chronic liver disease [30].

Tobacco Use Disorder

Epidemiology: Tobacco is the second most used substance among older adults. An epidemiologic study looking at the lifetime prevalence showed that about 52% of older adults had used tobacco in their lifetime and in the past 12 months about 14% had used a form of tobacco [37]. Other epidemiological studies show that older adults that smoke tend to be male and single and long-term smokers [38]. Tobacco use not only is a factor in cardiological and pulmonary diseases in all ages but in older adults has a negative impact on cognition and is linked to dementia [41]. Smoking is considered especially risky in older women with an increased risk for osteoporosis and breast cancer [42]. Older adults with life mood or personality disorder have increased tobacco use and adults with personality disorder have past-year alcohol use disorder [64].

Screening: There have not been specific tools to screen for tobacco use in older adults. The alcohol, smoking, and substance involvement screening test (ASSIST) has been developed by the World Health Organization but not validated in older adults [43].

Treatment: Unfortunately there are limitations in effective treatment for older adults. There are small studies which show motivational interviewing to be effective in older adults [44]. Older adults in this study were seen as more engaged to discuss the negative effect of smoking.

Pharmacological interventions: There are many interventions for nicotine cessation but less studied in older adults. There are many products that are available over the counter including nicotine gum, lozenge, and patch. In older adults the lozenge is easier than the gum as gum may get caught in people with jaw injuries and temporo-mandibular dysfunction. A nicotine patch may be considered in persons with cognitive impairment [2].

Combination NRT is considered effective in the general population but there is limited evidence in older adults [45]. In terms of common drugs Bupropion (dopamine-norepinephrine reuptake inhibitor) is not more effective than NRT in older adults [46]. Varenicline is a nicotinic agonist that is now widely used to aid smoking cessation but not studied in older adults [47].

Illicit Drug Use

The National Survey on Drug Use in 2012 showed the rate of substance use has almost doubled for persons aged 50 and older [48]. In 2012, 19.3% of adults older than 65 reported any instance of substance use and 47.6% of adults between 60 and 64 had lifetime drug use [33]. Results tend to primarily show much higher rates of illicit drug use in ages 50–64 than 65 plus [53].

Cannabis is the most common drug among illicit substances used. About 3.9% of older adults above 50 had past-year cannabis use from 2008 to 2012 [49, 50]. The data from NSDUH also indicate that people who continue to use cannabis are people that have begun to use it at a younger age of 18. Cannabis users also to be male and Caucasian. 132,000 older adults used marijuana and 4300 older adults used cocaine. All drugs act on various neurotransmitters in the brain and given age-related changes in the brain; older adults remain at high risk for adverse events [58]. About 90% of persons that use illicit drugs after the age of 50 have early onset of use [3, 33].

Past-year marijuana use among adults aged 50+ years is estimated to increase from 1.0% in 1999–2000 to 2.9% in 2020. Use of any illicit drug is expected to increase from 2.2% to 3.1% [52].

According to the study, the baby boomer generation has a more favorable attitude toward legalizing cannabis. Changing attitude has also come with having more positive views of the medicinal effect of Cannabis [51].

Risk in Older Adults: Marijuana use in older adults can cause increased heart rate, respiratory rate, and increased risk of a heart attack [33].

Screening: There are no format screening tools for screening illicit substance use in older adults; however, the consensus panel of the treatment improvement protocol recommended that all older adults be screened for illicit drug use [54].

Emergency room visits: In a study of 3000 plus people in an inner-city population around 3% tested positive for an illicit substance. Cocaine was the most used substance, followed by opioid and marijuana [61].

Treatment: One study done in 2009 indicated that opioids/heroin, cocaine, and marijuana are the drugs most commonly sought in treatment systems. Most older adults have comorbid diagnosis and tend to be referred from the criminal justice system.

Treatment for older adults per guidelines indicates that the least intensive route be taken including cognitive behavioral work, case management, and group therapy. 12-step programs may not be appropriate for all older adults. A non-confrontational method of improving self-esteem may be best [54, 55]. Some guidelines include a supportive and holistic stance which is flexible to needs such as gender and cultural differences [59].

Prescriptions Drug Misuse

In 2012, 2.9 million people above the age of 50 reported psychotropic prescription use [33]. About 1.4 million people of people above the age of 50 have reported misuse of drugs. The nonmedical use of prescription drugs (opioids, sedatives, tranquilizers, and stimulants) is projected to increase from 1.2% (911,000) to 2.4% (2.7 million) in 2020 [53, 2]. In 2020, the age distribution is estimated to be 48% of people in their 50's and 37% in their 60's (Book reference-substance use in older adults). National studies have shown that 72% of persons between ages 50 and 59 started illicit drug use around 30 [3].

Factors for prescription drug use include female gender, history of prior substance use, co-occurring mental health disorder, and isolation. Prescriptions of psychoactive medications also may increase the user's risk for nonmedical use, abuse, or dependence [56, 57].

Benzodiazepines are among the most prescribed psychiatric medications (Grohol, 2010). There are several medical drawbacks to the same, however this continues to be widely prescribed [56]. Benzodiazepines are fat-soluble substances with longer half-lives. The pharmacokinetics (the way our body breaks down drugs) changes as we age and benzodiazepines can remain longer in the body of older adults given slow metabolization. Benzodiazepines increase the risk for falls, fractures, and increase the risk of delirium and sleep disturbances [58]. Of note, past-year benzodiazepine and opioid misuse is associated with past-year suicidal ideation in adults above 50 [65].

Screening: Older adults often present with physical symptoms. However, there are common signs and symptoms which include but are not limited to frequent falls, bruises, burns, headaches, memory loss, poor hygiene, etc. One way of screening includes following the time follow back method, i.e., prospective monitoring, recording drug use, and then using a time frame to calculate substance use [4].

The US drug and substance use network data has shown consistently that there have been increasing visits to the emergency room for illicit substance use. In adults above 55, opioid use is most common and followed by benzodiazepines [24]. Also, in another study 1 in 4 elderly patients had a positive toxicology screen in psychiatric emergency room services notably that elderly patients with comorbid psychiatric illness have a high prevalence of ongoing drug use [63].

Treatment: Treatment for illicit substance use in older adults continues to be conservative. More non-pharmacological, supportive, and brief intervention therapy is usually preferred over the use of medications.

Special Populations

1. Lesbian, Gay, Bisexual, Transgender, Queer: There are approximately 1 million older adults that identify as LGBTQ [67]. Notably they are at higher risk for both substance use as well as affective disorders. The rate of substance use among the LGBTQ community tends to be higher than age-matched controls [68] for all adults. However, no specific studies have been conducted specifically in the older population.
2. Homeless Older Adults: The average age of single adults that are now homeless is above 50. A study conducted in Oakland California showed that more than two-thirds had ongoing substance use that met criteria for moderate to severe substance use disorder. About a fourth had met criteria for alcohol use disorder [66]. The study called for more integrated care for older adults with more training and development for geriatric training.
3. Older Incarcerated Adults: There have been limited studies that have been conducted on prison inmates [62]. Overall the conclusion has been that older inmates are chronic substance users, however hardly a third of them receive treatment. The inmates also tend to have chronic persistent mental illness. Opioid and cocaine appeared to be substances of choice [4, 62].
4. *Nursing Home*: There is a general consensus that older adults in nursing homes have substance use be it misuse or over-prescription [70]. Few studies have looked at the prevalence, however two studies have reported 29% to 49% of personnel have ongoing substance use [69]. There are few programs that work exclusively with older adults and substance use, the Jewish Home Lifecare in New York is the first one of its kind [71].

Conclusion

Alcohol and other substance use continue to be an ongoing public health issue among older adults and will continue to be so for the next many years. Traditional thinking continues to tend toward the understanding of decreased substance use as adults age, however recent epidemiological studies have continued to show use.

During routine screening in primary care offices, it is important to question and screen for ongoing substance use. Clinicians are encouraged to routinely screen use and understand the variable signs and symptoms that may be seen in older adults as compared to younger and middle-aged adults.

It is important to note that most studies exclude adults over 65 and most randomized controlled trials looking at treatment for older adults include adults above 50 which tend to be more prevalent. There continues to be more need for research in older adults. Factors such as physical comorbidities and mental health comorbidities need to be taken into account. There is more emphasis on non-pharmacological treatment that is supportive in nature, community-based, and integrated into primary care and other facilities.

Lastly, there will continue to be a significant number of adults who may identify with other sexuality, identify within a minority, may continue to be placed in long-term care or may be incarcerated. This chapter has not addressed older adults with HIV and substance use where there is more need for treatment. There is almost no data on these subtypes of population and epidemiological trends continue to show an uptrend increasing for need for research for the same.

It would be remiss not to speak about the impact of the ongoing pandemic on both mental health and substance use in older adults. Social isolation and anxiety around contracting the disease has increased in the older adult population which has in turn led to more substance use [72]. There is ongoing research which will come to fruition in the next several months discussing the toll of COVID-19 pandemic and treatment of both mental illness and substance use particularly in the population at risk ie older adults. (book reference- Ankit Jain Kamal Kant Sahu Paroma Mitra 2021 Coronavirus Disease - COVID-1910.1007/978-3-030-63761-3_42 Treatment of Patients with Mental Illness Amid A Global COVID-19 Pandemic).

References

1. US Census Bureau. Census.gov. The baby boom cohort in the United States: 2012 to 2060. Current Population reports. By Sandra L. Colby and Jennifer M. Ortman. Issued may 2014.
2. Maree RD, Ricelli CA. Substance related and addictive disorders. Psychiatric Disorders Late in Life- A Comprehensive Review.
3. Han B, Gfroerer JC, Colliver JD, Penne MA. Substance use disorder among older adults in the United States in 2020. Addiction. 2009b;104(1):88–96.
4. Mavandadi S, Oslin DW. substance related and addictive disorders. The American Psychiatric Publishing Textbook of Geriatric Psychiatry. 2015.
5. Cummings SM, Bride B, Rawlins-Shaw AM. Alcohol abuse treatment for older adults: a review of recent empirical research. J Evid Based Soc Work. 2006;3(1):79–99.
6. US. Department of Health and Human Services Substance Abuse and Mental Health Services Administration (SAMSHA). Results from the 2013 national survey on drug use and health: summary of national findings. Rockville, MD; 2013.
7. Borok J, Galier P, Dinolfo M, Welgreen S, Hoffing M, Davis JW, Ramirez KD, Liao DH, Tang L, Karno M, Sacco P, Lin JC, Moore AA. Why do older unhealthy drinkers decide to make changes or not in their alcohol consumption? Data from the healthy living as you age study. J Am Geriatr Soc. 2013;61(8):1296–302.
8. Thun MJ, Peto R, Lopez AD, et al. Alcohol consumption and mortality among middle-aged and elderly U.S. adults. N Engl J Med. 1997;337(24):1705–14.
9. Kennedy GJ, Efremova I, Frazier A, et al. The emerging problems of alcohol and substance abuse in late life. J Soc Distress Homel. 1999;8(4):227–39.
10. Kirchner J, Zubritsky C, Cody M, et al. Alcohol consumption among older adults in primary care. J Gen Intern Med. 2007;22:92–7.
11. Rehm J, Hasan O, Black SE, Shield KD, Schwarzinger M. Alcohol use and dementia: a systematic scoping review. Alzheimers Res Ther. 2019;11(1):1. https://doi.org/10.1186/s13195-018-0453-0.
12. Moore AA, Whiteman EJ, Ward KT. Risks of combined alcohol-medication use in older adults. Am J Geriatr Pharmacother. 2007;5:64–74.
13. Blazer DG, Wu L-T. The epidemiology of alcohol use disorders and subthreshold dependence in a middle-aged and elderly community sample. Am J Geriatr Psychiatry. 2011;19(8):685–94.
14. American Psychiatric Association. Diagnostic and Statistic Manual DSM 5.
15. Han B, Moore A. Prevention and screening of unhealthy substance use by older adults. Geriatr Med. 2018;34:117–29.
16. Yoast RA, Wilford BB, Hayashi SW. Encouraging physicians to screen for and intervene in substance use disorders: obstacles and strategies for change. J Addict Dis. 2008;27(3):77–97.
17. Ewing JA. Detecting alcoholism. The CAGE questionnaire JAMA. 1984;252(14):1905–7.
18. Stewart D, Oslin DW. Recognition and treatment of late-life addictions in medical settings. J Clin Geropsychol. 2001;7(2):145–58.
19. Babor TF, Higgins-Biddle JC, Saunders JB, et al. The alcohol use disorders identification test (AUDIT): guidelines for use in primary care. 2nd ed.
20. Gómez A, Conde A, Santana JM, Jorrín A, Serrano IM, Medina R. The diagnostic use- fulness of AUDIT and AUDIT-C for detecting hazardous drinkers in the elderly. Aging Ment Health. 2006;10(5):558–61.
21. Blow FC, Brower KJ, Schulenberg JE, et al. The Michigan alcohol screening test: geriatric version (MAST-G): a new elderly specific screening instrument. Alcohol Clin Exp Res. 1992;16:172.
22. Blow FC, Gillespie BW, Barry KL, et al. Brief screening for alcohol problems in elderly populations using the short Michigan alcoholism screening test-geriatric version (SMAST-G). Alcohol Clin Exp Res. 1998;22(Suppl):131A.
23. O'Connell H, Chin A, Hamilton F, et al. A systematic review of the utility of self-report alcohol screening instruments in the elderly. Int J Geriatr Psychiatry. 2004;19(11):1074–86.
24. Chapman SL, Wu LT. Epidemiology and demography of illicit drug use and drug use disorders amongst adults. Substance Use and Older People. 2014.
25. Alcoholics Anonymous, editor. Twelve steps and twelve traditions. New York: Alcoholics Anonymous; 2004.
26. Merrick EL, Horgan CM, Hodgkin D, et al. Unhealthy drinking patterns in older adults: prevalence and associated characteristics. J Am Geriatr Soc. 2008;56:214–23.

27. Moore AA, Blow FC, Hoffing M, et al. Primary care-based intervention to reduce at-risk drinking in older adults: a randomized controlled trial. Addiction. 106(1):111–20.
28. Schonfeld L, King-Kallimanis BL, Duchene DM, et al. Screening and brief intervention for substance misuse among older adults: the Florida BRITE project. Am J Public Health. 2010;100(1):108–14.
29. Ayalon L, Jin C, Mcculloch CE, et al. Integrated specialty mental health care among older minorities improves access but not outcomes: results of the PRISMe study. Int J Geriatr Psychiatry. 2008;23(August):1086–92.
30. Stahl S. Stahl's essential psychopharmacology - prescriber's guide. 5th ed. New York: Cambridge University Press; 2014.
31. Substance Abuse and Mental Health Services Administration. Incorporating alcohol pharmacotherapies into medical practice treatment improvement protocol (TIP) series, no. 49. Rockville, MD; 2009.
32. Caputo F, Vignoli T, Leggio L, Addolorato G, Zoli G, Bernardi M. Alcohol use disorders in the elderly: a brief overview from epidemiology to treatment options. Exp Gerontol. 2012;47(6):411–6.
33. Kuerbis A, Sacco P, Blazer DG, Moore AA. Substance abuse among older adults. Clin Geriatr Med. 2014;30(3):629–54.
34. Berlin R, Butler P, Perloff M. Gabapentin therapy in psychiatric disorders: a systematic review. Prim Care Companion CNS Disord. 2015;17(5).
35. Mason BJ, Quello S, Shadan F. Gabapentin for the treatment of alcohol use disorder. Expert Opin Investig Drugs. 2017;27(1):113–24.
36. Hock B, Schwarz M, Domke I, et al. Validity of carbohydrate-deficient transferrin (%CDT), gamma-glutamyl transferase (gamma-GT) and mean corpuscular erythrocyte volume (MCV) as biomarkers for chronic alcohol abuse: a study in patients with alcohol dependence and liver disorders of non-alcoholic and alcoholic origin. Addiction. 2005;100(10):1477–86.
37. Moore AA, Karno MP, Grella CE, Lin JC, Warda E, Liao D, Hu P. Alcohol, tobacco and non-medical drug use in U.S. adults aged 65 years and older: data from the 2001-2002 National Epidemiologic Survey of alcohol and related conditions. J Am Geriatr Soc. 2009;57(12):2275–81.
38. Hall SM, Humfleet GL, Munoz RF, et al. Extended treatment of older cigarette smokers. Addiction. 2009;104:1043–52.
39. Oslin DW, Pettinati H, Volpicelli JR. Alcoholism treatment adherence: older age predicts better adherence and drinking outcomes. Am J Geriatr Psychiatry. 2002;10(6):740–7.
40. Oslin DW, Liberto JG, O'Brien J, et al. Naltrexone as an adjunctive treatment for older patients with alcohol dependence. Am J Geriatr Psychiatry. 1997;5(4):324–32.
41. Anstey KJ, von Sanden C, Salim, A.,& O' Kearney, R. Smoking as a risk factor for dementia and cognitive decline: a meta-analysis of prospective studies. Am J Epidemiol. 2007;166:367–78.
42. Rapuri PB, Gallagher JC, Smith LM. Smoking is a risk factor for decreased physical performance in elderly women. J Gerontol A Biol Sci Med Sci. 2007;62(1):93–100.
43. Humeniuk R, Henry-Edwards S, Ali R. et al. Geneva (Switzerland): World Health Organization; 2010. The alcohol, smoking, and substance involvement screening test (ASSIST).
44. Hokanson JM, Anderson RL, Hennrikus DJ, et al. Integrated tobacco cessation counseling in a diabetes self-management training program: a randomized trial of diabetes and reduction of tobacco. Diabetes Educ. 2006;32:562–70.
45. Hartmann-Boyce J, Aveyard P. Drug for smoking cessation. Br Med J. 2016;352(571):1–5.
46. Cawkwell PB, Blaum C, Sherman SE. Pharmacological smoking cessation. Drugs Aging. 2015;32(6):443–5.
47. Garrison GD, Dugan SE. Varenicline: a first-line treatment option for smoking cessation. Clin Ther. 2009;31(3):463–91.
48. Han BH, Sherman S, Mauro PM, et al. Demographic trends among older cannabis users in the United States, 2006-2013. Addiction. 2016;112(3):516–25.
49. Kaskie B, Ayyagari P, Milavetz G, Shane D, Arora K. The increasing use of Cannabis among older Americans: A public health crisis or viable policy alternative? The Gerontologist. 2017;57(6):1166–72.
50. Choi NG, Di Nitto DM, Marti CM, Choi BY. Relationship between marijuana and other illicit drug use and depression/suicidal thoughts among late middle-aged and older adults. Int Psychogeriatr. 2015;27:1–13.
51. Black P, JosephL J. Still dazed and confused: midlife marijuana use by the baby boom generation. Deviant Behav. 2014;35:822–84.
52. Colliver JD, Compton WM, Gfroerer JC, Condon T. Projecting drug use among aging baby boomers in 2020. Ann Epidemiol. 2006;16:257–65.
53. Wu LT, Blazer DG. Illicit and nonmedical drug use among older adults: a review. J Aging Health. 2010;23(3):481–504.
54. Center for Substance Abuse Treatment. Substance abuse relapse prevention for older adults: A group treatment approach. Rockville, MD: Substance Abuse and Mental Health Services Administration, U.S. Department of Health and Human Services; 2005.
55. Center for Substance Abuse Treatment. Substance abuse among older adults; treatment improvement protocol (TIP) series 26. Rockville, MD: Substance Abuse and Mental Health. Services Administration, U.S. Department of Health and Human Services; 1998.

56. Achildi O, Leong SH, Maust DT, et al. Patterns of newly-prescribed benzodiazepines in late life. Am J Geriatr Psychiatry. 2013.
57. Culberson JW, Ziska M. Prescription drug misuse/ abuse in the elderly. Geriatrics. 2008;63(9):22–31.
58. Dowling GJ, Weiss SR, Condon TP. Drugs of abuse and the aging brain. Neuropsychopharmacology. 2008;33:209–18.
59. Schutte K, Lemke S, Moos RH, Brennan PL. Age-sensitive psychosocial treatment for older adults with substance use. In: Substance use and older adults. 1st ed; 2015.
60. Three-year incidence and predictors of first-onset of DSM-IV mood, anxiety, and substance use disorders in older adults: results from Wave 2 of the National Epidemiologic Survey on Alcohol and Related Conditions. J Clin Psychiatry. 2011:72(2);144–55.
61. Schlaerth KR, Splawn RG, Ong J, Smith SD. Change in the pattern of illegal drug use in an inner city population over 50: an observational study. J Addict Dis. 2004.
62. Arndt S, Turvey CL, Flaum M. Older offenders, substance abuse, and treatment. Am J Geriatr Psychiatr. 2002;10:733–9.
63. Woo BK, Chen W. Substance misuse among older patients in psychiatric emergency service. Gen Hosp Psychiatry. 2010;32(1):99–101.
64. Lin JC, Karno MP, Grella CE, Ray LA, Liao DH, Moore AA. Psychiatric correlates of alcohol and tobacco use disorders in U.S. adults aged 65 years and older: results from the 2001– 2002 National Epidemiologic Survey of alcohol and related conditions. Am J Geriatr Psychiatry. 2014;22(11):1356–63.
65. Ty S. Schepis, Linda Simoni-Wastila, Sean Esteban McCabe. Prescription opioid and benzodiazepine misuse is associated with suicidal ideation in older adults. Int J Geriatr Psychiatry. 2019;34: 122–9.
66. Spinelli MA, Ponath C, Tieu L, Hurstak EE, Guzman D, Kushel M. Factors associated with substance use in older homeless adults: results from the HOPE HOME study. Subst Abus. 2016;38(1):88–94.
67. Yarns BC, Abrams JM, Meeks TW, Sewell DD. The mental health of older LGBT adults. Curr Psychiatry Rep. 2016;18:60.
68. McCabe SE, Hughes TL, Bostwick WB, West BT, Boyd CJ. Sexual orientation, substance use behaviors and substance dependence in the United States. Addiction. 2009;104(8):1333–45.
69. Blow FC, Barry KL. Substance misuse and abuse in older adults: what do we need to know to help? Generations. 2014;38(3):53–67.
70. Sorrell JM. Substance use disorders in long-term care settings: a crisis of care for older adults. J Psychosoc Nurs Ment Health Serv. 2017;55(1):24–7.
71. Plotkin AF 2015, January 21. Jewish Home launches first in nation nursing home based geriatric substance abuse program.
72. Derek D, Satre Matthew E, Hirschtritt Michael J, Silverberg Stacy A. Sterling Addressing Problems With Alcohol and Other Substances Among Older Adults During the COVID-19 Pandemic. Am J Geriatr Psychiatr. 2020;28(7):780–783. https://doi.org/10.1016/j.jagp.2020.04.012.

Recommended Reading

Substance Use and Older Adults First Edition John Wiley and Sons 2015.

Psychiatric Disorder Late in Life: A Comprehensive Review 2016.

The Mental Health and Substance Use Workforce for Older Adults: In whose hands? 2012.

The American Publishing Textbook of Geriatric Psychiatry.

Treatment of Patients with Mental Illness Amid A Global COVID-19 Pandemic.

Child and Adolescent Substance Abuse Disorders

4

Jeffery J. Wilson and Michael Ferguson

Background

Even under the most favorable of circumstances, adolescence (ages 12–17) remains a tumultuous developmental time in the life of a young adult. During these formative years it is expected that many young adults will be exposed to and experiment with various recreational substances such as nicotine, alcohol, and illicit drugs. Data from the ongoing national survey conducted by the Substance Abuse and Mental Health Services Administration (SAMHSA) show that 23.9% of adolescents admitted to experimenting with at least one form of illegal drug. Experimentation with recreational drugs below the threshold of dependence can be considered a part of normal adolescent development as the child seeks to individualize and gain autonomy. Of these, only a relatively small percentage will go on to develop early onset substance use disorders. Early onset substance use disorders are associated with an increase in psychiatric comorbidity along with an overall worse prognosis than adult onset substance use disorders. Risk taking is a normative part of adolescence that is reflected in the rituals of many cultures, including our own. Only 20% are free from any risk-taking behaviors. Forty five percent engage in moderate to low risk behaviors and 35% of adolescents are involved in three or more risk-taking behaviors (very high or high risk). Ultimately, risk-taking behavior accounts for most of the preventable adolescent morbidity and mortality [10]. Examples of common morbidities and mortalities include motor vehicle accidents, homicide, delinquency, suicide, and substance abuse.

The DSM-V defines substance use disorder (SUD) as a cluster of cognitive, behavioral, and physiological symptoms indicating that the individual continues using the substance despite significant substance-related problems. Substance use disorder is a general term which is given specificity by association to one or more of 10 classes of drugs. These are alcohol, cannabis, hallucinogens (not including phencyclidine), inhalants, opioids, sedatives, hypnotics, anxiolytics, stimulants, and other/unknown substances. While these categories do not perfectly categorize all substances, they do serve to identify the major substances and classes of substances most commonly represented in abuse and misuse.

J. J. Wilson (✉) · M. Ferguson
Department of Psychiatry and Behavioral Medicine,
Virginia Tech Carilion School of Medicine,
St. Roanoke, VA, USA
e-mail: Meferguson@carilionclinic.org

E. Akerele (ed.), *Substance and Non-Substance Related Addictions*,
https://doi.org/10.1007/978-3-030-84834-7_4

Etiology and Availability

Many adolescents will experiment with drugs such as nicotine, alcohol, and marijuana before graduating from high school. It is important to differentiate between substance use and abuse in adolescents. Legality is not further considered here because in the United States at the time of this writing it is illegal for minors (age under 18) to use recreational substances such as alcohol which are legal for adults. Differentiating between use and abuse is also necessary because occasional "use" of drugs is not strongly correlated with the development of a substance use disorder. For example, over 80% of adolescents admit to trying alcohol before graduating from high school but fewer than 7% will go on to develop an alcohol use disorder (SAMHSA).

Until recently the primary means by which an adolescent could obtain illicit substances were believed to be limited to exposures in the home, the school, and with their peer groups. Today adolescents have access to far greater numbers of people through social media, online video games, and other similar internet-based tools. It was hypothesized that this massive increase in interconnectivity might make it easier for adolescent populations to obtain illicit substances. Interestingly, multiple investigations have failed to find statistically significant increases in prevalence in recent decades that would lend support to this theory.

Gender and Ethnic Factors

In the adult population, men have nearly twice the rate of substance abuse as compared to women, however, in adolescence the prevalence for both genders is equal at 6.9%. There has been little significant data to show that there exist any differences based on race or ethnicity. The current rates of male and female substance abuse hospital admissions for the non-Hispanic White population have been 58.2% and 66.4% respectively. Rates for Hispanic and non-Hispanic Black populations were similar.

Familial and Environmental Factors

Genetic influences are a significant consideration in risk stratifying a person's likelihood of developing a SUD. Studies have found that family members of dependent persons have an eightfold risk of SUD and that sibling influences (10–14 times) are even more robust than parental influences. Evidence is present for substance-specific risk heritability as well. Children of alcoholics were found to be 4–5 times more likely to meet the criteria for alcohol use disorder. Similarly elevated rates have been found in adolescents whose parents suffer from cocaine and opioid use disorders [11, 20]. Interestingly, there appears to be a non-specific heritable risk pattern of substance abuse as an increased risk of alcohol and nicotine use has been found in family members of persons with cannabis use disorder [14]. Similarly, an increase in the rates of nicotine and cannabis use has been demonstrated in family members of alcoholics.

There is widespread agreement that family factors (environmental, genetic, or both) play a significant role in the risk stratification for substance use disorders. The children of adults with substance abuse problems are at an increased risk for health problems, both medical and psychiatric. Data show that the risk of alcohol and illicit drug use was doubled for children with parents with alcohol abuse for all drugs except marijuana. Conversely, children of parents with non-alcohol substance abuse disorders were more likely to also abuse non-alcoholic substances. This suggests that there may be a more specific modeling effect of adolescent substance abuse as it relates to parental examples. Beyond this potential for mirrored substance abuse behaviors, children of parents with substance abuse issues are most likely to be neglected which places them at an increased risk of abuse. Research also shows that a child is at an equally increased risk of developing a substance abuse disorder by bearing witness to physical and sexual abuses, even if they themselves are not the direct victim. Witnessing violence is among the most powerful individual risk factors for a child developing a substance use disorder. The National Center for Addiction and Substance Abuse based at Columbia University reports that these children face a near three-fold increase in physical and sexual abuse. Overall, children of parents with substance abuse disorders are themselves eight times more likely to develop a substance use disorder. The rates of substance use disorders in adolescents who live in group homes are significantly higher than in the general population. Multiple investigations have shown that between 20% and 33% of these adolescents meet the criteria for substance use disorder and that over 50% admit to experimenting with illicit substances in the past. Lastly, in considering adolescents who are detained in juvenile detention facilities, the prevalence of substance use disorders is so high that it is the rule rather than the exception. It is worth noting that the prevailing opinion about substance abuse in these populations does not identify these high-risk environments and the primary risk factor. Rather it is most commonly an underlying psychiatric condition which is responsible for the increase in negative behaviors. Most commonly, this is identified as conduct disorder.

Comorbid Disorders

Substance use disorders occur with greater frequency in adolescents with comorbid psychiatric conditions. Data from adolescence clinical populations in treatment centers can report comorbid mental illness and substance use disorders at rates as high as 72%. The presence of a comorbid mental health disorder may explain why these adolescents are more likely to develop chronic substance use disorders compared to peers who will experiment with recreational substances but who will not go on to develop a dependency. Attempts to self-medicate undiagnosed or poorly controlled psychiatric conditions can explain the increased risk of continued use leading to dependency in this population.

Attention-Deficit Hyperactivity Disorder

The current gold standard for the pharmacologic management of ADD/ADHD are amphetamines. These drugs do come with associated risks and side effects such as insomnia, weight loss (or failure to gain appropriately), and tachycardia. ADHD is known to be a risk factor for tobacco usage later in life, however recent years have seen the emergence of the sensitization/dependence hypothesis. This concept emerged from parents of children with ADD/ADHD who feared that giving their children prescription amphetamines would put them at an increased risk for illegal amphetamine abuse. More specifically, the sensitization hypothesis suggests that the early exposure to therapeutic amphetamines causes a remodeling of the dopaminergic pathways in the brain which in turn leads to an increased sensitivity to these stimulants. Early research in rodent models did support this theory as the subjects showed convincing dependence and sensitivity to amphetamines however, these findings have not been observed or recreated in any human population. Numerous studies looking into this relationship have found the opposite to be true in humans. Longitudinal studies have found that children receiving early intervention for their ADD/ADHD were less likely to develop a substance use disorder as compared to those forgoing amphetamine treatments. Public perception about amphetamine abuse is not unfounded. There has been an increase in the abuse of prescription amphetamines in recent years, however this increase is in the setting of an overall increase in prescription drug abuse in the United States and not specifically within the population of adolescents with ADD/ADHD receiving amphetamine therapy.

Conduct Disorder

Conduct disorder has repeatedly been identified as the most strongly predictive psychiatric condition for present or future substance use disorder in adolescents. Conduct disorder is commonly comorbid with ADD/ADHD and has likely contributed to the misconception that ADHD therapy increased the risk of substance use disorder discussed previously. Not only was the diagnosis of conduct disorder itself predictive of substance use disorder but the severity of the illness was as well. This can be quantified by the number of potential symptoms of conduct disorder as outlined in the DSM-V.

Post-traumatic Stress Disorder

Attempting to correlate PTSD with substance use disorder in adolescents is inherently difficult because the symptoms of PTSD can frequently remain dormant until many years after adolescence. Additionally, those symptoms of PTSD which can manifest more acutely can be controlled relatively well with medications that belong to the same drug families as abusable or illicit drugs. For example, the symptoms of increased arousal, intrusive ideation, and avoidance can be modulated by the effects of alcohol in the short-term. It is therefore possible for patients with PTSD and a secondary risk factor for substance use disorder to effectively self-medicate the symptoms of PTSD using the sedative properties of the alcohol. This can reduce the clinical symptoms of PTSD below the threshold of what might be perceived by the clinician. Even so, studies have found an association between PTSD and an increased risk for tobacco and illicit drug dependence.

Anxiety Disorders

Of all the psychiatric conditions considered, the anxiety disorders were the most loosely associated with the development of substance use disorders. Experiments found rates which ranged from 7% to 40%, although the latter was an outlier with the average being approximately 16%.

Depressive Disorders

Numerous studies have found strong associations between rates of adolescent depression and the substance use disorders, particularly alcohol use disorder. Rates of depression in adolescents who claimed abstinence from alcohol were approximately 5% while those who consumed alcohol regularly reported rates of depression at nearly 24%. Similar rates of depression were found in adolescents taking other illicit substances.

Neurobiological Developmental Change

In the past two decades significant progress has been made in our understanding of adolescent developmental neurobiology. Much of this progress is attributed to the development and increasing use of functional MRI (fMRI) technologies. This has advanced our understanding of both the normal developmental changes that occur throughout adolescence into adulthood as well as pinpointing the neurological changes caused by different pathologies. While use of the fMRI and other advanced imaging technologies developed in recent years has paved the way for a greater understanding of the brain and behavior, it is important to remember that this technology has only emerged in the past two decades which places a hard cap on the number and duration of studies that track neurobiological changes over time. In the future, long-term studies like the Adolescent Brain Cognitive Development (ABCD) study hope to provide valuable information on this issue as they track neurodevelopment of over 10,000 children in 21 locations. While studies like this will certainly help to advance our understanding, there will always be intrinsic limitations to how fast this field can develop due to the ethical barriers to experimentation in this population.

Nevertheless, we have learned much in recent years about the developing brain. Most notably is that the adolescent brain does not undergo growth and maturation in all areas simultaneously. The central nervous system (CNS) consists of the brain and spinal cord which can be broken down into two types of neuronal tissue. The grey matter consists of the nerve cell bodies with their associated dendrites and synapses. Also included in the grey matter are the supporting glial cells and capillary supply. The white matter by contrast is represented by the myelinated axonal tracts that connect the areas of grey matter. Imaging studies have shown that the ratio of these two neuronal tissues shifts in development from higher concentrations of grey and fewer myelinated tracts at birth. The process through which redundant grey matter is reduced and myelination increases as a part of normal development is referred to as synaptic remodeling. An excellent clinical example of this process can be seen in the primitive reflexes. Low levels of CNS myelination at birth cause infants to have a positive Babinski reflex where stroking the sole of the foot causes the great toe to extend up, and the remaining toes to fan out. This reflex naturally fades in the first 2 years of life as CNS myelination increases. It can re-emerge in later life as a result of numerous neurodegenerative conditions that cause demyelination. During this time of increasing myelination, specific regions of the brain are known to mature earlier than others. Unfortunately, it appears as though the asynchronous development of different areas of the brain predispose the adolescent brain to increased risks. An in-depth review of all the relevant neuroanatomy would be beyond the scope of this text, however a basic understanding of several key areas is essential to understanding the association between the developing brain and the predisposition to increased risk-taking behavior. The evidence on nicotine, amphetamines, inhalants, MDMA, and polysubstance abuse is limited. The evidence examining the effects of amphetamines had increased striatal dimensions and was found to have a correlated increase in novelty and risk-taking behaviors. Adolescent MDMA users showed decreased reaction times and hyperactivity of the left hippocampus during working memory with verbal prompts.

Developmental Consequences of Alcohol and Marijuana

Multiple studies have shown that the area of the brain most affected in development by alcohol abuse is the frontal lobe. This conclusion is based primarily on fMRI analysis, however these findings can be easily conceptualized. The frontal lobe is one of the last areas of the brain to mature under normal circumstances. In the absence of a mature frontal lobe an adolescent would lack the impulse control and executive level decision-making capacities that are facilitated by the prefrontal cortex. Furthermore, any area of the brain that develops at a slower rate will be more susceptible to external forces by virtue of the increased exposure potential. Conversely, the areas of the brain that are known to mature earlier (hippocampus and amygdala) are associated far less with alterations in adolescents who abuse alcohol. Alcohol is also associated with temporal and parietal changes but to a lesser degree.

Chronic marijuana use has long been associated with learning and memory, executive function, processing speed, and attention. Alterations to normal neuroanatomy follow a similar distribution as does alcohol use, favoring change to the frontal lobe followed by the temporal and parietal lobes. In the case of the cannabinoids the distribution of receptors in the CNS must also be considered. Areas of the brain that are more heavily saturated with cannabinoid receptors include the basal ganglia, hippocampus, cerebellum, and frontal cortex. Not surprisingly, this receptor pattern correlates with the above symptoms observed in chronic marijuana use.

The anterior cingulate cortex (ACC) is a neuroanatomical region that has been increasingly examined in adolescent substance use disorders. With high levels of connectivity to the limbic system and the prefrontal cortex, it has implications with regard to emotional regulation and executive function respectively. When the functional connectivity of this region is disrupted, a decreased ability to access inhibitory control has been observed. This loss of inhibitory control is believed to contribute to ongoing patterns of substance abuse. Decreased functional connectivity in the ACC has been demonstrated in adolescents with cannabis use disorder during longitudinal fMRI studies. In an 18-month longitudinal study, not only was a lower ACC functional connectivity at the onset associated with increased cannabis use over the duration, but high levels of reported cannabis use during the study was associated with decreases in cognitive functioning and IQ testing at the conclusion.

Having now considered the regions of the brain most heavily impacted by marijuana and alcohol abuse in adolescent brains, it should not be surprising that these teens tend to have poorer cognitive functioning on tests of verbal memory, visuospatial functioning, psychomotor speed, working memory, attention, cognitive control, and overall IQ.

Substances of Abuse

The adolescent population data are inconsistent with this overall trend as they presently favor marijuana as the primary substance of abuse with 80.7% of male and 60.8% of female respondents identifying marijuana as their primary substance of abuse. Alcohol by contrast shows a 21.7% rate of abuse in adolescent females and 10.5% in adolescent males. Data from individuals aged 18–24 years of age show a dramatic decrease in marijuana use in both genders with a 33.4% usage rate in males and a 22.1% rate in women. Over time, these numbers continue to decline in favor of other drugs, primarily alcohol. The proportions of male to female usage of other commonly abused drugs were more consistent with overall lifetime rates. Primary amphetamine/methamphetamine use in adolescent females was reported at 4.2% and 1.3% in men. Primary abuse of prescription pain killers was also similar with 3.1% use reported in females and 1.7% reported in males.

The Gateway Drug Theory

Data show that most adolescents will begin their experimentation in drugs with alcohol, tobacco, and/or marijuana. This led to the notion of the gateway drug which proposed that the use of any of these substances places a person at an increased risk toward further experimentation with additional substances of abuse. There have been studies which would appear to support this theory, however in one review it has been found that these studies failed to consider other explanations for increased substance use. Once a person has experimented with marijuana, they are more likely to continue experimenting with additional drugs as compared to someone who has not. While exposure to marijuana is one possible explanation for this progression others must also be considered. For example, is there an underlying diagnosis of conduct disorder which would predispose them to substance abuse? Does the child have a positive expectation of drug use or another risk factor associated with substance abuse and addiction? While it remains possible that there is real merit to the gateway theory of drug abuse, this observation may be exaggerated by failing to account for adolescent demographics that are at an increased risk for substance abuse.

Marijuana

Marijuana has long been the most abused substance in the adolescent population, surpassing even alcohol which predominates in the adult population. Its popularity can be attributed to its widespread availability, relatively low cost, and more favorably perceived risk compared to other drugs. Its relatively low potency allows the average person to use marijuana recreationally with only a minority developing an addiction or dependency. The notion that marijuana carries a lower risk of addiction when compared to other drugs can be falsely reassuring. While it is true that other drugs have higher rates of addiction and can cause fatal overdose or withdrawal symptoms in excess of what is seen with marijuana, that does not qualify marijuana as a benign substance.

Understanding the relative risks of marijuana use necessitates an understanding of the chemical composition of marijuana and marijuana-containing products. The primary psychoactive component of marijuana and marijuana-derived products is delta-9-tetrahydrocannabinol, commonly known as THC. THC belongs to a family of compounds called cannabinoids, so named because they mediate their effects through action at cannabinoid receptors in the body. Two cannabinoid receptors have been studied in detail, CB1 and CB2. It has been determined that the binding of the CB1 receptor yields the psychoactive effects desired by many users [2]. The potency of any marijuana product can therefore be evaluated based on its concentration of THC which has equal binding affinity at both CB1 and CB2 receptors. The tremendous variability in THC concentration across the spectrum of marijuana products can result in users receiving significantly greater concentrations of the primary psychoactive substance than intended. Concentrated THC products are available as oils or waxes which can be smoked, vaped, or consumed as edibles. Products such as these have been found to contain THC concentrations of 95% and higher. Furthermore, as many of the edible marijuana products are fashioned into candies, pastries, and drinks, there has been a surge in accidental ingestion and exposure by young children who consume these by mistake. The notion that edibles and oils are the only sources of concentrated doses of THC is also incorrect. The THC content in marijuana has been steadily increasing for years due to selective growing practices. Between the 1960 and 1980 the average THC concentration and marijuana was approximately 2%. Starting in the early 1990s, the concentration doubled to 4%. From that time the concentration has steadily increased so that the average marijuana plant seized in the United States had a THC concentration of approximately 12% [4]. Certain popular strains that are sold legally in marijuana dispensaries have had THC concentrations as high as 28%.

Understanding the consequences of marijuana use in adolescence is especially relevant now that the legality of marijuana is being reconsidered in the United States. The legality of marijuana use in the United States is a dynamic issue and already numerous states have taken steps to either legalize or decriminalize recreational marijuana use. Current laws differ significantly from state to state. Marijuana may be considered legal for recreational use or strictly for supposed medical benefit when use is overseen by a licensed physician. Some states have also chosen to simply decriminalize marijuana possession. In these cases marijuana possession is still unlawful, however being found in possession of a small quantity does not result in criminal liability and does not result in legal action or potential incarceration. Critically, state law legalizing marijuana use in any capacity is currently in direct conflict with federal laws under which marijuana remains classified as a schedule 1 controlled substance. Substances in this classification are deemed to have no medical benefits and carry a high potential for abuse. The federal government does not currently prosecute cases of marijuana use in states that have legalized or decriminalized marijuana use. Instead, they have taken the position that they will monitor the states for more concerning violations such as the involvement of criminal enterprises in the distribution of marijuana for profit. This can give providers in these states the flexibility to prescribe or endorse marijuana use for adult patients. However, the federal government has also identified marijuana use by minors as a similarly concerning violation of federal policy. Therefore, regardless of state policy change related to the legalization of marijuana in adults, it is unlikely to become available to the adolescent population.

The perception of cannabis has changed as a result of marijuana legalization. Survey data from adolescents showed a 14–16% decrease in perception of marijuana harmfulness after their states passed laws legalizing recreational use. This change in perception was also reflected in a 2–4% increase in marijuana use over the same interval. Critically, even students in states where no legalization laws were passed also showed a 4–7% decrease in perceived risk of harm. There is also the evolving issue of legality of marijuana use in the United States and if the trend of legalization continues the number of adolescents who use marijuana is expected to further increase.

Nicotine – Tobacco and Vaping

The statistics on nicotine abuse in the adolescent population can be falsely reassuring. Thanks to sweeping changings in where and how tobacco can be advertised along with extensive public health campaigns educating the public about the consequences of smoking, adolescent cigarette smoking is at an historic low of 2.7%. NSDUH survey data show a continuous decline in the prevalence of adolescent cigarette use in the United States from 2002 to present. Monitoring the future survey data also reports historic lows in both current cigarette users and initiation of smoking. This provides strong evidence to suggest that efforts to reduce cigarette use in adolescents have been successful with over a decade of consistent decline in use. However, nicotine use in adolescents is rapidly rising as a result of vaping technology which has become extremely popular in the United States. Monitoring the future included questions specific to vaping nicotine products starting in 2017. Since then, data show the following dramatic increases in vaping prevalence:

Grade	Prevalence increase from 2017 to 2019	Current prevalence
8th	9.0%	16.5%
10th	14.9%	30.7%
12th	16.5%	35.5%

Johnston et al. [26]

MTF identifies these increasing trends in vaping as among the greatest recorded in the 45 years that the survey has been collecting data. If these trends continue, it is expected that vaping will reverse the progress made against cigarettes in adolescent nicotine use.

Electronic nicotine delivery systems (ENDS) like e-cigarettes and vaporizers are available in several device configurations, however the common feature in this new technology is that a battery-powered heating element is used to vaporize a solid or liquid nicotine source which is then inhaled similarly to traditional cigarettes. The key difference, and primary selling point used by companies offering these devices to the public, is that there is no combustion reaction responsible for delivering the nicotine. By utilizing a vapor-based system as opposed to releasing nicotine by burning tobacco leaves, ENDS have a much lower carcinogen burden delivered to the lungs in each puff. This emphatically does not result in a safe product that allows users to achieve a risk-free nicotine high.

Diagnosis and Treatment

As discussed previously, the current DSM-5 criteria for substance use disorder are less likely to exclude adolescents as diagnostic orphans for failing to meet the full criteria for either substance use or abuse. The diagnosis is made clinically and can be helped by certain laboratory tests. Confirmatory lab work however is not required and may be of greater clinical value during treatment to assess for ongoing use or relapse. Treatment should be tailored to the individual and must consider variables such as the length of habit, severity of physiologic dependence, and the complex balance of risk vs protective factors present. Given that psychosocial stressors related to family, peers, and environment are often implicated as precipitating factors, they are often involved in treatment planning. Medical management of withdrawal and maintenance can be indicated and must be considered on an individual basis. Treatment programs which incorporate multiple treatment facets tend to have greater success rates than monotherapies.

Laboratory Screening Methods

An important part of the prevention process has been the implementation of both voluntary and involuntary drug testing. Starting in the late 1980s with a federal mandate establishing workplace guidelines for drug screens for government employees, today there are an estimated 120 million screening tests for drugs conducted annually. Mandatory drug screening has evolved into common practice for certain demographics such as athletes, parolees, and pre-employment screenings. Random drug screens can also be related to employment; however, they are increasingly utilized by parents to monitor their children. While the increased availability of these screens allows for better surveillance of higher risk populations, the incorrect administration of these tests and/or the misinterpretation of the results can have serious consequences. Federal agencies and private employers that are subject to federal guidelines are required to follow the guidelines laid out by SAMHSA. This includes having trained medical personnel issue the tests and specimen analysis is done in federally approved labs/facilities. The five illicit drugs that are SAMHSA mandated for federal screening are amphetamines, THC, cocaine, opioids, and PCP. This corresponds to most basic drug screens offered at testing and medical facilities. This basic template can be expanded upon to include barbiturates, benzodiazepines, and methaqualones. Specific testing is available for inhalants, hallucinogens, anabolic steroids, hydrocodone, and MDMA. Ideally, all parties who issue any drug screen would be compelled to follow the same guidelines and standards. However, nonfederal agencies have surprising autonomy in testing protocols and parents using at-home tests conduct these tests without oversight or training. Today there are several biological samples currently used for drug testing. These include urine, breath, blood, saliva, hair, and sweat. Each of these testing modalities has strengths, weaknesses, and testing vulnerabilities which can lead to inaccurate results. Table 4.1 shows some of the more commonly tested substances and the typical estimates of how long they are detectable using currently available screening tools.

Table 4.1 Detection windows for commonly tested substances

Windows of detection in urine for various substances				
	Detection windows by drug test type			
Substance	Urine	Hair	Oral fluid	Sweat
Alcohol	10–12 h ETG, up to 48 h	N/A	Up to 24 h	N/A
Amphetamines	2–4 d	Up to 90 d	1–48 h	7–14 d
Methamphetamine	2–5 d	Up to 90 d	1–48 h	7–14 d
Barbiturates	Up to 7 d	Up to 90 d	N/A	N/A
Benzodiazepines	Up to 7 d	Up to 90 d	N/A	N/A
Cannabis (marijuana)	1–30 d	Up to 90 d	Up to 24 h	7–14 d
Cocaine	1–3 d	Up to 90 d	1–36 h	7–14 d
Codeine (opiate)	2–4 d	Up to 90 d	1–36 h	7–14 d
Morphine (opiate)	2–5 d	Up to 90 d	1–36 h	7–14 d
Heroin (opiate)	2–3 d	Up to 90 d	1–36 h	7–14 d
PCP	5–6 d	Up to 90 d	N/A	7–14 d

National Center on Substance Abuse and Child Welfare/ Substance Abuse and Mental Health Services Administration. Drug testing practice guidelines

Urine Drug Screen

The urine drug screen (UDS) is the oldest and most commonly used drug screen today. The versatility of this test is due to the ease of administration, relatively low cost, and the effectiveness of the test and detecting commonly used substances of abuse. Urine drug screens are based on the detection of drug metabolites that are detectable beyond the physiologic effects of the drugs themselves. This gives the UDS an advantage over serum testing as the typical progression of most substances is to be present first in the serum and then excreted into the urine. This allows for a greater window of detection for urine screens over serum. The ability to detect metabolites beyond the scope of clinically observable effects is both a strength but can also lead to misinterpretation. Not all substances detectable on a UDS are illegal for personal use, and a positive test only indicates the presence of metabolites above a certain minimal detectable threshold which is not an indication of degree of intoxication past or present. The most common approach to urine drug screens is to use either a qualitative one-step method where a drug metabolite is listed as either present within the detectable range or absent. Less commonly, a sample which tests positive for the presence of detectable metabolites will have a second, gas chromatography mass spectrometry (GC-MS) analysis which serves both as a confirmatory test as well as providing a quantitative measurement of the substance [8]. The benefit of the confirmatory GC-MS testing over the SAMHSA-5 UDS is that the increased accuracy is both beneficial to clinicians and protective to patients against false positives. A basic UDS is highly sensitive for the presence of drug metabolites but offers a relatively low sensitivity. Two common examples are Wellbutrin (Bupropion) which can cause a false positive for amphetamines and dextromethorphan (common ingredient in cough syrups) which can cause a false positive for PCP. Practitioners also benefit from the quantitative data provided by GC-MS because it allows them to trend concentrations in their patients, which can suggest whether a person has ongoing drug use vs residual metabolites. This is especially valuable in substances like THC which has high lipid solubility and can be detectable for weeks after use. Lastly, without the use of GS-MS it is not possible to differentiate between similar drugs belonging to the same pharmacologic class. Standard of care medications for comorbid psychiatric conditions such as ADHD need to be able to be differentiated from similar substances of abuse on screening tests. Similarly, patients with a history of substance use disorders who are now on maintenance therapies like suboxone (buprenorphine-naloxone) or methadone may require quantitative screens to ensure both compliance with prescribed medications as well as abstinence from illicit substances.

Although generally effective overall as a screening tool, the UDS is particularly vulnerable to tampering. Broadly, methods which can be used to affect the outcome of a UDS can be divided into three categories. First, in-vivo tampering involves a person ingesting another substance to influence the test result. In-vitro tampering involves the addition of another substance into the urine sample after it has been collected. Lastly, a substitution of samples can occur when the individual submits a clean urine sample that is not their own. While each of these methods can be successful in confounding legitimate test results, there is significant variability in effectiveness from one person to another, especially when it comes to in-vitro and in-vivo tampering. The concentration of metabolic byproducts in the urine is dependent on numerous variables pertaining to time, quantity of substance ingested, and individual metabolism and enzyme polymorphisms. Close observation of the patient as they provide the sample is the most effective way to reduce results tampering. Unfortunately, this is something many providers find difficult as it by design, violates a person's privacy and challenges the provider's own perception on what is socially normative and appropriate. There have been developments in chemical and technical deterrents to sample tampering, however currently direct observation of sample production offers the greatest protection against tampering.

Serum Analysis

Testing a patient's blood for the presence of drugs is a practice most commonly encountered in a hospital environment. Diagnostically it differs from the UDS in that instead of testing for drug metabolites excreted by the body, serum sampling looks for active components present in the bloodstream. The advantage of a serum sample is that it provides a snapshot at the real-time content of a person's blood. This form of testing is most valuable in an emergency room setting where a person can present acutely intoxicated and a UDS is not feasible either because the patient is unwilling/unable to produce a urine sample, or because the body has had insufficient time to metabolize detectable quantities of the drug. In an outpatient scenario however, serum testing has the potential to lose significant value. Unless the patient has actively used drugs in the hours leading up to a serum drug screening, it is more likely that they will have metabolized the active drugs into metabolic byproducts by the time they are tested, yielding falsely negative results.

The technical requirements of blood tests are prohibitive to routine outpatient or home use. Blood samples can only be safely drawn by trained medical personnel such as a phlebotomist, and even trained personnel can have difficulty obtaining IV access from chronic IV drug users due to poor venous access. Once collected, blood samples require laboratory analysis. Most hospitals will have in-house labs capable of running these tests, but smaller clinics will need to send the samples out for analysis which creates a delay providing clinicians with information needed to guide further treatment planning.

Drug Screening Using Hair, Saliva, and Sweat

Screening for drugs of abuse using saliva, hair, and sweat samples is used far less commonly than urine and blood testing, largely due to cost and lack of access to labs to perform the analysis. While these methods are utilized less by current providers, there are some noteworthy advantages to using these samples which may result in an increased prevalence in the future.

Saliva testing offers several advantages over blood and urine testing due to the completely non-invasive nature of collecting a saliva swab. The process is pain free and causes no issues with invasion of privacy during collection. Additionally, this technology allows for analysis at the point of care. An additional advantage of salivary analysis over a UDS is that it is resistant to tampering and interference. It has been shown that rinses/mouthwashes do not confound results so long as they are not used within 30 minutes of sample collection [3]. Another promising option that has become available recently is a sweat sampling patch which is applied to the skin for up to a week before being sent for analysis. This test can detect drug metabolites for substances taken shortly before and during when the patch is worn. The patch design is also intended to reduce tampering by showing device puckering or deformity if it is removed and reapplied prior to completion. Limitations to sweat analysis are cost, absence of point-of-care analysis, and at this time the patch can only detect SAMHSA-5 substances.

Analysis of hair follicles can provide a practitioner with the longest period of detection of samples. While it may take over a week for substances to be detectable by follicle analysis, they can remain identifiable for 3 months [1]. There are numerous limitations to using hair follicles to test for substance use. The obvious shortcoming based on the detection window is that follicle analysis cannot be used to detect substance use within the first week after use. Other limitations of this technology relate to how the information about a person's drug use is obtained. In short, substances taken into the body are eventually deposited in the core of the hair follicles. However, there are multiple factors which can affect this process including how much a person sweats and the ethnicity of the patient. People with darker hair due to increased melanin can have potentially higher detectable concentrations of substances during follicular analysis. A person can also alter the chemistry of the hair by using any number of common coloring and cleaning products that are commercially available. This method of testing is particularly vulnerable to tampering and interference. Because substances are deposited as the hair grows, the most recent drug use will be detected in the portion of the follicle shaft closest to the body. It is a simple task to cut the hair close to the body prior to providing a sample, and in this way conceal any subacute drug use that would have been detected. While sampling can be done on any hair taken from the body, removing body hair does not provide a meaningful deterrent to a determined patient [22]. There also exists a significant practical limitation with hair follicle testing in that laboratory testing is the only means of analysis with no point of care options currently available.

Evidence-Based Treatments for Adolescent Substance Use

Evidence-based psychosocial interventions for adolescents have only recently become a viable treatment option. This is not to say that nonpharmacologic treatment options for adolescents were historically unavailable, but rather they met with mixed success [6]. The realization that there were inadequate substance use treatment programs for adolescents in this country fueled a wave of research and development into effective adolescent treatment programs. A recent meta-analysis of this new generation of treatment options has identified motivational enhancement/motivational interviewing, brief interventions, cognitive behavioral therapy, and family-based treatments all as effective methods to treating substance use disorders in adolescent populations [24].

The first step in selecting an appropriate treatment plan for substance use disorder in an adolescent is to assess the level of care that is necessary. This will depend on individual factors relating not only to the physiologic level of addiction and risk of complicated withdrawal, but also the level of readiness to facilitate change by both the adolescent and their family. To aid in this decision-making, the American Society of Addiction Medicine (ASAM) has outlined six dimensions to consider when the need for and intensity of adolescent substance use treatment.

American Society of Addiction Medicine: the six dimensions of multidimensional assessment

Level	Description	Content
Dimension 1	Acute intoxication/risk for withdrawal	Examines past and present experiences with substance use and withdrawal
Dimension 2	Biomedical conditions and complications	Examining past medical history and current physical status
Dimension 3	Emotional, behavioral, or cognitive conditions/complications	Examining thoughts, emotions, and any mental health issues
Dimension 4	Readiness to change	Examining the current level of readiness to change
Dimension 5	Relapse, continued use, continued problem potential	Examining any history of relapse or continued use/ongoing problems
Dimension 6	Recovery/living environment	Examining factors related to living situation, personal contacts, and environmental risk factors

Psychosocial Interventions

In 1997, the Center for Substance Abuse Treatment formed the cannabis youth treatment (CYT) program with the intention of funding research to study existing adolescent substance use treatment programs to find effective, short-term outpatient treatment programs for adolescents who struggled with cannabis use. Those selected to be included in the study were chosen based on expert opinion that they were based on best practices, previously demonstrated effectiveness, and widespread applicability based on generalizability and financial considerations. Motivational Enhancement Therapy/Cognitive Behavioral Therapy, Family Support Network, Adolescent Community Reinforcement Approach (ACRA), and Multidimensional family therapy. The CYT study ultimately found that these programs were all effective in treating adolescent cannabis use disorders over 90 days or less, and only ranked the programs based on cost. Cost was determined primarily by the number of treatment sessions required by each program. While this research was commissioned in the name of advancing treatment methods for adolescent cannabis use disorder, the programs have become more broadly applied to helping overcome other substances of abuse in the adolescent population.

Motivational Interviewing

Motivational interviewing is a form of goal-directed therapy that is based on the adolescent resolving ambivalence toward their decision-making. This is accomplished by building motivation and empowering the adolescent to remain committed to their goals [17]. Many techniques central to the effectiveness of motivational interviewing share a commonality with other therapeutic techniques. They include features such as judgement-free treatment environment, expressing empathy toward the adolescent, and demonstrating acceptance. Motivational interviewing also places the adolescent the therapist on an equal level and does not advance based on the notion that the therapist is teaching or guiding the healing. This form of leading or instructing is believed to increase resistance in the adolescent population and ultimately this can be damaging the therapeutic alliance [18]. The role of the therapist with motivational interviewing is to draw out the adolescent's internal motivations for change.

Brief interventions as the name suggests are shorter in duration and less extensive than the average treatment programs for substance use disorder. Shorter duration therapies such as motivational enhancement therapy may not be as effective in addressing long-term substance use disorder, but they have been shown to be effective in shorter term addictions which are more common in adolescents [7]. That is because the goal of the brief intervention therapy is to address and enhance the adolescent's current motivation to change [23]. A motivational enhancement approach employs a harm reduction approach to substance use as opposed to an abstinence or zero-tolerance method. Motivational enhancement therapy is based on assisting and guiding the adolescent through the stages of change. There are six stages of change that occur in psychotherapy [12] (Table 4.2).

Motivational enhancement builds upon this model by first determining where the adolescent is with regard to their problem and assisting them in progressing toward successful maintenance and remission. The most critical stages for a therapist utilizing motivational enhancement are contemplation and determination. First, the patient is guided to consider the ramifications of their substance use. They must consciously consider how their substance use is affecting their lives and how this poses a problem for their success and stability going forward [16]. The small investment of time for modest return on improved outcomes makes the brief intervention a versatile treatment tool and may be especially valuable for situations where time with the patient may be limited, such as in emergency rooms, juvenile correction centers, and with primary care providers.

Cognitive Behavioral Therapy

Cognitive behavioral therapy (CBT) is based on the principle that substance use disorders and similar behaviors are learned behaviors that

Table 4.2 The six stages of change

Precontemplation	The individual is not at a point where they are considering making any change in their behavior, regardless of consequence
Contemplation	The individual is aware of the problem and has begun to consider making a change. During this time, they may reflect on the feasibility and cost of making this change
Determination	The individual has decided to act and make the change
Action	The individual has actually taken concrete steps to address the problem. Normally this phase can last from 3 to 6 months
Maintenance	The individual has successfully taken action and addressed the original problem
Relapse	This occurs if the efforts of the individual fail in which case the cycle starts again

originate and persist in the setting of environmental stressors [25]. This concept can be traced back to the idea of classically conditioned behavioral responses where craving control can be induced with an external stimulus. This thinking has fostered treatment models that emphasize identifying and avoiding triggering environments and stressors to combat substance use disorders. Once the triggers have been identified, treatment focuses on recruiting strategies for avoidance such as rewarding competing behaviors, promoting self-control, and developing coping skills. Behavioral modification can also focus on identifying the perceived benefits of substance use. Acutely, intoxication can be effective for acute stress reduction, social enhancement, and regulation of mood states. Identifying the individual's specific motivations for ongoing substance use, apart from physiologic dependence, can provide treatment targets for ongoing therapy. There is no all-inclusive model for cognitive behavioral therapy and there are numerous psychiatric conditions beyond substance use which respond well to CBT. Most often, CBT for substance use disorders will include aspects of self-monitoring, avoidance of triggering stimuli, altering reinforcement, and development of coping skills [25].

Multidimensional Family Therapy

Multidimensional family therapy (MFT) is a form of family-based therapy that recognizes that adolescent substance use is complex and multifactorial in etiology, owing to individual, social, familial, and environmental factors. The use of this structured familial therapeutic method is derived from earlier work involving the adult heroin use population. The adaption to adolescent substance use treatment comes from recognizing that advances in understanding of developmental psychology and psychopathology can be utilized in treatment planning. The goal for treatment is to incorporate normal developmental processes into the adolescent's life. This treatment program is divided into phases.

Phase 1: This begins with the therapist developing relationships with the adolescent and the members of the treatment network. This includes not only the parents or caregivers but also the other family members and other care providers in the environment like teachers, coaches, etc. In the second phase, the therapist makes a global assessment of risk from each area of the adolescent's life and determine the level of involvement/willingness to change of the providers in each area. This first phase is considered complete when a clear outline of mutually acceptable goals is outlined and accompanied by a strong commitment to restoring function to the parent-adolescent relationship.

Phase 2: Treatment begins to target the goals outlined in phase 1. Individual sessions with the adolescent work on behavior modification, skill-set development, coping skills, and identifying those factors which separate them from achieving normal psychosocial development. Skill-set development is highly customizable and commonly involves skills like learning to avoid high-risk peers and places but can also include vocational training and working to earn a GED. During individual sessions with the parent the therapist focuses on improving the wellbeing of the parent and improving parenting style. This includes addressing any existing stressors the parents have beyond their child in addition to improving parenting technique. Parents come to understand the difference between controlling vs influencing their child and learn to reconcile that not everything they see in their children can or should be fixed by them. The biggest transition in this phase of therapy is that of the role of the therapist from more passive assessment and information gathering to active intervention.

Adolescent Community Reinforcement Approach (ACRA)

The Adolescent Community Reinforcement Approach (A-CRA) method functions by substituting positive influences into the family, social, and education environments of the adolescent to help them achieve and maintain sobriety. The structure of the therapy involves 10 sessions of individual therapy with the adolescent, 4 sessions of group therapy with the caregiver circle of which two must include the entire family. Case management services are also provided over the treatment duration to a limited extent. With adolescent substance use, peer and environmental factors are believed to play a significant role in continued use, therefore ACRA therapy functions on an operant conditioning model with supporting skills therapy to teach adolescents how to cope with stress without turning to substance use. The therapist helps the adolescent to realize that substance use is in direct conflict with their long-term goals such as personal success and parental approval. As the therapist builds this realization in the adolescent, they are advocating for their patient by recruiting positive factors in the schools, jobs, community programs, etc. During family and caregiver treatment sessions, the therapist works to educate the family on parenting strategies and practices that are more likely to support the adolescent than they are to cause relapse.

Treatment sessions are structured around three techniques which are continuously updated throughout the treatment course. It begins by analyzing the causes which lead to substance abuse. This includes both internal factors that are revealed through ongoing therapy as well as any external factors which placed that at increased risk for use. The adolescent will also regularly quantify their level of happiness using a 14-point assessment tool. This allows for both the longitudinal tracking of progress over treatment as well as using the specific content to identify specific areas for improvement during therapy. These first two steps are combined to form the third tenet of ACRA, the treatment plan. Identifying the risks and consequences of their behaviors, coming up with a plan to overcome them, and tracking overall life satisfaction in real time allows for a dynamic treatment plan tailored to that adolescent's individual.

Pharmacotherapy

The opioid epidemic in the United States claimed over 700,000 lives by overdose between 1999 and 2017 (www.cdc.gov). In 2017 SAHMSA estimates that 214,000 adolescents were misusing opiates while only 2000 were using heroin. Finding an effective means of helping people overcome opioid addiction has appropriately become a priority for the medical community. Although withdrawal from opiates is not associated with significant mortality it is extremely unpleasant and without medical assistance opioid addiction has one of the highest rates of relapse [13]. Placing patients on agonist therapies to control cravings without delivering the potent high of illicit opiate use has been effective in long-term remission for many people with opiate use disorder. Currently, agonist therapies may be broadly grouped into methadone and buprenorphine-based treatment programs. Methadone is a weak opiate agonist, has been approved for use in opioid withdrawal since 1972. Buprenorphine is a partial agonist at opioid receptors and is available both as a monotherapy and a combination (buprenorphine-naloxone), sold under the brand name Suboxone. Suboxone contains both buprenorphine and as a protection against abuse, naltrexone which is an opiate antagonist to protect against abuse/misuse.

While both methadone and buprenorphine have been shown to improve rates of remission in opiate use disorder, buprenorphine offers several advantages over methadone treatment. Rigid federal regulations require that methadone therapy be conducted in highly regulated programs and facilities [15]. A new methadone patient will be required to return to such a clinic daily to receive their methadone treatment. This can be a logistical challenge for patients with childcare needs, limited transportation, and conflicting work schedules. Over time, patients can graduate to higher levels of trust and may be given methadone prescriptions on a weekly to monthly basis. Buprenorphine also requires additional certification and training on the part of the provider however after that, it can be dispensed from that doctor's office or clinic. While the data are unequivocal that agonist therapies reduce rates of relapse and decrease comorbid illness and crime, there are multiple barriers to using these therapies in the adolescent population ([19]; Institute of Medicine (US) Committee on Federal Regulation of Methadone Treatment, [9]). Practitioners must contend with issues of ability to consent to treatment, confidentiality, and assuming the responsibility of supervising maintenance therapy. FDA regulations of agonist therapy in adolescents require either two previous failed attempts at a medication taper or short-term rehabilitation stay in order to prescribe methadone [5] whereas the use of buprenorphine has no such requirement, provided that the adolescent is at least 16 years of age [21]. There are currently no FDA-approved pharmacologic treatments for adolescent substance use disorder under the age of 16, largely due to the paucity of empiric data available on treatment outcomes in this population.

References

1. Boumba V, Ziavrou K, Vougiouklakis T. Hair as a biological indicator of drug use, drug abuse or chronic exposure to environmental toxicants. Int J Toxicol. 2006;25:143–63.
2. Cooper ZD, Haney M. Actions of delta-9-tetrahydrocannabinol in cannabis: relation to use, abuse, dependence. Int Rev Psychiatry (Abingdon, England). 2009;21(2):104–12. https://doi.org/10.1080/09540260902782752.
3. Dams R, Choo RE, Lambert WE, et al. Oral fluid as an alternative matrix to monitor opiate and cocaine use in substance-abuse treatment patients. Drug Alcohol Depend. 2007;87:258–67.
4. ElSohly MA, Mehmedic Z, Foster S, Gon C, Chandra S, Church JC. Changes in Cannabis potency over the last 2 decades (1995–2014): analysis of current data in the United States. Biol Psychiatry. 2016;79(7):613–9. https://doi.org/10.1016/j.biopsych.2016.01.004.
5. Galanter M, Kleber HD. Textbook of substance abuse treatment. 4th ed. Washington, D.C.: American Psychiatric Publishing, Inc.; 2008.
6. Grella, C. (2006). The drug abuse treatment outcomes studies: outcomes with adolescent substance abusers. Adolesc Subst Abuse Res Clin Adv, 189 384–392.
7. GROUP, P. M. R. Matching patients with alcohol disorders to treatments: clinical implications from project MATCH. J Ment Health. 1998;7(6):589–602.
8. Hadland SE, Levy S. Objective testing: urine and other drug tests. Child Adolesc Psychiatr Clin N Am. 2016;25(3):549–65.
9. Institute of Medicine (US) Committee on Federal Regulation of Methadone Treatment; Rettig RA, Yarmolinsky A, editors. Federal regulation of methadone treatment. Washington, D.C.: National Academies Press (US); 1995. Executive Summary. Available from: https://www.ncbi.nlm.nih.gov/books/NBK232111/.
10. Jessor R, editor. New perspectives on adolescent risk behavior. Cambridge: Cambridge University Press; 1998.
11. Luthar SS, Merikangas KR, Rounsaville BJ. Parental psychopathology and disorders in offspring: a study of relatives of drug abusers. J Nerv Mental Dis. 1993;181:351.
12. McConnaughy EA, Prochaska JO, Velicer WF. Stages of change in psychotherapy: measurement and sample profiles. Psychotherapy Theory Res Pract. 1983;20(3):368.
13. Meltzer B, Masry A. The pharmacotherapy of adolescent opioid dependence. Child Adolesc Psychopharmacol News. 2010;15(2):1–7.
14. Merikangas KR, Stolar M, Stevens DE, Goulet J, Preisig MA, Fenton B, et al. Familial transmission of substance use disorders. Arch Gen Psychiatry. 1998;55(11):973–9.
15. Methadone. Retrieved February 02, 2020, from https://www.samhsa.gov/medication-assisted-treatment/treatment/methadone. 2020, January 16.
16. Miller WR. Motivational enhancement therapy with drug abusers. Albuquerque: University of New Mexico Press; 1995.
17. Miller WR, Moyers TB. Eight stages in learning motivational interviewing. J Teach Addict. 2006;5(1):3–17.
18. Miller WR, Rollnick S. Motivational interviewing: preparing people for change. 2nd ed. New York: The Guilford Press; 2002.
19. National Institute on Drug Abuse. Treatment approaches for drug addiction. *NIDA InfoFacts,* September 1–5. 2009.
20. Rounsaville BJ, Kosten TR, Weissman MM, Prusoff B, Pauls D, Anton SF, Merikangas K. Psychiatric disorders in relatives of probands with opiate addiction. Arch Gen Psychiatry. 1991;48(1):33–42.
21. Squeglia LM, Fadus MC, McClure EA, Tomko RL, Gray KM. Pharmacological treatment of youth substance use disorders. J Child Adolesc Psychopharmacol. 2019;29(7):559–72.
22. Substance Abuse and Mental Health Services Administration. Clinical drug testing in primary care. Technical assistance publication (TAP) 32. Rockville (MD): Substance Abuse and Mental Health Services Administration; 2012. HHS publication No. (SMA) 12–4668.

23. Tevyaw TOL, Monti PM. Motivational enhancement and other brief interventions for adolescent substance abuse: foundations, applications and evaluations. Addiction. 2004;99:63–75.
24. Tripodi SJ, Bender K, Litschge C, Vaughn MG. Interventions for reducing adolescent alcohol abuse: a meta-analytic review. Arch Pediatr Adolesc Med. 2010;164(1):85–91.
25. Waldron HB, Kaminer Y. On the learning curve: the emerging evidence supporting cognitive–behavioral therapies for adolescent substance abuse. Addiction. 2004;99:93–105.
26. Johnston LD, O'Malley PM, Bachman JG. Monitoring the future: national results on adolescent drug use: overview of key findings. Focus. 2003;1(2):213–34.

Part II

Nonsubstance Addictions

Compulsive Sexual Behavior

5

Samantha Swetter, Ralph Fader, Tiffany Christian, and Brentt Swetter

Introduction

For over a century authors have endeavored to categorize sexual behaviors and drives deemed to be in excess of the norm. The terms nymphomania for females [1] and Don Juanism [2] or satyriasis [3] for males have been used to describe a pattern of maladaptive and excessive sexual acts which include intercourse, masturbation, and pornography consumption. In more recent years, the phenomenon of out of control sexual behavior is variably described as hypersexual disorder, sexual impulsivity, sex addiction, compulsive sexual behavior, and dysregulated sexual behavior [4], often depending on the disease etiology to which the author subscribes. The term "psychosexual disorder not otherwise specified" was introduced in the third edition of the Diagnostic and Statistical Manual of Mental Illnesses (DSM-III) and defined as "distress about a pattern of repeated sexual conquests with a succession of individuals who exist only as things to be used" [5]. DSM-III-R was the first to introduce the concept of a "sexual addiction" [6]; however, the addiction phrasing was removed from subsequent editions due to lack of evidence and consensus supporting the addiction model and was instead replaced with the original DSM-III phrasing [7]. A diagnosis of hypersexual disorder was considered for DSM-5 [8], and the International Classification of Diseases 11th Revision (ICD-11) recently included a diagnosis of compulsive sexual behavior disorder (CSBD) [9].

Disinhibition of sexual behavior is observed across a number of medical and psychiatric conditions. Neurologic conditions include those in which normal inhibitory controls are impaired such as in frontal lobe lesions, dementia, and traumatic brain injury [10]. This behavior has also been associated with temporal lobe epilepsy [4] and as a side effect of antiparkinsonian agents [11]. Hypersexuality may also be found in the diagnostic criteria for bipolar mania as well [12]. Whether excessive sexual behaviors exist as an entity independent of trait impulsivity or deficits in affect regulation is an ongoing topic of discussion in the literature [13].

A need for avoiding pathologizing normal variant sexual behaviors in the name of sociocultural mores has also been discussed [8].

S. Swetter (✉)
Dartmouth's Geisel School of Medicine, Hanover, NH, USA
e-mail: Samantha.Swetter@dartmouth.edu

R. Fader
The Mount Sinai Hospital, New York, NY, USA
e-mail: ralph.fader@mountsinai.org

T. Christian
Mount Sinai Morningside Hospital, New York, NY, USA
e-mail: tiffany.christian@mountsinai.org

B. Swetter
Tarrytown, NY, USA

E. Akerele (ed.), *Substance and Non-Substance Related Addictions*,
https://doi.org/10.1007/978-3-030-84834-7_5

Categorizations of anomalous sexual behavior that rely on frequency of intercourse must be conscientious of misidentifying normal variations in behavior as pathological. Notably, a Swedish study on compulsive sexual behavior found that high-frequency sexual activity with a stable partner was associated with indicators of better psychological functioning whereas high-frequency solo or impersonal sexual behaviors correlated with measures of life dissatisfaction and negative health indicators [14]. Conversely, definitions that rely on perceived distress may identify individuals who incorrectly assume that their behavior or thoughts are in excess of norms. For example, individuals who endorsed higher levels of religiosity and moral disapproval of pornography were more likely to perceive addiction to internet pornography regardless of the actual degree of use [15].

The addiction model is one of the more popular conceptual frameworks used to consider dysregulated sexual behavior [16]. Central to this framework is the notion that, similar to illicit substances, sex derives pleasure, and problematic sexual behavior must therefore be mediated by an addictive process that involves recurrent failure to control sexual behavior despite harmful consequences [17]. Whether tolerance and withdrawal are experienced in sex addiction is a topic of debate, although some hypothesize that negative affective states when decreasing sexual behaviors may reflect withdrawal [18]. Some of the neurobiological pathways associated with addiction have been demonstrated to play a role in hypersexual behaviors [19].

As an alternative hypothesis, some argue that hypersexual behavior may become habitual through its ability to take away negative affective states such as depression, anxiety, and shame, thus making it more similar to a compulsion than an addiction [4]. Others consider impulse dysregulation, rather than desire or negative reinforcement, as a possible mechanism for excessive sexual behavior, positing that individuals have an inability to resist sexual drives even if they are harmful [20]. Models implicating adult attachment styles [21] and executive function have also been described [22]. Hypersexual disorder (HD) is a neutral term that does not prescribe to an underlying pathophysiology.

For the purposes of this chapter we will primarily use the term compulsive sexual behavior (CSB), although readers should keep in mind the complexity of this diagnosis and the possible heterogeneity of pathology. For a thorough review on the subject refer to Walton et al. [4], Montgomery-Graham [16], Kingston and Firestone [23], or Kraus et al. [24]. CSB in this chapter will be used to refer to persistent difficulties in controlling sexual thoughts, urges, and behaviors which cause distress or impairment of function. It is essential to note that this label distinguishes non-paraphilic behaviors from the paraphilic conditions listed in the DSM-5, although the conditions can exist comorbidly. Paraphilic behaviors are distinguished from non-paraphilic behaviors in that the former are considered to be "socially deviant" and the latter are not [25]. Paraphilic disorders include voyeuristic disorder, exhibitionistic disorder, frotteuristic disorder, sexual sadism, sexual masochism, pedophilic disorder, fetishistic disorder, and transvestic disorder [12]. Non-paraphilic behavior is conventional sexual behavior, although taken to the extremes in the context of CSB. Behaviors may include masturbation, use of sexual accessories such as drugs or objects, pornography use, promiscuity, telephone sex [26], or cybersex [27].

Epidemiology

Epidemiological data for compulsive sexual behavior is limited worldwide, with most of the data coming from the United States and Europe. While it was recently incorporated into the ICD-11, it is not a formal diagnosis in the DSM-5 and there is no consensus on screening measures or diagnostic criteria, although many have been proposed [7, 28, 29]. This lack of consensus combined with the stigmatization of perceived aberrant sexual behavior [30] and poor societal awareness [31] make acquiring epidemiological data difficult. Furthermore, the stigma associated with people seeking treatment likely leads to a higher severity of illness at the time of presentation and could skew study results [32]. In this section, we provide a brief overview of proposed screening measures and diagnostic criteria. We will then use this framework to describe the epidemiology of the disorder around the world.

Evolution of Epidemiological Characterization

In an early description of male sexual behavior, Kinsey and colleagues found that 7.6% of males up to age 30 had over seven total orgasms from any outlet (TSOs) per week for more than 5 years [33]. Further studies have found anywhere from 1% to 5% of males have over seven TSOs [34, 35]. These as well as other studies led Kafka to suggest that ≥7 TSOs for six consecutive months should define hypersexual behavior in males [36]. This definition, notably, does not have any criteria regarding impairment or distress, and there has been discussion about this definition pathologizing high-frequency sexual behavior [33]. Others have focused definitional taxonomy on the associated distress or impairment rather than the frequency of orgasms [37]. Although as discussed above, there should be a balance between the two so as not to conflate subcultural norms with pathology.

Table 5.1 Proposed diagnostic criteria for hypersexual disorder for inclusion in the DSM-5, as proposed by Martin Kafka. Reprinted by permission from Springer Nature. Archives of Sexual Behavior. Hypersexual Disorder: A Proposed Diagnosis for DSM-V, Martin P. Kafka, 2009 [7]

Proposed diagnostic criteria for hypersexual disorder
A. over a period of at least 6 months, recurrent and intense sexual fantasies, sexual urges, or sexual behaviors in association with 3 or more of the following 5 criteria.
A1. Time consumed by sexual fantasies, urges or behaviors repetitively interferes with other important (non-sexual) goals, activities, and obligations.
A2. Repetitively engaging in sexual fantasies, urges, or behaviors in response to dysphoric mood states (e.g., anxiety, depression, boredom, irritability).
A3. Repetitively engaging in sexual fantasies, urges, or behaviors in response to stressful life events.
A4. Repetitive but unsuccessful efforts to control or significantly reduce these sexual fantasies, urges, or behaviors.
A5. Repetitively engaging in sexual behaviors while disregarding the risk for physical or emotional harm to self or others.
B. There is clinically significant personal distress or impairment in social, occupational, or other important areas of functioning associated with the frequency and intensity of these sexual fantasies, urges, or behaviors.
C. these sexual fantasies, urges, or behaviors are not due to the direct physiological effect of an exogenous substance (e.g., a drug of abuse or a medication), a co-occurring general medical condition, or to manic episodes.
Specify if: Masturbation, pornography, sexual behavior with consenting adults, cybersex, telephone sex, strip clubs, other

Hypersexual Disorder in the DSM-5

To fully categorize the disorder for further study, Kafka proposed criteria for the inclusion of "Hypersexual Disorder" in the DSM-5 [7]. These criteria are in Table 5.1. While not accepted into the DSM-5 due to lack of research and concern for false positives [38], they have been field tested with good preliminary evidence of their validity [39], and the American Psychiatric Association has developed a screening tool – the Hypersexual Disorder Screening Inventory (HDSI) – for screening of this proposed disorder in line with these criteria [40]. The HDSI pertains to behavior over the last 6 months and includes five statements asking if the participant has had the symptoms listed in proposed criterion A of hypersexual disorder and two statements addressing distress and impairment (proposed criterion B) [29, 41]. The responses available are "never true," "rarely true," "sometimes true," "often true," and "almost always true" [29, 41]. This screening tool has shown to be a reliable screening measure in the United States, Brazil, and Sweden, although further investigations are needed to fully validate it, to delineate cut-off scores, and to identify specific behaviors [29, 40–42].

Compulsive Sexual Behavior Disorder in the ICD-11

While there have been recent advancements in screening and diagnosis as pertaining to the DSM-

5, these diagnostic criteria are not used around the world [43]. The World Health Organization (WHO) uses the ICD-11, where distressing hypersexual behavior is included as CSBD in the impulse control disorders section. The description is summarized as over 6 months of failure to control sexual impulses or urges to the point of neglecting interests, activities, or responsibilities with unsuccessful efforts to reduce behavior and causing distress or impairment not entirely from moral judgments. The description has an exclusion of paraphilic disorders [44].

There is also a self-report Compulsive Sexual Behavior Inventory-13 (CSBI-13) to screen for compulsive sexual behavior that has been used as well [45–47]. This instrument rates participants on 13 screening items ranging from 1 (never) to 5 (very frequently). A sum of 35 or more has good sensitivity and specificity for compulsive sexual behavior [47]. The queries ask about trouble controlling sexual urges, inability to control sexual behavior and feelings, using sex to deal with problems, feeling guilty or shameful, concealment of behavior, attempts to change behavior, interference of thoughts in relationships, excuses to justify behavior, missed opportunities, financial problems, emotionally distant during sex, and a greater frequency than intended [47].

The Sexual Compulsivity Scale (SCS) and the Sexual Inhibition Scale/Sexual Excitation Scale (SISSES) are also validated screening tools [7], although there are over 17 other instruments or scales that have been used [48]. In a recent analysis, the HDSI had the strongest psychometric support [16].

These advancements are the first steps to clarify diagnosis for further inquiries into epidemiology, treatment, and etiology. It should be noted that there is currently no consensus, resulting in data based on various measures, as described below.

Prevalence and Primary Regional Diagnosis Around the World

As the majority of the data regarding sexual behavior stems from studies in the United States, this region will be discussed in detail first and then similarities and differences in other global regions will be explored.

United States

Prevalence and Sociodemographics

In the United States, the prevalence of sex addiction is estimated to be 3–6% and has a male predominance [49, 50]. In a recent prevalence study based on community survey data from 2325 adults aged 18–50 throughout the United States, 10.3% of men and 7.0% of women reported clinically significant levels of distress or impairment from sexual feelings, urges, or behaviors [46].

It has been hypothesized that men are more susceptible to CSBs [7, 30, 51]. In comparison to females, males have increased sexual fantasy [52], increased frequency of masturbation, and more permissive attitudes toward masturbation and casual sex [53]. However, the majority of these effect sizes are decreasing in a more recent 2010 meta-analysis, although most did not change in clinical significance and larger effect sizes were seen in ethnic groups with lesser gender equity [54]. There was one area that was found to have a likelihood greater than chance – approval of sexual intercourse in a committed relationship – which went from a higher approval in men to higher approval in women [54].

In quantitative studies, the percentage of women among those that are afflicted is 20%, throwing support toward this hypothesis [30, 41]. However, there is some evidence to contrary, suggesting that the prevalence in females is underreported [55], and a more recent prevalence study found that women accounted for 40.8% of a large community sample [46].

There is also evidence that problematic sexual behavior can present differently in men and women. Women are more likely to call themselves “love addicts” [30]. This may present as multiple failed relationships, using sex as a business, fantasy sex, or sado-masochism [49]. Men are more likely to have compulsive masturbation, paraphilias, paying for sex, or anonymous sex [56].

There is also evidence that gay or bisexual men have a higher prevalence when compared to heterosexual males [57]. This is further expanded upon in the 2018 survey data above, where persons that identified themselves as gay or lesbian were 2.92 times more likely to endorse distress or impairment related to difficulty with sexual feelings, urges, or behaviors. Individuals that self-identified as bisexual were 3.02 times more likely, and people that identified as "other" were 4.33 times more likely to endorse distress or impairment [46].

Persons with less than a high school education, income of less than $25,000, income between $75,000–$100,000, and income over $150,0000 also have higher odds of endorsing clinically relevant levels of distress and impairment related to CSBs [46].

CSB has been found to be more common in Caucasians as compared to other races in treatment-seeking samples [39], however this data may be confounded by higher socioeconomic status and greater access to care [24, 39]. In contrast, national community survey data showed individuals that identify as black, Hispanic, or other were 2.50 times more likely to report distress and impairment associated with CSBs than those that identify as white [46]. This may reflect differences in treatment-seeking populations.

Family History

Substance use disorders are common in the family members of those with CSB; with 40% having at least one parent with a substance use disorder. Furthermore, 36% had a parent with CSB, 30% with a parent that had an eating disorder, and 7% with a parent that had problematic gambling [58].

Comorbidity

As is the case with many other psychiatric disorders, there is a high comorbidity of CSBD with other medical/psychiatric conditions as well as with characterologic traits. When treating CSBD, care must be taken to treat all other comorbid conditions and address possible predisposing or perpetuating traits.

There are high rates of psychiatric comorbid conditions with CSB, with 100% of one sample meeting criteria for an Axis-I disorder at some point in their lifetime [51]. It has been found to be associated with mood and anxiety disorders (up to 76.7% and 46.7% respectively) [25, 59, 60] and attention-deficit/hyperactivity disorder (ADHD) [25]. There is high comorbidity with personality disorders as well, at 44–46% [30, 51].

The overlap with substance use disorders is 38–71% [30, 51, 61], and with other behavioral addictions is 30–50% [25, 30, 62, 63]. Perhaps surprisingly, there is also a high prevalence of sexual dysfunctions in these populations at 46%. The comorbidity with a paraphilia is 8% [51].

CSB has also been associated with various character traits, such as impulsivity and compulsivity [30, 51], risk-taking behaviors [59, 64], loneliness [65, 66], insecure attachment styles [21], personal distress [26], and shame [59]. Mindfulness has also been inversely correlated with CSB [67]. Lastly, afflicted persons are more likely to have a history of childhood sexual abuse [30] although no causality has been established.

Sexual compulsivity has been associated with medical comorbidities as well. Afflicted persons have higher rates of unwanted pregnancies, sexually transmitted diseases including HIV, and physical trauma from sexual acts [32, 50, 62, 68, 69]. Furthermore, sexually transmitted diseases in women result in increased risk of cervical cancer and ectopic pregnancy [70].

Differential Diagnosis

When considering a diagnosis of CSBD, one must be careful not to conflate excessive sexuality without distress or CSB due to another underlying psychiatric illness, such as bipolar disorder, substance use disorder, obsessive-compulsive disorder, neurocognitive disorder, ADHD, autism spectrum disorders, or depressive disorders [71]. Dopamine agonist medications have also been shown to cause hypersexual behavior in people being treated for Parkinson's or restless leg syndrome [11], and it is prudent to treat address these iatrogenic causes before diagnosing the disorder if pertinent.

Outside of the United States

Prevalence and Sociodemographics

In the other regions of the world for which there is data on CSB, the diagnostic quandaries have paralleled those in the United States, with the terms sex addiction [72, 73], compulsive sexual behavior [74–76], and hypersexuality [4, 14, 41, 77] all being used. The only prevalence data is a New Zealand survey, where 13% of men and 7% of women reported perceived out-of-control sexual experiences, although only 3.8% of men and 1.7% of women felt that the experiences were interfering with their lives [78]. There is no other prevalence data for community samples, although some demographical associations have been reported.

CSB has been associated with male sex, neuroticism, extroversion, low agreeableness, and low conscientiousness in Norway [72] and Australia [4]; although in Norway it was also correlated with higher education [72] and in Australia correlated with lower inhibition from threat of consequences [4]. Germany also had an overlap with neurosis [79] and Spain with higher socioeconomic status [80]. In Britain, males that identify as gay or bisexual may have a higher prevalence of symptomatology [81]. In Sweden, symptoms were more likely for men and women with younger age, separation of parents in childhood, younger age of first vaginal intercourse, history of sexual abuse, ever having a sex-same partner, more easily aroused, arousal from seeing a stranger's genitals, arousal from spying on others' sexual activity, using pain deliberately, history of a sexually transmitted infection (STI), and history of asking professional for sexuality advice. They were more likely for men with urban living or ever having paid for sex [14]. In China, these behaviors have been related to high-risk sexual behavior, lower educational level, unemployed status, unsure HIV status, older age, not being a student [82], higher number of partners, higher likelihood of STI, inconsistent condom use, and sex with female sex workers [76].

There are some discrepancies above between high and low socioeconomic status and low education as well as younger and older age. More thorough investigations will need to be conducted to solidify these associations and sort out whether the discrepancies are culturally based.

There is also some literature supporting that when sexual guilt and encouragement of female abstinence is transmitted to children in Latino cultures, this delays sexual behavior in the United States and Mexico [83]; although it is unclear if this translates to a decrease in hypersexual behaviors. There may be other unknown cultural factors that affect CSB as well, such as religion and access to sexual partners.

Comorbidity

Comorbid psychiatric disorders, particularly mood and anxiety symptoms, have been reported in Spain [80], Brazil [75], Australia [4], and Denmark [77]. There is also a demonstrated association with substance use disorders in Germany [79] and Sweden [14] and with gambling in Spain [80] and Sweden [14]. Sexual dysfunction also appears to be a cross-cultural comorbidity as shown in Germany and Croatia [84], and eating disorders are comorbid in Germany [79].

One would postulate that the overlap with medical comorbidities, such as STIs and HIV, would also be problematic in other regions of the world, especially given an increased prevalence of STIs and HIV in many other areas around the globe [85].

Differential Diagnosis

The same differential diagnosis exists for other cultures as well, including for iatrogenic causes. An association with dopamine replacement therapy in Parkinson's disease has also been reported in Denmark [77], Russia [86], and Germany [87]; and there is a case report of aripiprazole, a partial dopamine agonist, causing compulsive sexuality in France [88].

Resource Poor Settings

There are many countries that are characterized by low incomes and high morbidity and mortality from communicable diseases and malnutrition. This can result in mental health being a low priority [89]. While CSB has not been studied in these regions, it is likely that it exists given the cross-cultural nature as demonstrated above and the transcultural addiction rates [90]. One could postulate that those afflicted in these regions may be at a higher risk of HIV given a higher local prevalence [85], and have reduced access to care, increasing the economic burden in these areas from higher morbidity and mortality due to associated diseases and disorders, although there is no data from these regions as of yet.

Treatment Around the World

A clear conceptual understanding of a disease can elucidate potential avenues for treatment. As you have read thus far, there is still significant debate on how to best conceptualize CSBD. Accordingly, there is still significant debate in how CSBs should be treated. This section will attempt to synthesize a framework for understanding the current evidence for treatment of CSBs, including work-up as well as pharmacologic, hormonal, surgical, and psychotherapeutic interventions. We then discuss variations in treatment around the world and provide a set of treatment guidelines that were most consistently recommended in the available literature.

General Concepts

Although there are significant clinical and legal burdens associated with CSBs, the literature relating to effective treatment recommendations is surprisingly heterogenous and scant. The reasoning for this is multifaceted. Firstly, as reviewed earlier in this chapter, CSB is not consistently well-defined as a clinical entity. The names and definitions of these behaviors change dramatically depending on when and where the study or review is conducted. In particular, the lack of a clearly defined neurobiological model for CSBs limits the generalizability of treatments. More recent studies distinguish CSBs as paraphilic and non-paraphilic, although it remains unclear whether there is a neurobiological difference between these two categories. Given that this distinction is made in the literature, we continue use of the distinction in this chapter. However, there are problems from maintaining this distinction. Namely, the most robust evidence on CSBs, the World Federation of Societies on Biological Psychiatry (WFSBP) 2010 treatment guidelines, is specific to paraphilic CSBs. We use the WFSBP guidelines because of the dearth of significant evidence for treatment of non-specific CSBs and also due to the lack of evidence for a neurobiological distinction between paraphilic CSBs and non-paraphilic CSBs.

The second reason that the evidence for treatment is so scant is that many types of CSBs are significantly criminalized. This leads to an overrepresentation of incarcerated populations, often men, as compared to non-incarcerated populations in study cohorts. This selection bias presents two specific problems. One is the obvious limitation in demographic generalizability when it comes to treatment. The other, which is subtler, is that oftentimes incarcerated populations are diagnosed with CSBs for purposes of sentencing, which creates a kind of selection bias intrinsic to the study population [91, 92]. Thirdly, owing to the criminalized nature of CSBs, study populations tend to be small and tend to have high drop-out rates. This means that we as providers must often extract clinical significance from studies with small samples and low power.

Finally, there is no ubiquitous legal standard for which interventions are used to treat CSBs, which makes generalizing treatment recommendations difficult [93]. Oftentimes, the strongest data comes from meta-analyses and systematic reviews of conglomerated case reports, case series, retrospective studies, and prospective trials. It should be noted that in spite of all these limitations, there is one point on which the literature is fairly clear: treatment for CSBs is more effective across outcome measure than no treatment at all. In particular, amongst sex offenders, the rates of recidivism with CSB treatment drop from roughly 17% to 11% [91, 94, 95]. The discussion of the literature below attempts to consolidate the available research on this difficult topic and present it in a way that offers guidance on clinical management of CSBs.

Work-Up for CSBs

The first step in any treatment protocol is to ensure that you know what you are treating. As previously discussed, the lack of a clearly defined neurobiological model makes this difficult. However, expert consensus on management of CSBs does agree on a certain evaluation pathway, both to help with diagnostic clarity and to inform treatment recommendations [91, 93, 95, 96].

A thorough psychiatric interview and assessment should be completed for any patient presenting with a complaint concerning for CSB [91, 93, 95, 96]. Concerted effort should be made to determine the extent of diagnostic criteria met as well as the severity of impairment. Investigation into the timeline of these symptoms, as well as any associated complaints, psychiatric or otherwise, may clarify underlying or associated conditions contributing to the current presentation. Special attention should be paid to psychiatric comorbidities, medical history, and psychosexual development.

The patient should also undergo physical examination and laboratory testing in the initial work-up for CSBs [91, 93, 95, 96]. Laboratory testing should include a complete blood count (with attention to hemoglobin and hematocrit), a basic metabolic panel (with attention to creatinine), TSH (to rule out underlying metabolic causes of psychiatric complaints), and a pregnancy test (to rule out pregnancy in case pharmacologic treatment is indicated). Additionally, labs assessing sexual function should be performed, including luteinizing hormone, follicular stimulating hormone, serum testosterone, free testosterone, and prolactin.

If the patient is undergoing assessment for initiation of androgen deprivation therapy (ADT), additional assessment should be included in the initial work-up as well. Additional history-taking includes personal history of smoking and alcohol use, exercise and dietary habits, and family history of cardiovascular disease, osteoporosis, diabetes mellitus, and hypercholesterolemia. Supplemental physical examination components should include height, weight, and waist circumference. Further testing for ADT should consist of a fasting blood glucose, a lipid panel, calcium and phosphorus levels, an electrocardiogram, and a dual-energy X-ray absorptiometry (DEXA) scan if increased risk of osteoporosis or history of pathologic fracture [97].

If the patient meets criteria for a paraphilic disorder as outlined in the DSM-5, and if there is no concern for an underlying medical or psychiatric condition to better explain their symptoms, you can then review potential CSB treatment options.

Treatment of Compulsive Sexual Behaviors

Treatment in this chapter is divided into pharmacologic treatments (including psychotropic and hormonal) and non-pharmacologic treatments (including psychological and surgical).

Pharmacologic Treatment – Psychotropic Medications

As previously discussed under General Concepts, research into effective treatments for CSBs are limited in size and power. To date, there have been no randomized double-blind placebo-controlled trials assessing the efficacy of psychotropic medications for management of CSBs, only case studies and open-label trials [96]. As a result, the list of medications shown to be effective in specifically treating CSBs is quite small. There are currently no psychotropic medications that are FDA-approved to treat CSBs.

Serotonergic agents such as selective serotonin reuptake inhibitors (SSRIs), serotonin norepinephrine reuptake inhibitors (SNRIs), and tricyclic antidepressants (TCAs) have had modest benefits in treating non-paraphilic CSBs. Individual case studies and open-label trials indicated some promise of using serotonergic agents to reduce cravings and control sexual preoccupation [18, 93]; however, meta-analyses and systematic reviews examining treatment of paraphilic CSBs showed that there was little significant effect of serotonergic agents on outcome measures such as recidivism [91, 93, 95, 96]. There was also no appreciable benefit between agents within each class (i.e., sertraline, fluoxetine, citalopram, etc., all had equally little benefit) [91, 93, 96]. If benefits were seen in patients diagnosed with CSBs on serotonergic agents, the benefit seemed to be primarily from treatment of non-paraphilic CSBs and/or co-morbid psychiatric conditions such as depression, anxiety, and obsessive-compulsive disorder (OCD) [91, 93, 95]. In a literature review in 2009, Guay recommended using SSRIs/SNRIs over TCAs if opting for a serotonergic agent for treatment of CSBs due to a better-tolerated side-effect profile [91]. Although serotonergic agents are preferred over hormonal therapies in treating adolescents with CSBs, SSRIs and SNRIs still come with an increased risk of suicidality in those younger than 24 years old and this should weigh into any treatment decision-making [98].

In 2010, the World Federation of Societies of Biological Psychiatry (WFSBP) published a set of guidelines for the treatment of paraphilic CSBs. These guidelines determined that there was modest evidence studying serotonergic agents such as SSRIs/SNRIs for paraphilic CSBs and that this evidence showed little benefit, mostly in decreasing self-reported urges/cravings and subjective distress from symptoms of CSBs [93]. This same set of guidelines qualified that expert consensus among providers and professional societies (such as the Association for Treatment of Sexual Abusers [ATSA] and American Academy of Child and Adolescent Psychiatry [AACAP]) holds that for mild CSBs and low risk of re-offending, SSRIs/SNRIs are an appropriate treatment.

There has also been low quality and limited data on the efficacy of other psychotropic agents in the treatment of CSBs. Again, most are case studies and open-label trials. Other psychotropic agents that have been examined in treatment of CSBs include antipsychotics, mood stabilizers, stimulants, benzodiazepines, buspirone, and naltrexone [91, 93, 95, 96]. A Cochrane review in 2010 showed that anticonvulsants such as valproate, carbamazepine, and phenytoin decreased violent behaviors (including sexual aggression) in incarcerated patients as compared to placebo [99, 100]. However, this data was not obtained specifically from sex offenders or from patients determined to have CSBs. One open-label study showed resolution of CSBs with either lithium (dose = 900 mg/day) or fluphenazine decanoate (dose range = 12.5–27.5 mg/2 weeks IM) but only in half of patients treated [93, 101]. In trials of antipsychotics, one showed no statistically significant difference between chlorpromazine, benperidol, and placebo [93, 102]. An open-label study of juvenile male patients with CSBs showed that naltrexone (dose range = 100–200 mg/day) significantly reduced CSBs; these behaviors recurred in those who decreased naltrexone dose to lower than 50 mg/day [93, 103].

Although individual case reports and small trials seemed promising, the WFSBP guidelines determined that there is no evidence to support the use of non-serotonergic psychotropic medications in the treatment of paraphilic CSBs [93]. If these medications are used in patients with CSBs, most of the literature supports their use for treatment of co-morbid psychiatric conditions (e.g., antipsychotics for psychotic illness, mood stabilizers for significant mood disorders, stimulants for ADHD or treatment-resistant depression, etc.) [91, 93, 95, 100]. Some reviews seem to suggest that SSRIs and SNRIs are appropriate for the treatment of non-paraphilic CSBs in those who are at low risk of legal offense related to CSB symptoms [18, 31, 91].

Pharmacologic Treatment – Hormonal Therapies

For more debilitating or violent CSBs, particularly paraphilic CSBs, the current mainstay of treatment is hormonal therapy, or androgen deprivation therapy (ADT) [18, 31, 91, 93, 95, 96, 100, 104]. There are a few important points to review before discussing the literature supporting the use of ADT in treating CSBs. One, the vast majority of studies on pharmacologic interventions were done on incarcerated patients or patients in court-mandated treatment, which causes selection biases toward more violent or impairing CSBs as well as toward patients who are compelled to stay in treatment. Two, the heavy focus of patients with CSBs in the judicial system seems to be associated with a lack of information on treating patients whose CSBs do not rise to the degree of impairment necessitating legal intervention. The stated goal of many of the studies on this topic uses outcomes that are appropriate for patients in the judicial system (i.e., recidivism) but may not be appropriate for patients who are not in the judicial system (i.e., healthy sexual behaviors). Therefore, the medications that have been deemed "effective" for patients with CSBs in these studies are actually "effective" for a specific population with a specific outcome in mind and may not be applicable to the general population of patients with CSBs. Lastly, the use of ADT was developed in the context of historical precedent which held that CSBs could be significantly decreased by decreasing sex hormone production and activity. In the past, this was accomplished with bilateral orchiectomy or stereotaxic hypothalamotomy (surgical castration) and estrogens (chemical castration). As clinical and legal approaches to CSBs evolved, use of surgical techniques and estrogens fell out of favor due to the invasive and irreversible nature of the former and the significant side-effects associated with both treatments [95, 105]. These treatments were replaced by what the literature now refers to as ADT, which includes the use of synthetic progesterones (medroxyprogesterone acetate [MPA] and cypoterone acetate [CPA]) and gonadotropin-releasing hormone agonists (GnRH agonists) such as leuprolide, triptorelin, and goserelin. This portion of the chapter will focus primarily on modern ADT using synthetic progesterones and GnRH agonists.

Synthetic progesterones are thought to decrease CSB through their effect on sex hormone production. When administered, synthetic progesterones circulate through the body until they reach the pituitary gland, where they decrease luteinizing hormone (LH) and follicular-stimulating hormone (FSH) production. Decreased circulating LH and FSH levels leads to a decrease in serum testosterone and dihydrotestosterone (DHT) levels [96, 106]. Synthetic progesterones are also thought to reduce serum testosterone by increasing its metabolism via hepatic alpha-ring reductase activity as well as increasing its binding to testosterone binding globulin (TeBG) [93, 96, 106]. These two pathways decrease testosterone levels and are the primary mechanism by which synthetic progesterones exert their therapeutic effect in treating CSBs: decreasing libido and sexual function.

Synthetic progesterones are associated with numerous side effects. Use of MPA and CPA can cause bone demineralization and osteoporosis, feminization (decrease in face and body hair), decreased libido, erectile dysfunction, anorgasmia, increased insulin resistance and diabetes mellitus, hypertension, hyperlipidemia and redistribution of body fat, gynecomastia and galactorrhea, testicular atrophy, thromboembolic events, Cushing disease, and depression. CPA in particular has also been associated with transaminitis [106]. Routine evaluation (including physical exam and laboratory tests, detailed later in this section) is a crucial component of treatment with synthetic progesterones as a way to mitigate the risk of these side effects.

The evidence supporting the efficacy of MPA and CPA was detailed extensively in the 2010 WFSBP guidelines on the treatment of paraphilic CSBs. For MPA, there were 13 case reports (including 23 patients) and 13 clinical trials (3 double-blind crossover studies comparing MPA vs. placebo; 9 open-label studies; 1 retrospective study; 334 patients total). These case reports and clinical trials used with oral MPA (with dosing range of 50-300 mg/day) or IM depot MPA (with dosing range 100-900 mg/week) over a wide range of follow-up periods (6 months to 13 years). The patients assessed were all male sex offenders, between the ages of 14 and 75 years old, with CSBs; some of these patients had multiple CSBs and some were also noted to have serious mental illness (e.g., schizophrenia, intellectual disability, major neurocognitive disorder). The outcome measures were varied, including recidivism, self-reports, clinical interviews, FSH/LH/testosterone levels, and penile plethysmography. The guidelines indicated that for those who responded to MPA, the resolution in CSBs and sexual fantasies occurred after 3–4 weeks on the medication. Recidivism dropped in those who responded from 50% recidivism rate to 27%. Three of the studies reported increased recidivism rates after cessation of MPA [93]. One study, Gottesman and Schubert [107], reported that low dose oral MPA (60 mg/day) eliminated CSBs and may be a more appropriate treatment regimen for those with a lower risk of re-offense and an increased risk of side-effects.

For CPA, the 2010 WFSBP guidelines for paraphilia treatment reported that there were 10 case reports (including 15 patients) and 10 clinical trials (including 4 double-blind crossover studies comparing CPA vs. either placebo, ethinyl estradiol, or MPA; 1 single-blind study; 5 open-label studies; 887 patients total). Both oral CPA (with dosing range 50–300 mg/day) and IM depot CPA (with dosing range 275–600 mg every 1–2 weeks) were used. The range of follow-up was also wide, ranging from 4 weeks to 10 years. The patients were predominantly but not entirely male, predominantly but not entirely sex offenders, age range of 19–70 years old. Significant comorbidities, including serious mental illness, were not universally excluded. Outcome measures, like in the studies of MPA, were similarly varied, including recidivism, self-reports, clinical interviews, FSH/LH/testosterone levels, and penile plethysmography. The guidelines reported that for those who responded to CPA, resolution in CSBs and sexual fantasies occurred after 4–12 weeks of treatment. Head-to-head comparisons of CPA to MPA and ethinyl estradiol showed no statistically significant difference in treatment outcomes aside from decreased sexual response to visual stimuli in CPA as compared to ethinyl estradiol. The recidivism rate for those on CPA was noted to be 6%, as compared to 85% prior to treatment. A significant number of patients re-offended once CPA was discontinued [93]. CPA was noted to not have much effect on LH and FSH levels but was associated with a moderate decrease in serum testosterone [91].

The listed contraindications for MPA included: lack of consent, puberty prior to bone growth completion, adrenal disease, pregnancy and breastfeeding, severe hypertension, history of thromboembolic disease, breast or uterine diseases, diabetes mellitus, severe depression, MPA allergy, and active pituitary disease [93]. The listed contraindications for CPA included: lack of consent, puberty prior to bone growth completion, hepatocellular disease, liver carcinoma, diabetes mellitus, severe hypertension, carcinoma except prostate carcinoma, pregnancy or breastfeeding, history of thromboembolic disease, cardiac disease, adrenal disease, severe depressive or psychotic disorders, tuberculosis, cachexia, epilepsy, CPA allergy, sickle cell disease or trait, and pituitary disease [93].

The WFSBP guidelines reported that there was moderate level evidence for MPA and CPA in the treatment of CSBs. It highlighted the risk of serious side effects with both medications, in particular noting that the risk of side-effects in MPA was so significant that the WFSBP could not recommend its use in treating CSBs. Although CPA had issues with adherence, the WFSBP did not recommend against the use of CPA in CSBs [93].

The most recent addition to the pharmacologic arsenal in the treatment of CSBs is GnRH agonists (leuprolide, triptorelin, goserelin). These medications work by activating GnRH receptors in the pituitary, which transiently increase LH production and release. This leads to an initial testosterone flare, followed by a rapid decrease in LH and testosterone as the pituitary neurons become desensitized to GnRH [91, 93, 96]. Although this decreases total testosterone levels, the production of adrenal androgens is not impeded by GnRH analogs. There is an additional theoretical neuromodulatory effect mediated by GnRH-sensitive pituitary neurons which project to the amygdala, leading to a decrease in sexual aggression [93]. Each of these in combination is thought to contribute to the anti-libidinal effect of GnRH agonists in the treatment of CSBs.

There is significant overlap in the side effect profiles of synthetic progesterones and GnRH agonists due to their shared anti-androgenic activity. GnRH agonists are associated with increased bone demineralization and osteoporosis, feminization, decreased libido, erectile dysfunction, anorgasmia, testicular atrophy, gynecomastia and galactorrhea, thromboembolic events, weight gain, changes in blood pressure, and depression [91, 93, 96]. They are also associated with muscle tenderness, nausea, and irritation at the site of injection [93]. As with synthetic progesterones, initial and ongoing evaluation including physical examination and laboratory tests should accompany treatment with GnRH analogs to monitor for and treat these side effects [91, 93, 96].

The 2010 WFSBP guidelines reported on the evidence examining the use of GnRH agonists. In total, there were 13 case reports (including 28 patients; 1 patient on triptorelin, 6 patients on goserelin, and 21 patients on leuprolide) and 7 clinical trials (including 5 open-label or non-randomized trials and 2 retrospective studies; 157 total patients, 75 patients on triptorelin, 3 patients on goserelin, and 39 patients on leuprolide, the remaining patients received control interventions). Dosing ranges were as follows: triptorelin 3.75 mg/month IM, goserelin with unknown doses administered IM, and leuprolide 3.75–7.5 mg/month IM or 11.25 mg/3 months IM. In some studies, CPA or flutamide were co-administered with assessed GnRH agonist in the initial weeks of treatment to counteract the testosterone flare. In most studies, psychotherapy was also offered in addition to pharmacotherapy. The range of follow-up was 6 months to 10 years, with a mean follow-up time of 1 year. The patients were universally male sex offenders (although one study with $N = 5$ excluded prisoners) with paraphilic CSBs ranging in age from 15 to 61 years old. Serious mental illness was not an exclusion criterion for these studies; some patients had multiple paraphilic disorders. Outcome measures varied significantly between studies but included recidivism, self-reports, testosterone levels, and penile plethysmography. The WFSBP guidelines reported that there were significant response rates across outcome measures for all of the GnRH agonists in those who were adherent with therapy. Across all studies and case reports, there were only 2 cases of patients who re-offended while on GnRH agonists. A significant number of patients who had initially responded to GnRH therapy and subsequently discontinued the medication (either as part of non-adherence or under provider supervision due to side effects) had resurgence of sexual fantasies and urges and in some cases ended up re-offending. Those who re-initiated GnRH agonist therapy after developing resurgence of sexual fantasies and urges again achieved resolution of said sexual fantasies and urges [93]. A literature review from 2018 [100] reported on case studies and clinical trials published since 2004 examining GnRH agonists in treatment of paraphilic CSBs. Amongst the papers included in this review, there were 136 patients who took leuprolide, 16 patients who took triptorelin, 5 patients who took goserelin, and 121 patients who took an unspecified GnRH agonist. The studies that were examined did not use consistent outcome measures (varied from testosterone and LH levels to fMRI activation to recidivism to self-reports, etc.). The results across most outcome measures were positive, although there were some case reports in which patients did not respond to treatment. Most studies did not include information on side effects, but the ones that did report comparable side effects as those listed above [100]. Additionally, one study from Canada showed that treatment with leuprolide and CBT had significant lower rates of recidivism at 5-year follow-up than CBT alone [108].

The listed contraindications for GnRH agonists included: lack of consent, puberty prior to bone growth completion, severe hypertension, pregnancy or breastfeeding, severe cardiac or renal disease, severe osteoporosis, history of pathologic fractures, severe depressive disorder, GnRH agonists allergy, and active pituitary disease [93].

The 2010 WFSBP guidelines concluded that there was moderate level evidence reporting on the use of GnRH agonists in paraphilic CSBs. Although the evidence was scant and confounded by selection biases, the reported efficacy of the GnRH agonists was good. Even more notable is that the GnRH agonists lead to resolution of symptoms even in those who failed other interventions including psychotherapy, psychopharmacologic agents, and synthetic progesterones.

The guidelines recommended diligent assessment and ongoing evaluation while on GnRH agonists due to the severity of the side effects.

The use of anti-androgenic therapy in treatment of CSBs generally and paraphilic disorders specifically requires more robust investigation. Although these medications come with increased risk of serious side effects, the lack of equally efficacious interventions preclude their removal from treatment consideration. Furthermore, the legal and ethical ramifications of non-treatment are dire enough that use of these medications in spite of the side effect risk is warranted in more severe cases of CSB.

Non-Pharmacologic Treatment – Psychological Interventions

Despite the limited research on psychological interventions in CSBs, the general consensus in the literature is that psychotherapy should be integrated into any treatment offered [18, 28, 93–96]. The reasons for this are multifold. Providers experienced in treating CSBs by and large conceptualize CSBs as part of an addictive process, for which psychotherapeutic techniques are crucial for dealing with urges/cravings, improving distress tolerance, and encouraging healthy goal-oriented behaviors [10, 18, 28, 93, 95]. Additionally, the stresses experienced by patients with CSBs extend across multiple spheres of daily living. There are interpersonal, familial, social, romantic, professional, legal, and ethical dimensions to the behaviors with which patients struggle; helping patients feel like they have support in addressing their symptoms may help to bolster their success in treatment [18, 28, 93, 95]. Finally, as previously discussed, CSBs are associated with significant psychiatric comorbidity, some of which may also respond to psychotherapy [18, 28, 93, 95].

Although numerous psychotherapeutic modalities have been assessed, only cognitive behavioral therapy (CBT) has been shown to have positive effect on CSB symptoms [18, 28, 93, 94]. In a 2005 meta-analysis of multiple treatment modalities for paraphilic CSBs (including 22,000 total patients across 80 independent comparison studies), Lösel and Schmucker [94] showed that behavioral therapy and CBT both had a moderate and statistically significant improvement in CSB symptoms (OR = 1.45 for both modalities). However, the main outcome measure used in assessing treatment efficacy for this meta-analysis was recidivism; commentary on other potential treatment outcomes was not included.

In studies examining the efficacy of CBT or behavioral therapy, specific guidelines regarding techniques or timelines are not laid out in detail. Discussions of general goals and treatment concepts have been included in some literature reviews [28, 95]. Cognitive components of CBT therapy are thought to include challenging cognitive distortions that reinforce the CSB (e.g., that victims of sexual assault enjoy the experience of being sexually assaulted, or that hypersexuality is a healthy expression of "normal" human sexual needs) [28, 95]. Behavior-focused psychotherapeutic techniques may include covert sensitization (i.e., repeated imaginal consequences of CSB such as imprisonment, humiliation, vomiting, etc.), masturbatory satiation as a way to regulate arousal patterns in a healthier way, and relapse prevention strategies to use when confronted with triggers [95]. CBT may also entail aspects of sex therapy to help the patient reintegrate healthy and appropriate sexual behaviors into their daily life as a replacement for more destructive CSBs [28]. Finally, CBT therapy should also help the patient build their sense of self-esteem and ability to create and maintain healthy patterns of daily living [28]. In combination, these strategies may facilitate both greater engagement in treatment, which is associated with decreased recidivism risk in and of itself, as well as help to treat the underlying psychological and biological processes that contribute to the CSBs.

It should also be noted that there has been research on community-based support groups as a form of psychological treatment. Although the literature has shown some benefit with this treatment modality [28, 93, 95], the variation in quality, dynamics, and philosophy of each group makes standardization difficult. Additionally, much like pharmacological interventions, some of the literature on this modality was assessed in the context of incarceration and/or court-mandated treatment, which confounds the selection process as well as treatment adherence. These groups generally follow a 12-step format in which recovery is viewed as a spiritual experience [95]. Some of these groups include Sex Addicts Anonymous, Sexaholics Anonymous, and Sex Anonymous [28]. The strictness with which individual groups view abstinence from any sexual behaviors during recovery varies considerably [95].

Overall, the use of psychological interventions is a foundational aspect of the treatment of CSBs, regardless of severity [28, 93, 96]. Regardless of other benefits that may be gleaned from engagement in psychotherapy, the improvement in recidivism risk from psychological intervention is significant enough to warrant its recommendation to patients seeking care [109].

Non-Pharmacologic Treatments – Surgical Interventions

Historically, the ethical and legal justifications for surgical intervention in the case of CSBs were debatable at best. Oftentimes, prior to the first reported case of surgical castration used for a therapeutic purpose in 1892, castration was used as a punishment or form of social control by government entities around the world for centuries [105]. Even after it became more mainstream in its therapeutic use in the Western world, the procedures used to surgically castrate people were often performed on the incarcerated as part of a legally ordered punishment for crimes of a sexual nature [105, 110]. Surgical castration often had both punitive and eugenic purposes, and it was frequently performed without the consent of those who underwent the procedure [105, 111]. Surgical treatment of CSBs remained widely in use across Europe and the United States until the 1970s, at which point it fell drastically out of favor; now only a handful of countries including Germany, the Czech Republic, and the United States offer the intervention and even then with significant limitations and safeguards [91, 105, 112].

There have been two primary surgical techniques used to treat CSBs. The first and less commonly used was stereotaxic hypothalamotomy, which entailed using an electrode to ablate the ventromedial hypothalamus unilaterally. This procedure was used throughout the mid-twentieth century as treatment for sexual aggression and deviancy, often as part of a legal punishment. The evidence from this time is sparse and consisted almost entirely of case reports with poor follow-up [105, 111, 113]. This procedure fell out of favor with other forms of psychosurgery in the 1970s due to the significant risks of neurosurgery, the irreversible side effects often associated with such procedures, and the serious ethical concerns voiced by medical providers at the time [105, 111]. The second technique, which is still used today, is bilateral orchiectomy, or removal of the testes. The use of this procedure for therapeutic reasons in areas other than Europe and North America remains unclear due to a dearth of literature on the subject. Most research on its use is from case reports. The recidivism rate is low, reportedly between 2% and 5% [91]. The side effects of the procedure include risks of bleeding and infection as a result of the procedure, decreased libido, anorgasmia, erectile dysfunction, sterility, feminization, weight gain, osteoporosis, and hot flashes. Additionally, the use of exogenous testosterone can reverse the anti-libidinal effect of the procedure, facilitating re-offense [91, 110]. Of the literature reviews that do exist, conclusions are varied, with some advocating for broader therapeutic use and other expressing concerns that medical and ethical risks of the procedure outweigh any potential benefits that it may offer [91, 105, 110, 113, 114].

Variations in Treatment Around the World

Europe

Europe (which for this book also includes Russia) has some of the most robust literature on the treatment of CSB. A significant number of prospective and even double-blinded and/or randomized trials were performed in European populations [18, 91, 93, 95, 96, 100]. Many of these studies have been referenced in the discussions of various treatment modalities earlier in this chapter. Given that the literature from this region is the strongest of any other, the formal treatment protocol provided at the end of this chapter will mirror the recommendations from this region and from North America.

In 2017, Turner et al. [100] summarized the prevalence in the use of various pharmacologic treatment modalities in this region as determined by a survey of forensic providers across Europe, Canada, and the United States. In Western Europe, SSRIs were listed as the most common treatment, with synthetic progesterones, GnRH agonists, and antipsychotics all used with similar frequency but less than SSRIs. In Eastern Europe, antipsychotics and synthetic progesterones were both used most commonly and with similar frequency; SSRIs and GnRH agonists were used with similar frequency but less commonly than antipsychotics and synthetic progesterones. As of 2017, voluntary ADT use is legally permitted in Austria, Belgium, the Czech Republic, Denmark, Estonia, Finland, France, Germany, Hungary, Iceland, Italy, Latvia, Macedonia, Moldova, the Netherlands, Norway, Poland, Spain, Switzerland, Sweden, and the UK. Court-mandated ADT use is permitted in Russia.

The WFSBP treatment guidelines for paraphilic CSBs were written by a group of leading experts on CSBs based on the literature that was available as of 2010 [93]. As per these guidelines, all those who are presenting with paraphilic CSBs should be offered psychotherapy, preferably CBT and/or relapse-prevention therapy. Those at lower risk of re-offense and/or with co-morbid depression, anxiety, or OCD should be offered a serotonergic agent such as an SSRI or SNRI. Those with co-morbid bipolar disorder should be placed on a mood stabilizer as clinically indicated and those with a co-morbid psychotic disorder should be placed on an antipsychotic. Stimulants can be considered in those with co-morbid ADHD or if otherwise clinically indicated. If the patient is at an elevated risk of re-offense and is developmentally an adult, they should be offered ADT, preferably with a GnRH agonist or a synthetic progesterone. Long-acting injectable formulations should be considered in those who struggle with adherence to treatment. Initial work-up and ongoing evaluation should be completed as previously discussed.

North America

As with Europe, North America also has a significant foundation of literature on treatment of CSBs, particularly out of the United States and Canada [18, 91, 93, 95, 96, 100]. The evidence and recommendations from this literature are in line with the WFSBP treatment guidelines for paraphilic CSBs, discussed in the section above.

In the survey of pharmacologic treatment modality prevalence by Turner et al. [100], North America (which in this case consisted of forensic providers in the United States and Canada) used SSRIs with the greatest frequency of any pharmacologic intervention. Synthetic progesterones and GnRH agonists were used with equal frequency but with less overall use than the SSRIs. Antipsychotics were used least frequently for the treatment of paraphilic CSBs. Of note, in the United States, the only states that have a legal precedent for using ADT in the treatment of CSBs are California, Florida, Georgia, Iowa, Louisiana, Montana, Oregon, and Wisconsin [91, 100, 110]. The requirements for use in treatment vary significantly state-to-state. For example, in Georgia ADT must be voluntary while in Louisiana those who have committed a second sexual offense against a minor must undergo ADT [91]. In Texas, there is no legal precedent for the use of ADT; however, Texas is the only state in the United States where bilateral orchiectomy may be a court-mandated treatment for those with paraphilic CSBs who commit a sex crime [91].

In Central America and the Caribbean, there is very little literature on the treatment of CSBs. The only available evidence seems to be case reports. One such case report out of Mexico written in 2010 seems to conflate homosexuality and an unspecified paraphilic disorder, but reports that the patient's distress and symptoms responded to psychotherapy [115]. There are no set guidelines for this region of North America.

South America

South America does not seem to have much literature on region-specific treatment of CSBs. The only papers from the region on treatment are case reports from Brazil and treatment in these cases was selected based on theoretical neurobiological mechanisms for CSBs. There are no region-specific treatment guidelines [116]. Brazil seems to have a system for treating those who have committed sex crimes but the information on this in the literature is scant. One study listed the portion of the population in treatment for CSBs as 75% incarcerated with the other 25% in outpatient clinics; however, they add the caveat that some of those in the outpatient setting are currently facing legal action as a result of their CSB [117, 118].

Africa

Africa has no region-specific treatment guidelines. There has been research in South Africa on treatment for paraphilic CSBs, but the guidelines seem to hew closely to WFSBP treatment guidelines (e.g., recommending use of SSRIs if there are concerns about side effects of ADT, and using ADT if there are concerns about an elevated risk of recidivism) [119].

Asia

In Asia, the literature on region-specific treatment is generally sparse. Most countries do not have published research on CSBs, and those that do generally have information that comes from literature reviews, retrospective studies, and case reports.

Israel published a forensic review on pharmacologic treatment recommendations for patients with CSBs who have been convicted of sexual offenses [120]. The paper outlines that patients who committed offenses that did not involve physical contact with the victim are generally offered SSRIs while those who committed more serious offense are given GnRH agonists or CPA.

Turkey's legal system has psychiatric experts provide court-mandated treatment recommendations as part of their sentencing process, but these experts are not required to use any specific treatment guidelines as part of their decision-making [121]. There are also isolated case reports for those not involved in the legal system, such as one report discussing an adolescent with autism spectrum disorder and fetishism who was successfully treated with mirtazapine [122]. Otherwise, there does not seem to be any region-specific treatment guidelines that providers adhere to in Turkey when determining which interventions to use for patients with CSBs.

India similarly has case reports detailing various treatments of paraphilias, including with naltrexone and fluoxetine [123, 124]. Rationale for the treatment decisions made in these case reports seems consistent with the WFSBP guidelines and does not seem to be region-specific.

South Korea uses ADT as part of court-mandated treatment for paraphilic CSBs, but there is no mention of specific guidelines that are used in this kind of decision-making [125].

There is a single case report out of Japan on successful treatment of paraphilic CSB using carbamazepine and behavioral therapy, but again, no specific treatment guidelines were discussed in relation to this case [126].

Taiwan has numerous case reports on the treatment of CSBs, including those with comorbidity. One case report detailed an adolescent with paraphilic CSBs and ADHD who responded to long-acting methylphenidate [127]. Another adolescent with paraphilia responded to CBT and supportive and psychodynamic psychotherapies, but there was no long-term follow-up for this patient [128]. Additionally, there was a case report of a young man with paraphilia who did not respond to psychological interventions until he was titrated to topiramate 200 mg daily, at which point his symptoms decreased in intensity and severity [129].

Oceania

Research into treatment of CSBs in Oceania comes heavily from Australia, which adheres to WFSBP guidelines. Interestingly, there seems to be a body of research from Australia into the treatment of adolescents with CSBs who are involved in the legal system. Treatment guidelines for this population recommend multisystemic therapy (MST, psychotherapy that incorporates individual, group, school-based, and family therapies) [98]. SSRIs are recommended if MST alone does not lead to resolution of symptoms; however, adolescent patients on SSRIs should be closely monitored for suicidality given the increased incidence in suicidal ideation in those under 24 years old on SSRIs [98]. The research also recommends against GnRH agonists or synthetic progesterones unless the patient has significant risk of re-offense and confirmation of Tanner Stage V development and epiphyseal closure on long bone X-rays [98].

Treatment Protocol

The protocol provided below synthesizes recommendations provided in various literature reviews and meta-analyses, including the 2010 WFSBP treatment guidelines [18, 91, 93, 95, 96, 100, 104]. These recommendations were made specifically for treatment of paraphilic CSBs. However, given the dearth of evidence-based recommendations on treatment of CSBs, this protocol may also be helpful in informing treatment recommendations for those with non-paraphilic CSBs.

When a patient initially presents with a complaint suggestive of CSB, it is important to fully characterize the nature, duration, frequency, and severity of the behavior. Additionally, the patient should be asked to characterize the level of distress and impairment caused by the symptoms. A complete psychiatric and medical history should be obtained, with particular attention paid to associated psychiatric or somatic symptoms, substance use, developmental history, and family history [91, 93, 95, 96].

The provider should also obtain and review all relevant and available collateral to bolster diagnostic evidence and social supports for the patient. This should include a full assessment of risk of re-offense, which will help to guide treatment decisions further on in the process. The most concerning risk factors for recidivism are multiple victims, male victims, multiple paraphilias, deviant sexual interests (i.e., pedophilia), use of force, young age of onset, previous sexual offense, central nervous system dysfunction or history of brain injury, history of psychiatric illness including impulsive disorders or antisocial personality, and history of treatment failure [93].

Once you have this information, the patient should undergo a complete physical examination and basic lab work should be obtained to rule out any potential reversible and/or medical causes of CSB, as detailed in the sub-section above on Work-Up for CSBs. If the work-up is unremarkable, the patient should be informed of all the treatment options available to them and the goals of treatment should be reviewed [91, 93, 95, 96]. This section is crucial to obtaining consent for the treatment and will vary considerably depending on the context in which the patient is presenting for care (i.e., in the outpatient setting, in the inpatient setting, while incarcerated, pending trial, etc.).

Any patient, regardless of presentation, should be offered at a minimum CBT and relapse prevention therapy if it is available. Psychological interventions like CBT have consistent evidence of improving symptoms and decreasing recidivism, are generally low cost, and have less risk of concerning side-effects than pharmacologic or surgical interventions [91, 93, 95, 96].

Patients who are adolescents who are not responding to psychotherapy alone, are at lower risk of re-offense, or have co-morbid depression, anxiety, or OCD symptoms should be offered an SSRI as an initial pharmacologic agent. The medication should be given a full trial of at least 6–8 weeks at the lowest effective therapeutic dose. Other psychiatric co-morbidities should be treated as clinically appropriate (i.e., mood stabilizers for bipolar disorder, antipsychotics for psychotic disorders, stimulants for ADHD, etc.) [91, 93, 95, 96].

Patients who are adults at higher risk of re-offense or who have failed treatment with psychotherapy and SSRI should be offered ADT. The preferred initial agent should be a GnRH agonist, although in the absence of GnRH agonists, synthetic progesterones may also be beneficial. If you anticipate starting a patient on one of these medications, informed consent must be obtained and additional evaluation and laboratory testing should be pursued. This includes history of thromboembolic and osteoporosis risk factors, family history of hyperlipidemia and diabetes mellitus, BMI and body circumference measurements, calcium and phosphorus levels, lipid panel and fasting blood glucose, ECG, and (if concern for osteopenia/osteoporosis) a DEXA scan. If this additional work-up is within normal limits or if the benefits of treatment sufficiently outweigh the risks, then treatment with a GnRH agonist or a synthetic progesterone may be initiated [91, 93, 95, 96].

If the patient is at significantly elevated risk of re-offending and they have failed all other interventions, and if the governing body has a legal statute permitting its use, surgical intervention with bilateral orchiectomy may be considered [91, 93]. However, this treatment should be considered a last resort in the face of complete treatment failure, given its irreversibility and significant side-effects. Rules on consent for this procedure vary depending on the governing body, but if incarcerated patients are legally permitted to elect to obtain this procedure, careful and thorough review of indications, alternatives, risk and benefits should be performed [91, 93].

Prognosis

CSB typically starts in adolescence, with paraphilic behaviors beginning earlier than nonparaphilic behaviors [30, 61]. Young adults are more likely to develop more serious behaviors [130]. The behavior can be chronic or episodic [32], can start with abnormally high rates of masturbation or pornography use [131], and is progressive without treatment [132, 133]. Due to lack of consensus regarding definition, diagnostic criteria, stigma, and lack of awareness, there is limited data on the illness itself and therefore limited data about the economic and medical costs of untreated illness. Furthermore, due to the uncertain nature of diagnostic criteria, therapists have been reluctant to diagnose patients with significant behavioral indicators [79].

Many researchers have found high rates of distress or psychological impairment [4, 31, 134] as well as impairment in family relationships, occupational functioning, and other areas of life [30, 32, 135] in those meeting criteria for CSB. Those meeting criteria for CSB have many problems that affect quality of life [130], such as risky sexual behavior that results in higher rates of sexually transmitted diseases such as HIV [51, 136, 137]. High comorbidity with psychiatric illness as well as chronic medical conditions such as HIV and unwanted pregnancy, suggest high cost of lost productivity in the economy as well as cost of treatment for comorbid conditions. This cost may be especially high in areas where condoms are less available, HIV is more prevalent, and there is lower access to care, such as in low-resource settings.

Although it is too early to determine the most efficacious therapeutic intervention, it does appear treatment for CSBs is more effective across outcome measure than no treatment at all [91, 94, 95]. This highlights the importance for further definitional taxonomy clarity to guide diagnosis and treatment, as there is currently an unquantifiable and likely modifiable economic burden due to problematic compulsive sexual behaviors.

Conclusions and Future Directions

Problematic sexual behavior has been hypothesized and reported by physicians and psychologists for decades, leading to debate about the merits of using diagnostic criteria. Recently ICD issued diagnostic criteria for Compulsive Sexual Behavior Disorder, but a similar diagnosis was left out of the DSM-5 due to lack of empiric evidence supporting a unique diagnostic entity [8]. The lack of consensus is due to remaining ambiguity of the best conceptualization of compulsive sexual behavior, lack of a common nomenclature across researchers, the difficulty of ensuring symptoms are not caused by other conditions, and the difficulty of defining aberrant levels of sexual behavior. This combined with the stigmatization [30] and poor societal awareness [31] produce barriers to care and make acquiring data for diagnosis and treatment difficult. Non-paraphilic compulsive behaviors such as excessive masturbation, preoccupation with pornography, and ego-dystonic promiscuity causing frequent casual sex or multiple extramarital affairs are the most common manifestations of CSB [31].

From the limited data that is available, there may be up to 6–10% prevalence of non-paraphilic CSBs in the general population [46, 49, 50] with a male predominance [46, 49, 50]. There is also a high rate of comorbid medical and psychiatric conditions that must be identified and addressed to prevent conflation of compulsive sexual behavior due to another psychiatric or underlying medical or iatrogenic condition [11, 25, 51, 71].

Regarding therapeutic interventions, treatment has been shown to be more effective than no treatment [91, 94, 95]. Both pharmacological and nonpharmacological treatments have shown promise, but more studies need to be performed in order to verify their efficacy. SSRIs, SNRIs, and TCAs have shown modest benefits in treating non-paraphilic and paraphilic CSBs and are appropriate treatment for mild CSBs and low risk of reoffending [18, 31, 91, 93]. Although case reports and small trials have yielded some benefit for non-serotonergic psychotropic medications [91, 93, 95, 96, 100–103], the WFSBP guidelines reported that there was no evidence for non-serotonergic medications except to treat comorbid conditions with regards to paraphilic CSBs [91, 93, 95, 100].

For more debilitating or violent CSBs, particularly paraphilic CSBs, GnRH agonists have moderate level evidence according to the 2010 WFSBP guidelines, particularly with respect to persons with prior treatment failures. However, due to the severity of side effects with these medications, the guidelines recommended diligent ongoing evaluation [93].

The general consensus is that psychotherapy should be integrated into any treatment offered providing techniques that are crucial for dealing with urges/cravings, improving distress tolerance, encouraging healthy goal-oriented behaviors, and for treatment of comorbid or underlying psychiatric disorders [10, 18, 28, 93, 95].

Compulsive sexual behavior is progressive without treatment [132, 133]. There is little known about prognosis, but given the abundance of psychiatric and medical comorbidities [11, 25, 51, 71], one could speculate that the economic burden in lost productivity is high.

While there is increasing data in this field, there is still a paucity of information to help tailor definitional taxonomy for diagnosis and treatment. More research into the neurobiological underpinnings of compulsive sexual behavior would greatly help to determine the pathology of the disorder and help with defining diagnostic criteria. Once diagnostic criteria are established, large-scale epidemiology and treatment intervention studies can be conducted to further characterize these problematic behaviors to reduce psychological distress, increase quality of life, and reduce economic burden.

Bibliography

1. Ellis A, Sagarin E. Nymphomania. A study of the oversexed woman. New York: McFadden-Bartell Corporation; 1965.
2. Stoller RF. Perversion: the erotic form of hatred. 1st ed. New York: Pantheon Books; 1975.
3. Allen C. A textbook of psychosexual disorders. London: Oxford University Press; 1969.
4. Walton MT, Cantor JM, Lykins AD. An online assessment of personality, psychological, and sexuality trait variables associated with self-reported hypersexual behavior. Arch Sex Behav. 2017; https://doi.org/10.1007/s10508-015-0606-1.
5. American Psychiatric Association. DSM-III: diagnostic and statistical manual of mental disorders. Am Psychiatr Assoc. 1980; https://doi.org/10.1017/CBO9781107415324.004.
6. American Psychiatric Association. Diagnostic and statistical manual of mental disorders (3rd ed. revised) (DSM-III-R). Diagnostic Stat Man Ment Disord (3rd ed revised). 1987. https://doi.org/10.1176/ajp.145.10.1300.
7. Kafka MP. Hypersexual disorder: a proposed diagnosis for DSM-V. Arch Sex Behav. 2010;39:377–400.
8. Reid RC, Kafka MP. Controversies about hypersexual disorder and the DSM-5. Curr Sex Heal Rep. 2014;6:259–64.
9. Kraus SW, Krueger RB, Briken P, et al. Compulsive sexual behaviour disorder in the ICD-11. World Psychiatry. 2018;17:109–10.

10. Sadock B, Sadock V, Ruiz P. Kaplan & Sadock's comprehensive textbook of psychiatry. 10th ed. Philadelphia: Wolters Kluwer; 2017.
11. Weintraub D, Koester J, Potenza MN, Siderowf AD, Stacy M, Voon V, Whetteckey J, Wunderlich GR, Lang AE. Impulse control disorders in Parkinson disease: a cross-sectional study of 3090 patients. Arch Neurol. 2010;67:589–95.
12. American Psychiatric Association. DSM 5 diagnostic and statistical manual of mental disorders. Am Psychiatr Assoc. 2013; https://doi.org/10.1176/appi.books.9780890425596.744053.
13. Moser C. Hypersexual disorder: searching for clarity. J Treat Prev. 2013;20:48–58.
14. Långström N, Hanson RK. High rates of sexual behavior in the general population: correlates and predictors. Arch Sex Behav. 2006;35:37–52.
15. Grubbs JB, Exline JJ, Pargament KI, Hook JN, Carlisle RD. Transgression as addiction: religiosity and moral disapproval as predictors of perceived addiction to pornography. Arch Sex Behav. 2015;44:125–36.
16. Montgomery-Graham S. Conceptualization and assessment of hypersexual disorder: a systematic review of the literature. Sex Med Rev. 2017;5:146–62.
17. Goodman A. What's in a name? Terminology for designating a syndrome of driven sexual behavior. Sex Addict Compulsivity. 2001;8:191–213.
18. Garcia FD, Thibaut F. Sexual addictions. Am J Drug Alcohol Abuse. 2010;36:254–60.
19. Voon V, Mole TB, Banca P, et al. Neural correlates of sexual cue reactivity in individuals with and without compulsive sexual behaviours. PLoS One. 2014;9:e102419.
20. Reid RC, Berlin HA, Kingston DA. Sexual impulsivity in hypersexual men. Curr Behav Neurosci Rep. 2015;2:1–8.
21. Zapf JL, Greiner J, Carroll J. Attachment styles and male sex addiction. Sex Addict Compulsivity. 2008;15:158–75.
22. Mulhauser KRW, Struthers WM, Hook JN, Pyykkonen BA, Womack SD, MacDonald M. Performance on the Iowa gambling task in a sample of hypersexual men. Sex Addict Compulsivity. 2014;21:170–83.
23. Kingston DA, Firestone P. Problematic hypersexuality: a review of conceptualization and diagnosis. Sex Addict Compulsivity. 2008;15:284–310.
24. Kraus SW, Voon V, Potenza MN. Should compulsive sexual behavior be considered an addiction? Addiction. 2016;111:2097–106.
25. Kafka MP, Hennen J. A DSM-IV Axis I comorbidity study of males (n = 120) with paraphilias and paraphilia-related disorders. Sex Abus. 2002;14:349–66.
26. Kafka MP, Hennen J. The paraphilia-related disorders: an empirical investigation of nonparaphilic hypersexuality disorders in outpatient males. J Sex Marital Ther. 1999;25:305–19.
27. Delmonico DL, Carnes PJ. Virtual sex addiction: when cybersex becomes the drug of choice. Cyberpsychol Behav. 1999;2:457–63.
28. Rosenberg KP, Carnes P, O'Connor S. Evaluation and treatment of sex addiction. J Sex Marital Ther. 2014;40:77–91.
29. Womack SD, Hook JN, Ramos M, Davis DE, Penberthy JK. Measuring hypersexual behavior. Sex Addict Compulsivity. 2013; https://doi.org/10.1080/10720162.2013.768126.
30. Black DW, Kehrberg LL, Flumerfelt DL, Schlosser SS. Characteristics of 36 subjects reporting compulsive sexual behavior. Am J Psychiatry. 1997;154:243–9.
31. Derbyshire KL, Grant JE. Compulsive sexual behavior: a review of the literature. J Behav Addict. 2015;4:37–43.
32. Kuzma JM, Black DW. Epidemiology, prevalence, and natural history of compulsive sexual behavior. Psychiatr Clin North Am. 2008;31:603–11.
33. Kinsey AC, Pomeroy WB, Martin CE. Sexual behavior in the human male. Philadelphia: W. B. Saunders Company; 1948.
34. Atwood JD, Gagnon J. Masturbatory behavior in college youth. J Sex Educ Ther. 1987;13:35–42.
35. Laumann EO. The social organization of sexuality: sexual practices in the United States. Chicago: University of Chicago Press; 2000.
36. Kafka MP. Hypersexual desire in males: an operational definition and clinical implications for males with paraphilias and paraphilia-related disorders. Arch Sex Behav. 1997;26:505–26.
37. Black DW. Compulsive sexual behavior: a review. J Psychiatr Pract. 1998;4:219–29.
38. Kraus SW, Martino S, Potenza MN. Clinical characteristics of men interested in seeking treatment for use of pornography. J Behav Addict. 2016;5:169–78.
39. Reid RC, Carpenter BN, Hook JN, Garos S, Manning JC, Gilliland R, Cooper EB, McKittrick H, Davtian M, Fong T. Report of findings in a DSM-5 field trial for hypersexual disorder. J Sex Med. 2012;9:2868–77.
40. Parsons JT, Rendina HJ, Ventuneac A, Cook KF, Grov C, Mustanski B. A psychometric investigation of the Hypersexual Disorder Screening Inventory among highly sexually active gay and bisexual men: an item response theory analysis. https://doi.org/10.1111/jsm.12117.
41. Öberg KG, Hallberg J, Kaldo V, Dhejne C, Arver S. Hypersexual disorder according to the hypersexual disorder screening inventory in help-seeking Swedish men and women with self-identified hypersexual behavior. Sex Med. 2017;5:e229–36.
42. Scanavino M de T, Ventuneac A, Rendina HJ, et al. Sexual compulsivity scale, compulsive sexual behavior inventory, and hypersexual disorder screening inventory: translation, adaptation, and validation for use in Brazil. Arch Sex Behav. 2016;45:207–217.
43. Stein DJ, Lund C, Nesse RM. Classification systems in psychiatry: diagnosis and global mental health in

the era of DSM-5 and ICD-11. Curr Opin Psychiatry. 2013;26:493–7.
44. World Health Organization. ICD-11 beta draft. World Heal Organ. 2018; https://doi.org/10.1002/2013GL058769.
45. Coleman E, Miner M, Ohlerking F, Raymond N. Compulsive sexual behavior inventory: a preliminary study of reliability and validity. J Sex Marital Ther. 2001;27:325–32.
46. Dickenson JA, Gleason N, Coleman E, Miner MH. Prevalence of distress associated with difficulty controlling sexual urges, feelings, and behaviors in the United States. JAMA Netw Open. 2018;1:1–10.
47. Miner MH, Raymond N, Coleman E, Swinburne Romine R. Investigating clinically and scientifically useful cut points on the compulsive sexual behavior inventory. J Sex Med. 2017;14:715–20.
48. Hook JN, Hook JP, Davis DE, Worthington EL, Penberthy JK. Measuring sexual addiction and compulsivity: a critical review of instruments. J Sex Marital Ther. 2010;36:227–60.
49. Black DW. The epidemiology and phenomenology of compulsive sexual behavior. CNS Spectr. 2000;5:26–35,72.
50. Coleman E. Is your patient suffering from compulsive sexual behavior? Psychiatr Ann. 1992;22:320–5.
51. Raymond NC, Coleman E, Miner MH. Psychiatric comorbidity and compulsive/impulsive traits in compulsive sexual behavior. Compr Psychiatry. 2003;44:370–80.
52. Leitenberg H, Henning K. Sexual fantasy. Psychol Bull. 1995;117:469–96.
53. Oliver MB, Hyde JS. Gender differences in sexuality: a meta-analysis. Psychol Bull. 1993;114:29–51.
54. Petersen JL, Hyde JS. A meta-analytic review of research on gender differences in sexuality, 1993–2007. Psychol Bull. 2010;136:21–38.
55. Grant JE, Williams KA, Potenza MN. Impulse-control disorders in adolescent psychiatric inpatients: co-occurring disorders and sex differences. J Clin Psychiatry. 2007;68:1584–92.
56. Bancroft J, Vukadinovic Z. Sexual addiction, sexual compulsivity, sexual impulsivity, or what? Toward a theoretical model. J Sex Res. 2004;41:225–34.
57. Grant JE, Potenza MN. Sexual orientation of men with pathological gambling: prevalence and psychiatric comorbidity in a treatment-seeking sample. Compr Psychiatry. 2006;47:515–8.
58. Schneider JP, Schneider BH. Couple recovery from sexual addiction/coaddiction: results of a survey of 88 marriages. Sex Addict Compulsivity. 1996;3:111–26.
59. Kaplan MS, Krueger RB. Diagnosis, assessment, and treatment of hypersexuality. J Sex Res. 2010;47:181–98.
60. Kafka MP, Prentky RA. Compulsive sexual behavior characteristics. Am J Psychiatry. 2006;154:1632.
61. Kafka MP, Prentky R. A comparative study of non-paraphilic sexual addictions and paraphilias in men. J Clin Psychiatry. 1992;53:345–50.
62. Coleman E, Raymond N, McBean A. Assessment and treatment of compulsive sexual behavior. Minn Med. 2003;86:42–7.
63. Goodman A. Diagnosis and treatment of sexual addiction. J Sex Marital Ther. 1993;19:225–51.
64. Sussman S. Sexual addiction among teens: a review. Sex Addict Compulsivity. 2007;14:257–78.
65. Yoder VC, Virden TB, Amin K. Internet pornography and loneliness: an association? Sex Addict Compulsivity. 2005;12:19–44.
66. Butler MH, Pereyra SA, Draper TW, Leonhardt ND, Skinner KB. Pornography use and loneliness: a bidirectional recursive model and pilot investigation. J Sex Marital Ther. 2018;44:127–37.
67. Reid RC, Bramen JE, Anderson A, Cohen MS. Mindfulness, emotional dysregulation, impulsivity, and stress proneness among hypersexual patients. J Clin Psychol. 2014;70:313–21.
68. Kalichman SC, Cain D. The relationship between indicators of sexual compulsivity and high risk sexual practices among men and women receiving services from a sexually transmitted infection clinic. J Sex Res. 2004;41:235–41.
69. Wainberg ML, Muench F, Morgenstern J, Hollander E, Irwin TW, Parsons JT, Allen A, O'Leary A. A double-blind study of citalopram versus placebo in the treatment of compulsive sexual behaviors in gay and bisexual men. J Clin Psychiatry. 2006;67:1968–73.
70. Ebrahim SH, Peterman TA, Zaidi AA, Kamb ML. Mortality related to sexually transmitted diseases in US women, 1973 through 1992. Am J Public Health. 1997;87:938–44.
71. Grant JE. Compulsive sexual behavior: a non-judgmental approach. Curr Psychiatr Ther. 2018;17:34–46.
72. Andreassen CS, Pallesen S, Griffiths MD, Torsheim T, Sinha R. The development and validation of the Bergen-Yale sex addiction scale with a large National Sample. Front Psychol. 2018;9:144.
73. Dhuffar MK, Griffiths MD. Barriers to female sex addiction treatment in the UK. J Behav Addict. 2016;5:562–7.
74. Salmerón-Sánchez P, Ballester-Arnal R, Gil-Llario MD, Morell-Mengual V. Sexual compulsivity and sexual sensation seeking: a preliminary approach among male sex workers compared to gay men in Spain. J Sex Marital Ther. 2017;43:56–67.
75. Scanavino M de T, Ventuneac A, Abdo CHN, Tavares H, Amaral MLS do, Messina B, Reis SC dos, Martins JPLB, Parsons JT. Compulsive sexual behavior and psychopathology among treatment-seeking men in São Paulo, Brazil. Psychiatry Res. 2013;209:518–524.
76. Liao W, Lau JTF, Tsui HY, Gu J, Wang Z. Relationship between sexual compulsivity and sexual risk behaviors among Chinese sexually active males. Arch Sex Behav. 2015;44:791–8.
77. Callesen MB, Weintraub D, Damholdt MF, Møller A. Impulsive and compulsive behaviors among

Danish patients with Parkinson's disease: prevalence, depression, and personality. Parkinsonism Relat Disord. 2014;20:22–6.

78. Skegg K, Nada-Raja S, Dickson N, Paul C. Perceived "out of control" sexual behavior in a cohort of young adults from the Dunedin multidisciplinary health and development study. Arch Sex Behav. 2010;39:968–78.
79. Briken P, Habermann N, Berner W, Hill A. Diagnosis and treatment of sexual addiction: a survey among German sex therapists. Sex Addict Compulsivity. 2007;14:131–43.
80. Farré JM, Fernández-Aranda F, Granero R, et al. Sex addiction and gambling disorder: similarities and differences. Compr Psychiatry. 2015;56:59–68.
81. Warner J, McKeown É, Griffin M, Johnson K, Ramsay A, Cort C, King M. Rates and predictors of mental illness in gay men, lesbians and bisexual men and women: results from a survey based in England and Wales. Br J Psychiatry. 2004;185:479–85.
82. Xu W, Zheng L, Liu Y, Zheng Y. Sexual sensation seeking, sexual compulsivity, and high-risk sexual behaviours among gay/bisexual men in Southwest China. AIDS Care. 2016;28:1138–44.
83. Espinosa-Hernández G, Vasilenko SA, Bámaca-Colbert MY. Sexual behaviors in Mexico: the role of values and gender across adolescence. J Res Adolesc. 2016;26:603–9.
84. Klein V, Jurin T, Briken P, Štulhofer A. Erectile dysfunction, boredom, and hypersexuality among coupled men from two European countries. J Sex Med. 2015;12:2160–7.
85. UNAIDS. UNAIDS report on the global AIDS epidemic | 2012. MSF access to Essent Med. Doi: JC2502/1/E. 2011.
86. Nikitina AV, Fedorova NV. Impulsive-compulsive syndrome in Parkinson's disease. Zhurnal Nevrol i psikhiatrii Im SS Korsakova. 2013;113:32–8.
87. Poletti M, Logi C, Lucetti C, et al. A single-center, cross-sectional prevalence study of impulse control disorders in Parkinson disease association with dopaminergic drugs. J Clin Psychopharmacol. 2013;33:691–4.
88. Mété D, Dafreville C, Paitel V, Wind P. Aripiprazole, gambling disorder and compulsive sexuality. Encéphale. 2016;42:281–3.
89. Okasha A. Mental health in Africa: the role of the WPA. World Psychiatry. 2002;1:32–5.
90. World Health Organization (WHO) (2010) ATLAS on substance use (2010).
91. Guay DRP. Drug treatment of paraphilic and nonparaphilic sexual disorders. Clin Ther. 2009;31:1–31.
92. First M. DSM-5 and paraphilic disorders. J Am Psychiatry Law. 2014;42:191–201.
93. Thibaut F, La Barra FD, Gordon H, Cosyns P, Bradford JMW, WFSBP Task Force on Sexual Disorders. The World Federation of Societies of Biological Psychiatry (WFSBP) guidelines for the biological treatment of paraphilias. World J Biol Psychiatry. 2010;11:604–55.
94. Schmucker M, Lösel F. Does sexual offender treatment work? A systematic review of outcome evaluations. Psicothema. 2008;20:10–9.
95. Saleh FM, Guidry LL. Psychosocial and biological treatment considerations for the paraphilic and nonparaphilic sex offender. J Am Acad Psychiatry Law. 2003;31:486–93.
96. Bradford JM. The neurobiology, neuropharmacology, and pharmacological treatment of the Paraphilias and compulsive sexual behaviour. Can J Psychiatr. 2001;46:26–34.
97. Gooren L. Ethical and medical considerations of androgen deprivation treatment of sex offenders. J Clin Endocrinol Metab. 2011;96:3628–37.
98. Kasinathan J. Treatment for youth paraphilic disorders: opportunities to reduce harm. Australas Psychiatry. 2017;25:121–5.
99. Khalifa N, Duggan C, Stoffers J, Huband N, Völlm B, Ferriter M, Lieb K. Pharmacological interventions for antisocial personality disorder. Cochrane Database Syst Rev. 2010;(8):CD007667.
100. Turner D, Briken P. Treatment of paraphilic disorder in sexual offenders or men with a risk of sexual offending with luteinizing hormone-releasing hormone agonists: an updated systematic review. J Sex Med. 2018;15:77–93.
101. Bártová D, Náhunek K, Svestka J. Pharmacological treatment of deviant sexual behaviour. Act Nerve Super. 1978;20:72–4.
102. Murray M, Bancroft J, Anderson D, Tennett T, Carr P. Endocrine changes in male sexual deviants after treatment anti-androgens, oestrogens or tranquilizers. J Endocrinol. 1975;67:179–88.
103. Ryback R. Naltrexone in the treatment of adolescent sexual offenders. J Clin Psychiatry. 2004;65:982–6.
104. Hill A, Briken P, Kraus C, Srohm K, Berner W. Differential pharmacological treatment of paraphilias and sex offenders. Int J Offender Ther Comp Criminol. 2003;47:407–21.
105. Gordon H. The treatment of paraphilias: an historical perspective. Crim Behav Ment Health. 2008;18:79–87.
106. Gordon G, Southren A, Tochimoto S, Olivo J, Altman K, Rand J, Lemberger L. Effect of medroxyprogesterone acetate (provera) on metabolism and biological activity of testosterone. J Clin Endocrinol Metab. 1970;30:449–56.
107. Gottesman H, Schubert D. Low-dose medroxyprogesterone acetate in the management of the paraphilias. J Clin Psychiatry. 1993;54:182–8.
108. Gallo A, Abracen J, Looman J, Jeglic E, Dickey R. The use of leuprolide acetate in the management of high-risk sex offenders. Sex Abus. 2018;31:930. https://doi.org/10.1177/1079063218791176.
109. Hanson R, Gordon A, Harris A, Marques J, Murphy W, Quinsey V, Seto M. First report of the collaborative outcome data project on the effectiveness of psychological treatment for sex offenders. Sex Abus. 2002;14:169–94.

110. Codispoti V. Pharmacology of sexually compulsive behavior. Psychiatr Clin North Am. 2008;31:671–9.
111. Fuss J, Auer MK, Biedermann SV, Briken P, Hacke W. Deep brain stimulation to reduce sexual drive. J Psychiatry Neurosci. 2015;40:429–31.
112. Bilefsky D. Europeans debate castration of sex offenders. New York Times A1. 2009.
113. Dieckmann G, Schneider-Jonietz B, Schneider H. Psychiatric and neuropsychological findings after stereotactic hypothalamotomy, in cases of extreme sexual aggressivity. Acta Neurochir Suppl (Wien). 1988;44:163–6.
114. Rieber I, Sigusch V. Psychosurgery on sex offenders and sexual 'deviants' in West Germany. Arch Sex Behav. 1979;8:523–7.
115. Haasen C. Comorbidity of paraphilia and depression in Mexico. Ment Illn. 2010;2:e8.
116. Clemente J, Pillon S, Mari J, da Silva C, Santana P, Diehl A. Paraphilic thoughts, behaviors and sex addiction in a sample of patients who use drugs: a cross-sectional study. J Addict Med. 2017;11:377–85.
117. Oliviera Júnior W, Abdo C. Unconventional sexual behaviors and their associations with physical, mental and sexual health parameters: a study in 18 large Brazilian cities. Braz J Psychiatry. 2010;32:264–74.
118. Baltieri D, Boer D. Two clusters of child molesters based on impulsiveness. Braz J Psychiatry. 2015;37:139–45.
119. Lippi G, van Staden P. The use of cyproterone acetate in forensic psychiatric cohort of male sex offenders and its associations with sexual activity and sexual functioning. S Afr J Psychiatry. 2017;23:982.
120. Birger M, Bergman-Levy T, Asman O. Treatment of sex offenders in Israeli prison settings. J Am Acad Psychiatry Law. 2011;39:100–3.
121. Taktak Ş, Yılmaz E, Karamustafalıoglu O, Ünsal A. Characteristics of paraphiliacs in Turkey: a retrospective study - 20 years. Int J Law Psychiatry. 2016;49:22–30.
122. Coskun M, Mukkades N. Mirtazapine treatment in a patient with autistic disorder and fetishism. J Child Adolesc Psychopharmacol. 2008;18:206–9.
123. Usmani MK, Gaur R, Ahmad Azmi S, Gangwar S. Treatment of transvestic fetishism with fluoxetine: a case report. Iran J Psychiatry Behav Sci. 2002;6:100–1.
124. Firoz K, Nidheesh Sankar V, Rajmohan V, Manoj Kumar G, Raghuram T. Treatment of fetishism with naltrexone: a case report. Asian J Psychiatr. 2014;8:67–8.
125. Koo K, Shim G, Park H, Rha K, Choi Y, Chung B, Hong S, Lee J. Treatment outcomes of chemical castration in Korean sex offenders. J Forensic Legal Med. 2013;20:563–6.
126. Masuda K, Ishitobi Y, Tanaka Y, Akiyoshi J. Underwear fetishism induced by bilaterally decreased cerebral blood flow in the temporal occipital lobe. BMJ Case Rep. 2014; https://doi.org/10.1136/bcr-2014-206019.
127. Chang H, Chow C. The treatment of fetishism in an adolescent with attention deficit hyperactivity disorder. Chang Gung Med J. 2011;34:440–3.
128. Chiang Y, Yeh S, Hsiao C, Ree S. Treatment of a transvestic fetishist with cognitive-behavioral therapy and supportive psychotherapy: case report. Chang Ye Xue Za Zhi. 1999;22:299–312.
129. Shiah I, Chao C, Mao W, Chuang Y. Treatment of paraphilic sexual disorder: the use of topiramate in fetishism. Int Clin Psychopharmacol. 2006;21:241–3.
130. Blum AW, Chamberlain SR, Grant JE. Quality of life of young adults with non-paraphilic problematic sexual behaviors: an exploratory study. Addict Behav Reports. 2018;8:164–9.
131. Carnes P. Don't call it love : recovery from sexual addiction. New York: Bantam Books; 1991.
132. Carnes PJ. Addiction or compulsion: politics or illness? Sex Addict Compulsivity. 1996;3:22.
133. Bergner RM. Sexual compulsion as attempted recovery from degradation: theory and therapy. J Sex Marital Ther. 2002;28:373–87.
134. Fong TW, Reid RC, Parhami I. Behavioral addictions: where to draw the lines? Psychiatr Clin North Am. 2012;35:279–96.
135. Spenhoff M, Kruger THC, Hartmann U, Kobs J. Hypersexual behavior in an online sample of males: associations with personal distress and functional impairment. J Sex Med. 2013;10:2996–3005.
136. Coleman E, Horvath KJ, Miner M, Ross MW, Oakes M, Rosser BRS, Men's INTernet Sex (MINTS-II) Team (2010) Compulsive sexual behavior and risk for unsafe sex among internet using men who have sex with men. Arch Sex Behav 39:1045–1053.
137. Parsons JT, Rendina HJ, Ventuneac A, Moody RL, Grov C. CUNY academic works hypersexual, sexually compulsive, or just highly sexually active? Investigating three distinct groups of gay and bisexual men and their profiles of HIV- related sexual risk. City Univ New York. 2016;20:262–72.

Food Addiction

6

Oluwole Jegede and Tolu Olupona

Introduction

The concept of food addiction supposes that some types of foods could pose a particular strong addictive potential much like any substance. The conceptualization of the Food Addiction nosology has, however, been controversial even among addiction experts asking questions about its distinction from other forms of disordered eating, whether this is more like a substance use disorder or a behavioral addition. The enunciation of the types of foods that may result in addiction and determination of its consistent features are only just emerging [1]. Recent work on food addiction including a more acceptable characterization of its phenomenology has gained traction over the last few years especially following the work of Gearhardt et al.(2009) which developed the Yale Food Addiction Scale (YFAS), further strengthening the notion of the similarity between addictive properties of food and other psychoactive substances [2].

Food addiction is defined by a physical and psychological dependency on high fat and high sugar foods. This description derives strongly from experimental and epidemiological models of substance use disorders. In order to qualify as addiction, substances display a problematic pattern of use that include an inexplicable craving for the substance despite problematic social, occupational, or recreational issues that directly derive from such use. The DSM-5 does not recognize FA as a diagnosis but the YFAS 2.0 utilizes all 11 criteria for substance use disorder in creating the tool for clinicians to diagnose FA but unlike illicit substances, food may present particularly interesting from of addiction which may not be clear to the patient or the provider. Indeed, the line is not always clear between food addiction and other eating disorders such as Binge Eating Disorder (BED) and the manifestation of FA goes beyond physical characteristics of being overweight or obese, although- as we will see later in this chapter – these are important clinical considerations [3].

As described above, the development and validation of the Yale Food Addiction Scale (YFAS) have been instrumental to the increased understanding of FA including known epidemiologic data and associated correlates. The YFAS has been validated across several languages and cultures, with robust psychometric properties, including internal consistency reliability. More recently, updated versions of the YFAS (i.e., the YFAS 2.0 and the briefer mYFAS 2.0) have been developed to reflect DSM-5 criteria for substance use disorders. Both the YFAS 2.0 and the mYFAS 2.0 instruments display consistent and adequate psychometric properties [4, 5].

O. Jegede (✉)
Department of Psychiatry and Behavioral Sciences, Yale University, New Haven, Connecticut, USA
e-mail: oluwole.jegede@yale.edu

T. Olupona
Department of Psychiatry and Behavioral Sciences, Interfaith Medical Center, Brooklyn, NY, USA
e-mail: tolupona@interfaithmedical.org

E. Akerele (ed.), *Substance and Non-Substance Related Addictions*,
https://doi.org/10.1007/978-3-030-84834-7_6

The present framework of FA is supported by work in animal and human models. In the former, there is a consistent, behavioral response in rats exposed to high fat and high sugar foods for prolonged periods. In humans, as measured by the YFAS, highly processed sugars, and fats have been strong indicators in individuals meeting the criteria for FA diagnosis. The work of Robinson et al., (2015) showed the behavioral and neurobiological consequences of exposure to high sugars and fats and the resultant downregulation of striatal D2R mRNA regardless of the subjects' development of obesity [1, 6].

Epidemiology

The development of the Yale Food Addiction scale has provided a consistent diagnostic criterion based on the DSM. FA is identified in about 20% of the population. In a large meta-analysis, the weighted mean prevalence of YFAS food addiction diagnosis was 19.9% with the diagnosis found to be higher in adults aged >35 years, females, individuals with higher body mass indices (BMI), and among clinical samples.

According to the National Health and Nutrition Examination Survey, the prevalence of obesity in 2015–2016 among U.S. adults was 39.8% and 18.5% in youths. The observed prevalence was higher among non-Hispanic black and Hispanic adults than among non-Hispanic white and non-Hispanic Asian adults and youths. An increasing trend is seen among youths, making obesity a clear public health concern (Fig. 6.1) [8].

The prevalence and severity of FA diagnosis has been reported to be increased in females but decreases with increasing age [9, 10]. Reports on ethnicity have yielded conflicting reports with some reporting no ethnic variability while others

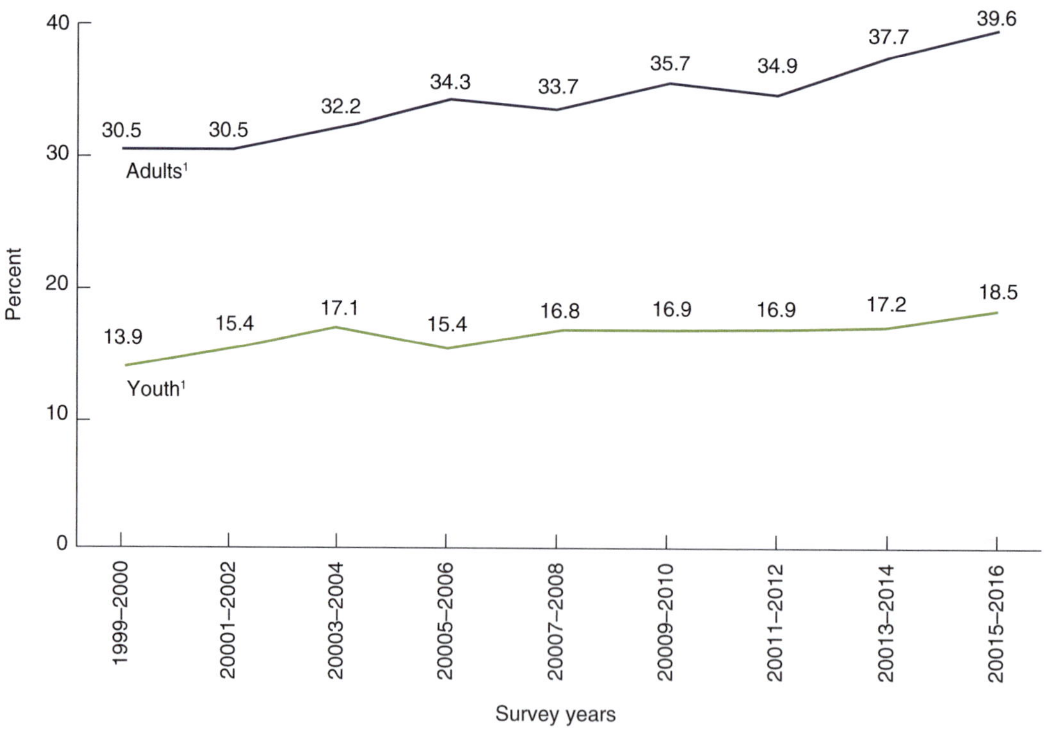

Fig. 6.1 Trends in obesity prevalence among adults aged 20 and over (age adjusted) and youth aged 2–19 years: United States, 1999–2000 through 2015–2016. (Source: NCHS, National Health and Nutrition Examination Survey, 1999–2016)

have reported higher FA scores in African Americans and others among white females [10].

Other associated factors identified include psychiatric diagnosis of schizophrenia, major depressive disorder, neuroticism, tobacco smoking and hypercholesterolemia as well as a decrease in physical activity [7, 10, 11].

The children adaptation of the YFAS (YFAS-C) was published in 2013 with a lower reading level and more appropriate content. Based on the YFAS-C, the prevalence of FA in African American obese adolescents was reported as 10% and in a Russian sample, reported at 4.5%. Possible explanation of these lower than expected values includes methodological differences and underreporting of distress experienced from addiction [1, 12].

The influence of cultural factors has also been studied especially as less developed countries undergo socioeconomic changes that shape their eating behaviors. One of such studies challenges the supposition that FA may be a problem only for developed countries, they reported a Food Addiction prevalence of 32.5% among men and women in India [13].

In summary, the risk factors for food addiction include the following:

1. Other specified eating disorders.
2. Higher BMI.
3. Psychiatric diagnosis such as schizophrenia, depressive disorders, body image dissatisfaction.
4. Age.
5. Gender.
6. Medical diagnosis.
7. Personality factors such as food preference susceptibility and neuroticism.

Neurobiology of Food Addiction

An increasing number of neurobiological researches continue to support the central premise of food addiction, they show consistently that prolonged consumption of high sugar foods results in predictable changes in the brain's reward pathway similar to those in drug addiction. Literature has shown results of functional magnetic resonance imaging (fMRI) in the assessment of neural responses to food cues showed a distinct correlation between FA diagnosis based on the YFAS score and brain activity in a similar pattern to substance use disorders [14, 15].

Highly interconnected central and peripheral signaling pathways are responsible for food addiction. The neurologic pathways identified to be primarily responsible for the feelings of pleasure and reward include dopaminergic, GABAergic, opioid, and serotonergic neural circuits in the striatum, amygdala, orbitofrontal cortex (OFC), and midbrain. Dopamine is however regarded as the most important mediator of addiction with projections throughout the brain and interactions with opioid-mediated GABAergic, cholinergic, and serotonergic circuits [16].

Four brain regions appear to be involved in the regulation of feeding:

1. Amygdala/Hippocampus.
2. Insula.
3. OFC.
4. Striatum.

The hypothalamus (Orexin and melanin) and the arcuate nucleus (neuropeptide Y and alpha-melanocyte-stimulating hormone) have been implicated in weight regulation. There are four gut and fat-derived hormones that facilitate the homeostatic regulation of feeding and provide feedback to the brain about satiety, including:

1. Ghrelin.
2. Leptin.
3. Insulin.
4. Peptide YY.

Ghrelin is released from the stomach and acts on the hypothalamus to increase food consumption, the hormone also stimulates dopaminergic reward pathways. Serum ghrelin levels typically rise during a fast and fall after feeding. Leptin relays information to the brain about the body's fat reserves, acting on the hypothalamus to decrease food intake and increase metabolic rate. Insulin (pancreas) and peptide YY (small intestine) relay information to the brain about acute changes in energy levels. Leptin and insulin inhibit dopaminergic circuits.

Animal Models and Human Clinical Studies

Animal model research and clinical studies show that foods might have reinforcing abilities similar to other drugs of abuse. As noted above, the role for mesolimbic dopamine pathways is implicated in the overlap between obesity and addiction [17]. Furthermore, lower levels of D2 receptor availability have been observed in obese humans. Studies have shown an association between higher food addiction scores and an increased activation of regions encoding the motivation in response to food cues, such as the amygdala, anterior cingulate cortex, and orbital frontal cortex. Stice et al. assessed the genetic factors that influence brain dopamine in humans in relation to neuroimaging and found that individuals with the DRD2 TaqIA A1 allele have weaker activation of the frontal operculum, lateral orbitofrontal cortex, and striatum in response to the imagined intake of palatable foods versus the imagined unpalatable foods or water, and that the presence of these alleles predicted future increases in body mass. Thus, individuals may overeat to compensate for hypofunctioning in reward-related brain regions, and this may be more apparent in those with genetic polymorphisms thought to attenuate the dopamine signaling in this region [18].

Clinical Presentation and Diagnosis

The Yale Food Addiction Scale (YFAS) operationalizes the construct of the Diagnostic and Statistical Manual for Mental Disorders (DSM-5) criteria for substance use disorder (Table 6.1). Originally the YFAS was based on the DSM-IV-TR but the tool has had multiple adaptations, including a briefer scale (mYFAS), the YFAS 2.0 was developed to reflect changes to diagnostic criteria in the DSM-5 and the YFAS-C was adapted for use in the pediatric population. The following is the criteria set for substance use disorder according to the DSM-5:

Table 6.1 The modified Yale Food Addiction Scale 2.0 (mYFAS 2.0) questions derived from general DSM-5 criteria [5]

DSM-5 SUD criteria	mYFAS 2.0 Question
Substance taken in larger amount and for longer period than intended	I ate to the point where I felt physically ill
Persistent desire or repeated unsuccessful attempts to quit	I tried and failed to cut down on or stop eating certain foods
Much time/activity to obtain, use, recover	I spent more time feeling sluggish or tired from overeating
Important social, occupational, or recreational activities given up or reduced	I avoided work, school, or social activities because I was afraid, I would overeat there
Use continues despite knowledge of adverse consequences	I kept eating in the same way even though my eating caused emotional problems
Tolerance	Eating the same amount of food did not give me as much enjoyment as it used to
Characteristic withdrawal symptoms; substance taken to relieve withdrawal	If I had emotional problems because I had not eaten certain foods, I would eat those foods to feel better
Continued use despite social or interpersonal problems	My friends or family were worried about how much I overate
Failure to fulfill major role obligations	My overeating got in the way of me taking care of my family or doing household chores
Use in physically hazardous situations	I was so distracted by eating that I could have been hurt (e.g., when driving a car, crossing the street and operating machinery)
Craving, or a strong desire or urge to use	I had such strong urges to eat certain foods that I could not think of anything else
Use causes clinically significant impairment	I had significant problems in my life because of food and eating. These may have been problems with my daily routine, work, school, friends, family, or health
Use causes clinically significant distress	My eating behavior caused me much distress

Substance-use disorder is defined as a maladaptive pattern of substance use leading to clinically significant impairment or distress, as manifested by two (or more) of the following, occurring within a 12-month period:

1. Recurrent substance use resulting in a failure to fulfill major role obligations at work, school, or home (e.g., repeated absences or poor work performance related to substance use; substance-related absences, suspensions, or expulsions from school; neglect of children or household).
2. Recurrent substance use in situations in which it is physically hazardous (e.g., driving an automobile or operating a machine when impaired by substance use).
3. Continued substance use despite having persistent or recurrent social or interpersonal problems caused or exacerbated by the effects of the substance (e.g., arguments with spouse about consequences of intoxication and physical fights).
4. Tolerance, as defined by either of the following:
   (a) Need for markedly increased amounts of the substance to achieve intoxication or desired effect.
   (b) Markedly diminished effect with continued use of the same amount of the substance (Note: tolerance is not counted for those taking medications under medical supervision such as analgesics, antidepressants, anti-anxiety medications, or beta-blockers).
5. Withdrawal, as manifested by either of the following:
   (a) The characteristic withdrawal syndrome for the substance (refer to Criteria A and B of the criteria sets for withdrawal from the specific substances).
   (b) The same (or a closely related) substance is taken to relieve or avoid withdrawal symptoms (Note: withdrawal is not counted for those taking medications under medical supervision such as analgesics, antidepressants, antianxiety medications, or beta-blockers).
6. The substance is often taken in larger amounts or over a longer period than was intended.
7. There is a persistent desire or unsuccessful efforts to cut down or control substance use.
8. A great deal of time is spent on activities necessary to obtain the substance, use the substance, or recover from its effects.
9. Important social, occupational, or recreational activities are given up or reduced because of substance use.
10. The substance use is continued despite knowledge of having a persistent or recurrent physical or psychological problem that is likely to have been caused or exacerbated by the substance.
11. Craving or a strong desire or urge to use a specific substance.

Although the YFAS is by far the most popular tool utilized for FA, other existing tools include

1. Food Craving Questionnaire.
2. Dutch Eating Behavior Questionnaire.
3. Three-Factor Eating Questionnaire.
4. Power of Food Scale.
5. Questionnaire of Eating and Weight Patterns—Revised.

Management of Food Addiction

The conceptualization that food has addictive potentials like other substances presupposes that the management of food addiction will follow similar concepts. The goals of treatment must be clearly defined with the patient. As with other conditions associated with disordered eating, patients with FA must have a medical, nutritional, and psychiatric evaluations and treatments tailored along these lines as well. Other than psychological treatments which are widely regarded as treatment of choice for eating disorders, the association of FA with obesity lends it to possible response to pharmacological management.

Psychotherapy Management

Psychotherapy for food addiction include

1. Cognitive Behavioral Therapy.
2. Interpersonal Psychotherapy.
3. Dialectical Behavioral Therapy.
4. Psychodynamic psychotherapy.
5. Problem-solving 12-step programs.

Pharmacotherapy

There are no FDA-approved pharmacologic treatments for food addiction but medications may have a role in the consequences of food addiction namely obesity and attendant comorbidities. It is also imperative to address other psychiatric or substance abuse disorders with which the patient may present.

References

1. Schulte EM, Jacques-Tiura AJ, Gearhardt AN, Naar S. Food addiction prevalence and concurrent validity in African American adolescents with obesity. Psychol Addict Behav. 2018;32(2):187.
2. Gearhardt AN, Corbin WR, Brownell KD. Preliminary validation of the Yale food addiction scale. Appetite. 2009;52(2):430–6.
3. Burrows T, Skinner J, McKenna R, Rollo M. Food addiction, binge eating disorder, and obesity: is there a relationship? Behav Sci. 2017;7(3):54.
4. Gearhardt AN, Corbin WR, Brownell KD. Development of the Yale food addiction scale version 2.0. Psychol Addict Behav. 2016;30(1):113.
5. Schulte EM, Gearhardt AN. Development of the modified Yale food addiction scale version 2.0. Eur Eat Disord Rev. 2017;25(4):302–8.
6. Robinson MJ, Burghardt PR, Patterson CM, Nobile CW, Akil H, Watson SJ, et al. Individual differences in cue-induced motivation and striatal systems in rats susceptible to diet-induced obesity. Neuropsychopharmacology. 2015;40(9):2113.
7. Pursey KM, Stanwell P, Gearhardt AN, Collins CE, Burrows TL. The prevalence of food addiction as assessed by the Yale food addiction scale: a systematic review. Nutrients. 2014;6(10):4552–90.
8. Hales CM, Carroll MD, Fryar CD, Ogden CL. Prevalence of obesity among adults and youth: United States, 2015–2016. NCHS data brief, no 288. Hyattsville: National Center for Health Statistics. p. 2017.
9. Eichen DM, Lent MR, Goldbacher E, Foster GD. Exploration of "food addiction" in overweight and obese treatment-seeking adults. Appetite. 2013;67:22–4.
10. Flint AJ, Gearhardt A, Corbin W, Brownell K, Field A, Rimm E. Food addiction scale measurement in two cohorts of middle-aged and older women. Am J Clin Nutr. 2014;99:578–86.
11. Goluza I, Borchard J, Kiarie E, Mullan J, Pai N. Exploration of food addiction in people living with schizophrenia. Asian J Psychiatr. 2017;27:81–4.
12. Borisenkov MF, Tserne TA, Bakutova LA. Food addiction in Russian adolescents: Associations with age, sex, weight, and depression. Eur Eat Disord Rev. 2018;26(6):671–6.
13. Wiedemann AA, Lawson JL, Cunningham PM, Khalvati KM, Lydecker JA, Ivezaj V, Grilo CM. Food addiction among men and women in India. Eur Eat Disord Rev. 2018;26(6):597–604. https://doi.org/10.1002/erv.2613. Epub 2018 Jul 12
14. Gearhardt AN, Yokum S, Orr PT, Stice E, Corbin WR, Brownell KD. Neural correlates of food addiction. Arch Gen Psychiatry. 2011;68:808–16.
15. Carter A, Hendrikse J, Lee N, Yücel M, Verdejo-Garcia A, Andrews ZB, Hall W. The neurobiology of "food addiction" and its implications for obesity treatment and policy. Annu Rev Nutr. 2016;36:105–28.
16. Blumenthal DM, Gold MS. Neurobiology of food addiction. Curr Opin Clin Nutr Metab Care. 2010;13(4):359–65.
17. Avena NM, Gold JA, Kroll C, Gold MS. Further developments in the neurobiology of food and addiction: update on the state of the science. Nutrition. 2012;28(4):341–3.
18. Stice E, Spoor S, Bohon C, Small DM. Relation between obesity and blunted striatal response to food is moderated by TaqIA A1 allele. Science. 2008;322:449–52.

7 Internet Addiction

Geoffrey Talis

Introduction

The internet has undoubtedly revolutionized the way we humans live in our daily lives. It has brought humanity conveniences never previously thought imaginable, readily controlled at our fingertips. The internet has found its way into our lives through our personal and professional lives and is primarily accessed through computers and cell phones. As a result, we are now able to communicate and connect at lightning fast speeds at any time of day and during almost any activity of our choice. The internet has allowed the development of applications, games, programs, hobbies, and an entire new world of human existence. The internet has clear benefits; however, it has the potential to be misused causing severe social and occupational dysfunction.

Internet addiction (IA), a term used interchangeably with problematic internet use (PIU) in the literature, has been on the rise worldwide with surveys estimating that up to half of adolescents worldwide are experiencing negative consequences of excessive internet use [25]. The variability in the literature in studying IA has made it difficult to have more accurate public health estimates. Most studies have not uniformly specified the particular use of the internet the participants engage in, such as gambling, gaming, social networking, smartphone, sex, shopping, and information gathering. Each of these categories of internet use may one day be considered for classification under their own disorder category or as subtypes of IA with further study [5, 7].

Neurobiological and genetic research has found common neural pathways and genes related between IA and substance use disorders, supporting classification IA as an addiction of behavior, as GD has in the DSM-V. Further targeted understanding of the neurobiology and genetic factors of IAD is required to compare differences and similarities among other substance use and behavioral addictions. The evidence currently points to various interconnected, overlapping neural networks in the brain are affected, though apparently differ slightly between which use of the internet the user is engaging in (GD vs. IGD) [23, 27].

The remainder of this chapter discuss the classification, diagnostic considerations, etiology, demographics, treatments, and neurobiology of behavioral addictions with attention to IAD.

Classification

PIU is a term used for individuals whose internet use has become problematic or pathologic, specifically because of one's inability to control their use of the internet despite adverse life

G. Talis (✉)
Rutgers NJMS University Hospital, Newark, NJ, USA
e-mail: talisga@njms.rutgers.edu

E. Akerele (ed.), *Substance and Non-Substance Related Addictions*, https://doi.org/10.1007/978-3-030-84834-7_7

consequences. The DSM-V does not currently categorize disorders under a category of behavioral addictions; however, conditions such as kleptomania and GD have been included in the DSM-V under the categories of impulse-control disorders and non-substance addiction. Internet addiction also shares similar features to these disorders. The culmination of the past decade of research into behavioral addictions, including internet addiction, has provided enough evidence to distinguish pathologic versus non-pathologic internet use. Continued elucidation of specific criteria for diagnosis of internet addiction is needed through further developing validated and standardized measures in collecting epidemiological data [23].

It is also important to consider a cultural context of internet use when formulating a new classification of mental illness. It is not uncommon for people today to use the internet, computers, or smartphones to perform any combination of activities including personal and professional use for a large portion of the day. Distinguishing the intentions and effects excessive internet use has on people is required when pathologizing a common behavior that many people have today. Intentions for use of the internet and the results or consequences of continued use should be evaluated carefully. The purpose of creating diagnostic criteria for disorders is to be able to identify individuals at risk and carefully and systematically define conditions in a reliable and valid manner so that they can be better understood and treated. A balance must be found where the criteria of the disorder are not too narrow to hinder generalizability and not too broad to obscure knowledge [26].

Diagnostic Considerations

Internet addiction does not have as precisely defined criteria as does gambling disorder or IGD. The criteria for IGD may appear to be adapted straight from gambling disorder; however, IGD does indeed have evidence-based support for its criteria, though further studies are needed to specify a threshold of criteria to officially rule-in a diagnosis of IGD. Disagreement remains in the literature with regard to the specific diagnostic criteria for IAD, which causes marked variability in prevalence reports. Future studies are required to more precisely define the criteria for IAD. Barriers to investigation include discrepancies in approach and scale measures used in large population-based studies. There have been several scales measuring the severity of IAD that have been created both in East-Asian countries and United States. Table 7.1 indicates an adapted version of proposed IAD criteria by using the DSM-V diagnostic criteria for another substance use disorder as published by Ascher and Levounis (2015).

Many types of rating scales have been used in the evaluation of IAD with different target cultures and varying areas of focus, some with unknown specificities and sensitivities. These include: the Young Internet Addiction Scale is the best validated tool to date [1]. Other scales such as the gaming addiction scale for adolescents (GASA), internet addiction scale (IAS), scale for the assessment of internet and computer game addiction (AICA, clinician and self-reports), the adolescent pathological internet use scale (APIUS), Beard's diagnostic questionnaire for addiction (BDQ), Internet addiction diagnostic questionnaire (IADQ), impulsive-compulsive internet usage disorder Yale-Brown Obsessive-compulsive scale (IC-IUD-YBOCS), online cognition scale (OCS) and the Internet overuse self-rating scale (IOSS) each have their strengths and weaknesses, however the common theme among these assessments is a lack of evidence supporting their individual validity [3].

Assessments such as the Korean-internet addiction scale (K-IAS) and Chinese Internet addiction scale (CIA) have been developed in their respective countries for the specific study of IAD as it presents in their cultures. Culture, context, and demographics have shown to be essential in understanding the holistic picture of an individual with problematic internet use. More studies are needed using one agreed-upon

Table 7.1 Proposed adapted diagnostic criteria for other (or unknown) substance use disorder: problematic internet use

A problematic pattern of use of the internet and other related technologies leading to clinically significant impairment or distress, as manifested by at least two of the following, occurring within a 12-month period:
1. Internet usage is in larger amounts of time or intensity than was intended.
2. There is a persistent desire or unsuccessful efforts to cut down or control use of the internet.
3. A great deal of time is spent in activities necessary to use or recover from use of the internet.
4. Craving, or a strong desire or urge to use the Internet.
5. Recurrent use of the internet resulting in a failure to fulfill major role obligations at work, school, or home.
6. Continued internet use despite having persistent or recurrent social or interpersonal problems caused or exacerbated by the effects of its use.
7. Important social, occupational, or recreational activities are given up or reduced because of internet use.
8. Recurrent internet use in situations in which it is physically hazardous.
9. Internet use is continued despite knowledge of having a persistent or recurrent physical or psychological problem that is likely to have been caused or exacerbated by internet use.
10. Tolerance, as defined by either of the following:
(a) A need for markedly increased amounts of internet use to achieve the desired effect.
(b) A markedly diminished effect with continued same amount of Internet use
11. Withdrawal, as manifested by the following: internet use is at times employed to avoid withdrawal symptoms.
Specify if: *In early remission*: After full criteria for problematic internet use disorder were previously met, none of the criteria for problematic internet use disorder have been met for at least 3 months, but for less than 12 months (with the exception that Criterion A4, "Craving, or a strong desire or urge to use the internet," may be met). *In sustained remission*: After full criteria for problematic internet use were previously met, none of the criteria for problematic internet use disorder have been met at any time during a period of 12 months or longer (with the exception that Criterion A4, "Craving or a strong desire or urge to use the Internet," may be met).
Specify if: *In a controlled environment*: This additional specifier is used if the individual is in an environment where access to the internet is restricted.
Specify current severity: *Mild*: Presence of 2–3 symptoms. *Moderate*: Presence of 4–5 symptoms. *Severe*: Presence of 6 or more symptoms.

Source: [34, 35]

standardized questionnaire in larger populations to elicit a more accurate estimate of IAD worldwide [3].

Differential Diagnosis

The first step in formulating a differential diagnosis of a patient with IAD is to understand whether the disorder is as a result of an underlying, comorbid psychiatric condition, or if it contributes or potentiates another illness. Patients with IAD who are treated for a mood, anxiety, obsessive-compulsive or substance use disorder and whose internet use reacts accordingly, we can conclude that the problematic internet use was as a result of the underlying condition. Having a thorough understanding of a timeline or pattern of occurrence may help the provider identify what internet use may be the result of. Does internet use change with an improvement in mood after a depressive episode, a stabilization of mood during a manic episode, alleviation of anxiety associated with social phobia or a reduction in the use of a substance?

Being able to identify the purpose of the internet use also becomes an essential component of specifying an appropriate diagnosis and treatment plan. A patient who uses social media as a mode of communicating without the pressure of having real-life, casual social encounters may require further work-up for social phobia. It is also possible for a patient with social phobia to have IAD, it is also important to categorize the amount of time the patient also spends watching pornography, using social media, gambling, shopping, or gaming (Balakrishnan and Griffiths 2018).

Epidemiology

Estimates of IAD range broadly (0.3–38%) as the prevalence and cultural context within each country are combined with the inconsistency and variability of scales measuring symptomatology ([10], Mihajlov et al. 2017). Standardization and agreement on basic criteria measures will be required to further strengthen the validity of prevalence reports. More confounding variables regarding reports of epidemiological data include failure to distinguish or specify what exactly the populations of individuals being studied were actually using the internet for (social media, smartphone use, gaming, shopping, pornography, gambling) as well as evaluating for the presence of other comorbid psychiatric disorders such as social anxiety, mood disorders, obsessive-compulsive and ADHD. In a comprehensive review of problematic internet gaming and internet gaming disorder, Gonzalez-Bueso and colleagues found that 92% of individuals have comorbid anxiety, 89% with depression, 85% with symptoms of ADHD, 75% with social phobia and obsessive-compulsive symptoms with IGD. Rates were clearly higher in males. As previously discussed, there are contradictions in the literature regarding these variables and require more longitudinal studies addressing the complex relationship of these comorbidities.

In a systematic review by Carli et al., males were the majority affected by PIU and most commonly had symptoms of depression and ADHD. As previously stated, the significant heterogeneity that is pervasive in the literature of IAD makes accurate conclusions less apparent. In other studies, IAD was found to be more common among young females and IGD more common among males [26].

Etiology

The etiology of IA may be looked at through a variety of lenses. Viewing IA through a biopsychosocial model may be most holistic, which is inclusive of analyzing genetic vulnerabilities or abnormalities in neurochemical processes, personality characteristics, demographic factors, and ease of accessibility. Other models of understanding the development and maintenance of IA are the triple A model (accessibility, anonymity and affordability), the cognitive-behavioral model, and the anonymity, convenience, escape model [8]. As discussed, the etiology of IA must be further specified to the specific intention or purpose the user is using the internet for.

Treatment (Pharmacotherapy and Psychotherapy)

IA lacks definition consensus, as previously mentioned, which directly impacts the quality of studies that address treatment methods. Both psychopharmacology and psychotherapy interventions have been studied independently and together as well described in a systematic review by [33]. Antidepressants such as escitalopram and bupropion were compared both head to head, with and without psychotherapy (cognitive-behavioral, motivational interviewing, family-based). These studies indicated statistically significant reductions in the Young Internet Addiction Scale score after 4–6-week trial of both antidepressant and CBT interventions in affected individuals from around the world. Inclusion criteria varied between these studies, some documenting change in time in hours spent online versus scale based. Studies were also of small sample sizes between 10 and 62 participants. Overall, the groups treated with bupropion with and without CBT were found to be more effective in reducing YIAS scores than escitalopram with and without CBT. Other medications that have been studied include psychostimulants such as methylphenidate and atomoxetine, which have been shown to reduce ADHD symptoms and internet use in a group of 62 medication-naïve children after 8 weeks of treatment [16].

As will be further explained, the phenomenology and neurobiology of IA shares similarities with other psychiatric disorders such as substance-use disorders, impulse control disorders, obsessive-compulsive disorders, and other mood and psychotic disorders. Studies using medications such as antipsychotics, mood-stabilizers opioid-receptor antagonists, and glutamate-receptor antagonists are limited in number and treatment effectiveness, though may be important to consider if another psychiatric disorder is suspected in the work-up of a patient affected with IA.

Psychotherapy techniques such as cognitive-behavioral therapy (CBT), motivational interviewing (MI), psychodynamic psychotherapy, family therapy, and mindfulness-based interventions have also been studied in IA as well as IGD. Most studies are limited due to lack of control groups and a consensual agreement on diagnosing IA.

Cognitive-behavioral therapy for internet addiction (CBT-IA), developed by Young includes maintaining a log of time spent online, development of time management skills, goal setting, and restructuring cognitive distortions. CBT period has been shown to be the most evidence-based method of reducing distress and improving functionality in IA to date [12].

IA affects the family dynamic at home, as the most likely sufferers of IA are currently adolescent males. Family therapy has been shown to be effective in reducing IA distress at both the level of the patient and family. Included in family therapy are three approaches: improving family communication through active listening, establishing limits on screen time and screen free zones, and enhancing family bonding through close examination of current relationships and through role playing.

Motivational interviewing has been shown to be helpful for IA. Adolescents typically have minimal desires to change their addictive or problematic behaviors and therefore it is the parents who typically present for help. Helping teens bring attention to the activities that are being missed is an effective exercise in the process of behavior change [9, 31].

Neurobiology of Behavioral Addictions

The definition of addiction has mostly been exclusive to substance use disorders in the twentieth century. There are defined neuroplastic changes that occur in those developing an addiction via alterations in glutamatergic signaling, altering the motivation, executive functioning, reward pathways in the brain leading to changes in the patterns of cognition, emotion, and behavior [20]. It is not surprising that after chronic use of substances as well as behaviors that the neural pathways are altered and strengthened to promote continued engagement with the substance and/or behavior. Their new neurobiological functioning predisposes individuals to experience irresistible cravings, developing tolerance, experiencing withdrawal syndromes when the substance or behavior is removed, leading to high rates of relapse after discontinued use and further engagement with the substance and/or behavior [30].

Regions of the brain that affect motivation, executive functioning, and reward pathways are the glutamatergic and dopaminergic neurons within the dorsal striatum, nucleus accumbens, ventral tegmental area, and prefrontal cortices (mesocorticolimbic system and extended amygdala pathways). MRI, fMRI, and PET studies of affected individuals indicate that altered functioning of these areas in the brain is shared among IAD, IGD, and substance-use disorders, thus, in favor of labeling internet use as an addiction. EEGs have been used to assess brain wave reactivity, such as reductions of inhibitory control and an increase in cue-reactivity; therefore, requiring increased levels of cognitive resources to complete tasks secondary to impulsivity and impaired executive functioning [20].

Smartphones and Social Media, Pornography, Gambling, and Gaming

Social Media and Smartphones

The smartphone has become one of the most accessible methods using the internet [21]. Problematic smartphone use and social media use have been found to be directly related and identified as the most common issue regarding smartphone use [19, 29]. Socializing via online social media platforms may present as an opportunity to those individuals who are fearful of real-life social situations or could present as evidence of a pathological coping mechanism for adult developmental transitions and crises. They use social networking to find psychological meaning to a deep and compelling need to feel emotionally close to others. In an online environment they can express themselves and find the acceptance missing in their lives [28]. Excessive smartphone usage also facilitates problematic pornography viewing and gambling [19].

Most frequently reported estimate of college students affected by smartphone addiction is between 10% and 20% [6]. As the internet and smartphones have infected the entire world, use of smartphones should especially be evaluated in the context they are being studied in. With relation to Asian society, there is commonly little time for in-person socialization which contributes to high usage of mobile devices [18].

Problematic smartphone use is not classified as addiction as no large studies have been conducted to evaluate the suitability of such a diagnosis. General lack of construct validity to "smartphone addiction studies" [24]. Current internet use may be a natural progression of the modern-day way of life, which researchers may only have a pathological explanation for this phenomenon [29]. This is another instance where it is especially important that mental health providers not pathologize normal behavior in a technologically developing society [13].

Online Gambling

Gambling disorder (GD) has been identified as a unique disorder and classified under the category of substance-related and addictive disorders in the DSM-V as it has been found to share more commonalities with substance use disorders (SUDs) rather than those of obsessive-compulsive disorders (OCD) or impulse control disorders. Concepts such as "chasing losses" and superstitious beliefs differentiate gambling disorder from SUDs. These findings have been based on multiple domains including diagnostic criteria, clinical characteristics, social factors, co-occurring disorders, personality features, behavioral measures, biochemistry, neurocircuitry, genetics, and treatments [27]. The dysregulation of dopaminergic tone is the neurobiological link gambling disorder and impulse control disorders. Games that are classified under the umbrella of gambling include games commonly found at casinos such as slots and card games, sports betting, dice, and lottery. The shift of these common casino games to an online platform has increased the access, availability, and exposed vulnerable individuals to gamble more frequently and with ease.

Gambling involves risking something of value in a game of chance in hopes of obtaining something of greater value. Online gambling has become immensely popular with tens of millions of dollars in quarterly earnings at many casinos nationwide. Online gambling features many enchanting, spectacular, and engaging displays of fun and suspense as the slots appear to be in traditional casinos, though with more customizable options and unique themes. Online gambling closely relates to internet gaming in that the flashing lights and engaging game play keep the player glued to the screen awaiting the next attractive sound or visual splendor.

In business and law, gambling is debated even within other online domains such as gaming. A mystery "loot box" found in some games offers the player to spend money on the contents within the box, which is unknown to the player. The contents of the box may be superior in some way, allowing the player to gain unique access to aspects of the game otherwise not available to others. Loot boxes have already been banned in some countries and are currently under investigation in the USA.

The South Oaks Gambling Screen is a validated tool that has been extensively used to identify pathologic gambling, though may be somewhat outdated with a high number of false positives. Gamblers Anonymous Survey has not yet been validated, though can provide useful clinical information and can be helpful to patients and families. The Lie/Bet Questionnaire is simply two questions to ask when evaluating a patient: "Have you ever had to lie to people important to you about how much you gamble?" and "Have you ever felt the need to bet more and more money?" This tool is highly sensitive and will signal the evaluator to investigate further about the patient's gambling tendencies.

Internet Gaming

Internet Gaming Disorder (IGD) has been added in Sect. 3 of the DSM-V as a condition for future study and is likely the closest of other behavioral addictions to be added to the next version of the DSM. In China, internet gaming has already been defined as an addiction. There continues to be a lack of a standard definition from which to derive prevalence data (diversity of assessment tools). Criteria for this disorder closely resemble that of gambling disorder (GD; previously known as pathological gambling, PG) and substance use disorders including aspects such as tolerance, withdrawal, cravings, preoccupation, and dysfunction in major life areas (school, work, relationships) [4].

It is estimated that the majority afflicted with IGD are adolescent men with comorbid psychiatric conditions such as depression, ADHD, OCD, and substance use disorders. Other disorders such as generalized and social anxiety, hypomania, obsessive-compulsive personality disorder, borderline personality disorder, avoidant personality disorder, and psychosis have been found to be higher in prevalence with individuals with IGD. Those most susceptible to developing the disorder are children and adolescents who have high impulsivity, lower social competence, and higher amounts of game play. These individuals tend to also have higher rates of aggression and poor relationships with parents and comorbid depression and ADHD symptoms. Males are almost twice as likely to suffer from IGD than females [14].

Affected individuals are typically drawn into games with team aspects and that are competitive in nature. They will play a game between 8 and 10 hours per day on average and exceed 30 hours of gameplay per week. Male adolescents and Asian populations tend to have been the most commonly studied populations to date.

Various types of psychotherapeutic approaches such as psychodynamic, cognitive-behavioral, family, and group-based interventions as well as psychopharmacologic interventions have been studied for treatment of IGD. It is of greatest importance to uncover what motivating factors are most salient to the individual who is suffering from excessive game play and tailor treatment specifically to that individual [14, 15].

Problematic Online Pornography Use

POPU fits the triple A framework (accessibility, affordability, anonymity) and thereby enhances the risk for prone individuals, to engage in various types of sexually related behaviors, most commonly including masturbation. Risk factors for developing POPU are being a novelty-seeking, young, religious man who uses the internet frequently, most commonly finding himself in negative mood states, prone to sexual boredom. Minors are a particularly vulnerable population as they are still in the process of sexual neurodevelopment. The clinical manifestations of POPU are sexual dysfunction and psychosexual dissatisfaction, which are reversible when the behavior is controlled. Out-of-control sexual behavior has been included in the

ICD-11 and will be of use when addressing patients that seek medical attention [2].

Love et al. [22] conclude that internet pornography addiction fits into the addiction framework and shares similar basic mechanisms with substance addiction, similarly to other behavioral addictions mentioned in this chapter. It stimulates the brain's reward system, and the person is searching for additional excitement online. The excessive use of internet pornography could also be explained from a neurobiological aspect, as there is an expectation of a more intense content the individual seeks further excitement by increasing the frequency of online sexual activities [11, 17].

Criteria most commonly proposed include concepts of loss of control, excessive time spent on sexual behavior, and negative consequences to self and others. A flexible assessment tool must be developed to aid in determining when a normal behavior becomes pathologic, which may require correlation with neurobiological evidence. Treatment is focused on the reduction or elimination of the behavior. Fortunately, it appears that clinical symptoms are reversible with reduction or removal of the behavior and normal functioning returns. Individual treatment course will be determined on case-by-case basis and may typically include elements of mindfulness and acceptance-based psychotherapy, which on occasion has been shown to be equally or more important than a pharmacological approach [2]. A pilot study for POPU with acceptance commitment therapy showed promising results teaching coping skills around distress tolerance or frustration intolerance may be useful [32].

Conclusions

The internet has evolved from simple personal and professional applications like text chatting and web browsing to include more spectacular and psychologically engaging activities such as gaming, gambling, pornography, and social media. The availability, access, and vulnerability model has opened the flood gates for people to use the internet excessively for these purposes, ultimately leading to problematic or addictive behaviors that have severe consequences in these individual's lives in all aspects. The first step is to identify the reason for usage and rule-out any underlying mental illnesses to be treated, as problematic internet use may subside or resolve upon treatment of any mood, anxiety, or psychotic disorders. Further work in this field will involve reaching a consensus for criteria for the above-mentioned disorders that do not pathologize behavior that may be considered normal in our technologically advancing society as to avoid negative consequences.

References

1. Aboujaoude E. Problematic internet use: an overview. World Psychiatry. 2010;9(2):85–90.
2. Alarcon R, Iglesia JI, Casado NM, Montejo AL. Online porn addiction: what we know and what we don't – a systematic review. J Clin Med. 2019;8(1):91.
3. Balhara YPS, Mahapatra A, Sharma P, Bhargava R. Problematic internet use among students in South-East Asia: current state of evidence. Indian J Public Health. 2018;62(3):197–201.
4. Balakrishnan J, Griffiths MD. Perceived addictiveness of smartphone games: a content analysis of game reviews by players. Int J Mental Health Addiction. 2019;17:922–34.
5. Banz BC, Yip SW, Yau YHC, Potenza MN. Behavioral addictions in addiction medicine: from mechanisms to practical considerations. Prog Brain Res. 2016;223:311–28.
6. Billieux J, Maurage P, Lopez-Fernandez O, Kuss DJ, Griffiths MD. Can disordered mobile phone use be considered a behavioral addiction? An update on current evidence and a comprehensive model for future research. Curr Addict Rep. 2015;2(2):156–62.
7. Carli V, Durkee T, Wasserman D, Hadlaczky G, Despalins R, Kramarz E, Wasserman C, Sarchiapone M, Hoven CW, Brunner R, Kaess M. The association between pathological internet use and comorbid psychopathology: a systematic review. Psychopathology. 2013;46(1):1–13.
8. Cash H, Rae CD, Steel AH, Winkler A. Internet addiction: a brief summary of research and practice. Curr Psychiatry Rev. 2012;8:292–8.
9. Cerniglia L, Zoratto F, Cimino S, Laviola G, Ammaniti M, Adriani W. Internet addiction in adolescence: neurobiological, psychosocial and clinical issues. Neurosci Biobehav Rev. 2017;76(Pt A):174–84.
10. Chakraborty K, Basu D, Kumar K. Internet addiction: consensus, controversies, and the way ahead. East Asian Arch Psychiatry. 2010;20(3):123–32.

11. Cooper A, Putnam DE, Planchon LA, Boies SC. Online sexual compulsivity: getting tangled in the net. Sex Addict Compuls. 1999;6(2):79–104.
12. Davis RA. A cognitive behavioral model of pathological internet use (PIU). Comput Hum Behav. 2001;17(2):187–95.
13. Elhai JD, Levine JC, Dvorak RD, Hall BJ. Fear of missing out, need for touch, anxiety and depression are related to problematic smartphone use. Comput Hum Behav. 2016;63:509–16.
14. González-Bueso V, Santamaría JJ, Fernández D, Merino L, Montero E, Ribas J. Association between internet gaming disorder or pathological videogame use and comorbid psychopathology: a comprehensive review. Int J Environ Res Public Health. 2008;15(4):668.
15. Grohol JM. Internet addiction guide. 2019 [updated 2019, May 17; cited 2019 September 29]. Available from: http://psychcentral.com/netaddiction/.
16. Han DH, Lee YS, Na C, et al. The effect of methylphenidate on Internet video game play in children with attention-deficit/hyperactivity disorder. Compr Psychiatry. 2009;50(3):251–6.
17. Hilton DL. Pornography addiction – a supranormal stimulus considered in the context of neuroplasticity. Socioaffective Neurosci Psych. 2013;3:20767.
18. Ito M. Mobile phones, Japanese youth, and the replacement of social contact. In: Ling R, Pedersen P, editors. Mobile communications: re-negotiation of the social sphere. London: Springer; 2005. p. 131–48.
19. Jeong SH, Kim H, Yum JY, Hwang Y. What type of content are smartphone users addicted to?: SNS vs. games. Comput Hum Behav. 2016;54:10–7. https://doi.org/10.1016/j.chb.2015.07.035.
20. Kuss DJ, Pontes HM, Griffiths MD. Neurobiological correlates in internet gaming disorder: a systematic literature review. Front Psych. 2018;9(166):1–12.
21. Lopez-Fernandez O, Kuss D, Romo L, Morvan Y, Kern L, Graziani P, Rousseau A, Rumpf HJ, Bischof A, Gässler AK, Schimmenti A, Passanisi A, Männikkö N, Kääriänen M, Demetrovics Z, Király O, Chóliz M, Zacaréc JJ, Serra E, Griffiths MD, Pontes HM, Lelonek-Kuleta B, Chwaszcz J, Zullino D, Rochat L, Achab S, Billieux J. Self-reported dependence on mobile phones in young adults: a European cross-cultural empirical survey. J Behav Addict. 2017;6(2):168–77.
22. Love T, Laier C, Brand M, Hatch L, Hajela R. Neuroscience of internet pornography addiction: a review and update. Behav Sci (Basel). 2015;5(3):388–433.
23. Mihajlov M, Vejmelka L. Internet addiction: a review of the first twenty years. Psychiatr Danub. 2017;29(3):260–72.
24. Panova T, Carbonell X. Is smartphone addiction really an addiction? *J Behav Addict.* 2018;7(2):252–9.
25. Paulus FW, Ohmann S, Von Gontard A, Popow C. Internet gaming disorder in children and adolescents: a systematic review. Dev Med Child Neuro. 2018;60:645–59.
26. Petry NM, Zajac K, Ginley MK. Behavioral addictions as mental disorders: to be or not to be? Annu Rev Clin Psychol. 2018;14:399–423.
27. Potenza MN. Clinical neuropsychiatric considerations regarding nonsubstance or behavioral addictions. Dialogues Clin Neurosci. 2017;19(3):281–91.
28. Smahel D, Brown BB, Blinka L. Associations between online friendship and Internet addiction among adolescents and emerging adults. Dev Psychol. 2012;48:381–8.
29. Smahel D, Blinka L, Ledabyl O. Playing MMORPGs: connections between addiction and identifying with a character. Cyberpsychol Behav. 2008;11:715–8.
30. Tereshchenko S, Kasparov E. Neurobiological risk factors for the development of internet addiction in adolescents. Behav Sci (Basel). 2019;9(6). pii: E62.
31. Winkler A, Dörsing B. Treatment of internet addiction disorder: a first meta-analysis [Diploma thesis]. Marburg: University of Marburg; 2011.
32. Young KS, Griffin-Shelley E, Cooper A, O'Mara J, Buchanan J. Online infidelity: a new dimension in couple relationships with implications for evaluation and treatment. Sex Addict Compuls. 2000;7(1–2):59–74.
33. Zajac K, Ginley MK, Chang R, Petry NM. Treatments for internet gaming disorder and internet addiction: a systematic review. Psychol Addict Behav. 2017;31(8):979–94.
34. Ascher MS, Levounis P. The behavioral addictions. Washington, DC: APP; 2015.
35. Diagnostic and statistical manual of mental disorders. 5th edn. Arlington: American Psychiatric Association; 2013.

Gambling Disorder

8

Evaristo Akerele

Introduction

Gambling is universal and has been in existence for several millennia, with lifetime gambling of approximately 78% in the United States [1].

Pathological gambling was initially recognized as a psychiatric disorder in 1980. At the time it was grouped under Impulse Control Disorders. Numerous data over the past decade suggest several similarities between pathological gambling and the substance use disorders, including some neurobiological overlap [2, 3]. More recently pathological gambling has been reclassified as "Gambling Disorder" in the addictions category of the *Diagnostic and Statistical Manual of Mental Disorders* (DSM-5) [4, 5, 6] The DSM-5 reclassified pathological gambling (renamed "disordered gambling") from the "Impulse Control Disorders Not Elsewhere Classified" category into the new "Substance-Related and Addictive Disorders" category. This new term and category lends credence to the concept that drugs are not necessary for individuals to be engaged in addictions. This is the concept of behavioral addictions; individuals may be compulsively and dysfunctionally engaged in behaviors without external drug administration, and these behaviors can be conceptualized within an addiction framework as different expressions of the same underlying syndrome. Its inclusion in DSM V reflects similarities between problem gambling and substance use disorders [7, 8].

Gambling is defined in DSM V as Persistent and recurrent problematic gambling behavior leading to clinically significant impairment or distress, as indicated by the individual exhibiting four (or more) of the following in a 12 month period:

(a) Needs to gamble with increasing amounts of money in order to achieve the desired excitement.
(b) Is restless or irritable when attempting to cut down or stop gambling.
(c) Has made repeated unsuccessful efforts to control, cut back, or stop gambling.
(d) Is often preoccupied with gambling (e.g., having persistent thoughts of reliving past gambling experiences, handicapping or planning the next venture, thinking of ways to get money with which to gamble).
(e) Often gambles when feeling distressed (e.g., helpless, guilty, anxious, depressed).
(f) After losing money gambling, often returns another day to get even ("chasing" one's losses).
(g) Lies to conceal the extent of involvement with gambling.

E. Akerele (✉)
Department of Psychiatry, New Jersey Medical School, Rutgers University, Newark, NJ, USA

E. Akerele (ed.), *Substance and Non-Substance Related Addictions*,
https://doi.org/10.1007/978-3-030-84834-7_8

(h) Has jeopardized or lost a significant relationship, job, or educational or career opportunity because of gambling.
(i) Relies on others to provide money to relieve desperate financial situations caused by gambling.

The gambling behavior is not better explained by a manic episode.

Disordered gambling is the only addictive disorder that is included in the main section of DSM-5. "Internet gaming disorder" another behavioral addiction has been flagged as a possible candidate for future inclusion in the addictions category. In the sections that follow, prevalence, global impact, public health relevance, risks factors, and treatment options are addressed.

Epidemiological studies that have employed screening instruments like the South Oaks Gambling Screen [9] have frequently generated higher prevalence estimates than have those employing DSM criteria [10, 11].

Meta-analytic data suggest that prevalence of past-year adult disordered gambling ranges from 0.1% to 2.7% [12] The estimated proportion of disordered gamblers among college students appears higher, estimated in one study at 7.89% [13].

DSM V criteria for disordered gambling are a guide in defining the characteristics of other behavioral disorders [14, 15]. For example, Young's Diagnostic Questionnaire [16] proposes the following criteria for Internet addiction: withdrawal, tolerance, preoccupation with the Internet, longer than intended time spent on the Internet, risk to significant relationships or employment relating to Internet use, lying about Internet use, and repeated, unsuccessful attempts to stop Internet use. Prevalence for data adolescents ranges from 4.0% to 19.1%, and for adults, from 0.7% to 18.3% [17]. Similarly, a range of prevalence estimates have been reported for problematic video-game playing among adolescent populations (4.2–20.0%), with adult estimates (11.9%) also falling in that range [17].

The relevance of gambling as a public health issue is of paramount importance. Gambling is often one of a variety of acceptable modalities of relaxation. It is mostly experienced as an enjoyable and innocuous activity. However, for a small group, it can become problematic with severe negative consequences. Therefore, the expansion of legalized gambling is an important public health concern [18]. In light of these concerns about gambling, it makes immanently good sense to study the epidemiology of this behavior. The epidemiological study provides information about the incidence of problem gambling. This will help inform efficacy of policies implemented to mitigate the public health issues associated with gambling [19].

The potential for negative public health impact globally has led to initiatives to reduce harm associated with this expansion. Generally, gambling disorder has not been given top priority as an urgent public health issue. However, a few jurisdictions have addressed it as a public health issue and focused on both prevention and treatment. Data from Australian and New Zealand suggest that the burden of harm due to gambling is approximately equal to that of major depressive disorder and alcohol use disorder [20]. Gambling-related burden of harm is approximately twice that of diabetes and three times that of substance use disorder. This burden is primarily due to the impact on finance, relationships, health, productivity, and education. This burden aggravates health and social disparities.

National current (past 12 months) gambling prevalence rates range from 0.1% to 6.0% [21]. These estimates are subject to the type of screening measures used and survey methodology. Williams and colleagues corrected for these methodological differences across global studies using applied weightings [19]. Their data suggest prevalence rates are generally low in Europe, high in Asia, and intermediate in Australasia and North America. The trend is regions with adequate data (Australia, Canada, and the United States) was an initial increase in problem gambling prevalence followed by a decrease over time. It is noteworthy that in these jurisdictions gambling availability increased throughout the period considered. In a meta-analysis of 34 Australian and New Zealand surveys conducted since 1990, the prevalence of problem gambling prevalence was found to both increase and decrease over time relative to the number of electronic gaming machines per capita in the year surveys were conducted [22]. Both relationships were strong, accounting for almost three-quarters of the prevalence variation. Therefore, these data support for both the availability and adaptation hypotheses. The availability hypotheses propose that increased gambling availability leads to increased participation and increased problem gambling. The adaptation proposes that over time adaptation due to "host" immunity and protective environmental changes, adaptation occurs. As a result there is a reduction in gambling participation and problem levels fall, in spite of increases in gambling availability. In general, greater gambling availability has led to increased consumption and increased problems globally. However, in both expanding and maturing markets, gambling consumption and problem gambling rates can decline, sometimes markedly, rather than increase. While reductions in gambling consumption and problems occur together in these situations, recent studies conducted in New Zealand, Sweden, and Australia have found a different pattern [23, 24]. Significant reductions in gambling participation occurred in these jurisdictions. However, prevalence rates remained unchanged. Data in two of these studies suggest increased gambling prevalence in spite of very large decreases in youth gambling participation [24]. These findings are not consistent with either availability or adaptation and cannot be elucidated simply by gambling exposure. Other factors that play a role in the onset and progression of problem gambling have to be considered. Although several factors contribute to the onset of problem gambling, both initially and in cases of relapse, gambling participation measures are the most strongly implicated [25]. Gambling frequently and the feeling of being skilled in these activities are strongly linked to the development of problem gambling. Participation in multiple gambling forms, high gambling expenditure, commencing gambling at a young age, and experiencing an early big win are additional risk factors.

Other factors related to gambling include but are not limited to having family members or friends who are regular and/or problem gamblers, gambling being the primary leisure activity and membership of rewards programs that encourage gambling. Men, young adults, low-income, and single individuals are almost universally found to be at elevated risk. Indigenous and some ethnic minority groups also have high incidence and prevalence rates. Additional risk factors identified in a number of groups include living in poor neighborhoods, membership of certain religious groups, lack of formal education, and unemployed status. Many of these high-risk groups live disproportionately in neighborhoods that are both deprived and have high concentrations of gambling venues. Living close to residential gambling venues is also associated with problem gambling. Some of these at-risk groups have low levels of gambling participation and limited prior exposure to more hazardous forms of gambling. A combination of increased vulnerability, low socio-economic disadvantage, and high gambling exposure plays a major role in the development of problem gambling [23]. This combination may also, in part, explain the plateauing of problem gambling prevalence rates in spite of falling general population gambling participation and spending rates. Another likely explanation for plateauing prevalence rates in the face of reduced gambling participation is that populations with many years of exposure to gambling will contain substantial numbers of past problem gamblers who are prone to relapse. Recent data [24–26] in populations of this type found that, of current 4 problem gamblers, at least fifty percent became problem gamblers during the preceding 12 months. Approximately thirty percent of these "new" problem gamblers were individuals who relapsed. Pathological and problem gambling are highly comorbid with a large number of other mental health disorders, especially substance use disorders [27]. They also suggest that problem gamblers also have significantly higher rates of mood, anxiety, and personality disorders. Problem gambling sometimes precedes the onset of the comorbid disorder and other times it is vice versa. Two of the recent studies suggest that substance abuse and dependence and behavioral addictions are significantly correlated with future problem gambling. These studies also identified other mental health disorders as predictors of problem gambling. Negative experiences early on in childhood, which include abuse and trauma are also correlated to later problem gambling development [28]. Furthermore, data genetics makes significant heritable contribution to problem gambling. The co-occurrence of gambling and alcohol use disorders appears to be partially attributable to genes that affect both disorders. Data from multiple studies suggest that cognitive characteristics and deficits and multiple neurotransmitter systems apparently play a significant role in emotional, cognitive, and behavioral aspects of problem gambling [7]. Problem gamblers are highly prone to cognitive distortions including over-rating their own gambling skill, illusions of control, illusory associations, superstitious beliefs, interpretive biases, e.g., the belief that a win will come after a number of loses and selective memory. Problem gambling prevalence is determined both by the inflow of new problem gamblers and outflow – through recovery, remission, migration, and death. From prospective general population studies, it is known that problem gambling prevalence rates usually remain much the same over a period of a few years. However, in any given year, around half move out of the problem gambling category and are replaced by "new" problem gamblers. As mentioned, this includes both first-time and relapsing cases. Adolescents are also avid gamblers.

Adolescent gambling is illegal, it is nonetheless relatively common [29]. Studies suggest that individuals under the age of 18 years often report taking part in a variety of gambling activities, and youth is often reported as a common risk factor for developing gambling disorder (GD) [30, 31]. The risk factors for gambling disorder are numerous. These include but are not limited to individual risk factors (alcohol use frequency, antisocial behaviors, depression, male gender, cannabis use, illicit drug use, impulsivity, number of gambling activities, problem gambling severity, sensation seeking, tobacco use, violence, and under-controlled temperament), relationship risk factor (peer antisocial behaviors), community risk factor (poor academic performance), individual protective factor (socio-economic status), and relationship protective factors such as parental supervision and social problems [32].

Although the prevalence of GD is higher in younger age groups, it is also a considerable problem for many older adults. Older individuals with GD were more likely to be single or divorced/separated [33]. One of the primary reasons for engaging in gambling in this group is an effort to minimize negative emotional states. Older individuals may either have limited access to other exciting activities or are unable to participate in these activities. These factors, along with having a fixed income and limited prospects of future earnings, make them an extremely vulnerable group [34]. However, risk factors for gambling disorder are multifactorial.

These factors include psychological risk factors such as impulsivity. This is a common feature in nearly all addictions, including GD [35–37]. Personality traits are associated with GD, yet no single profile can encompass all gamblers. However, there is a degree of consensus that harm avoidance, low self-directedness, and difficulties with decision-making and planning are, alongside impulsivity and sensation seeking, closely associated with the risk of developing a gambling problem [38].

In comparison with the general population, individuals with GD have an increased risk for suicide. A study in treatment-seeking individuals with GD suggests that approximately 32% of individuals had experienced suicidal ideation [39], whereas another study found that 30.2% of patients reported one or more suicide attempts in the 12 months preceding GD treatment [40]. Increased medical and psychiatric comorbidity leads to a significantly decreased quality of life because of GD, yet still only 10% of individuals with GD ever seek treatment for GD [41]. However, some reports indicate that treatment-seeking rates are higher for patients with greater disorder severity [42].

Reducing the prevalence of problem gambling, and to some extent associated harms, requires implementing primary prevention measures to lower the rate of problem onset, as well as treatment and other measures to accelerate recovery or remission and prevent relapse. While further research is required, it appears that many of the factors implicated in problem gambling development also contribute to problem chronicity and relapse. A variety of policy and prevention approaches have been developed to reduce the prevalence of problem gambling and gambling-related harm [20]. Those that focus on the agent gambling include measures intended to (1) reduce gambling supply, (2) reduce the potency of gambling activities and participation, and (3) reduce demand. Supply reduction interventions include legal and regulatory measures to: prohibit or reduce the number of gambling venues and outlets, either generally or selectively (e.g., in vulnerable neighborhoods); reduce access hours; impose access restrictions (e.g., based on age or resident status); and, implement venue exclusion. In the 5 cases of EGMs, the main contributor to gambling harm in most jurisdictions where they have been widely introduced, potency reduction measures include modifying game parameters such as speed of play, number of near misses, bet size and mandatory pay-outs; enforced breaks in play; static and dynamic messaging, self-appraisal messaging, monetary and time-based pop-up messaging; normative feedback and enhanced messaging; limit setting (precommitment), behavioral tracking tools; and prohibition and modification of note acceptors. Demand reduction measures include smoking bans; prohibiting or limiting alcohol use while gambling, restricting access to money (e.g., credit and ATMs); modifying venue design; restricting advertising, promotions and sponsorship; information and awareness campaigns, education regarding gambling and gambling harm; changing attitudes; changing cognitions; venue staff training and host responsibility programs; on-site information and/or counseling centers, helplines and on-line face-to-face interventions for problem gamblers and significant others. It is not known how effective most of the foregoing measures are and, as mentioned, it appears that those likely to be least effective are the ones most frequently deployed. This is perhaps not unexpected as problem gamblers account for a large proportion of gambling revenue, for instance, as much as 40% in the case of EGMs in Australia [43]. Governments and gambling providers seek to maximize revenue and profits; both of which are likely to fall, probably substantially, if prevention and harm reduction measures are fully and effectively implemented. Hancock and Smith [44] maintain that the widely followed Reno Model of responsible gambling intended to provide consumer protection and reduce gambling-related harm, paradoxically, is an impediment to implementation of effective prevention and harm reduction measures. In large part, this attributed to the model's emphasis on individual responsibility and problem gamblers. They call for this approach to be incorporated within broader framework that includes public health principles, consumer protection, duty-of-care, regulatory responsibility, and independent research. While much of the research and policy focus has been on problem gambling, as with a number of other public health issues, it has been shown that most of the harm associated with gambling participation is generated by gamblers other than problem gamblers (the "prevention paradox"). A recent Victorian study found that only 15% of harm was attributable to problem gamblers. Most harm was occasioned by people classified as low or moderate-risk gamblers [45]. This occurs because while problem gamblers and people associated with them experience high levels of harm, they are greatly outnumbered by subclinical gamblers. Consequently, it is important that this group is also the focus of regulatory and preventive interventions. Given the very high levels of gambling-related harm in some population sectors targeted as well as more universal approaches will be required to reduce harm and disparities between different ethnic, socioeconomic, and other social groups [46]. Many of the non-gambling risk and protective factors for at-risk and problem gambling are common to other mental health and addiction disorders. Reducing these risk factors and strengthening protective factors can be expected to have health and social benefits that extend beyond problem gambling and gambling-related harm.

Similarity Between Substance Use and Behavioral Disorders [47, 48]

Individuals with substance use and behavioral disorders generally score high on self-report measures of impulsivity and low on measures of harm avoidance [3]. However, some data suggest that individuals with gambling use disorder may exhibit high levels of harm avoidance [49]. Individuals with gambling disorder and obsessive-compulsive disorder (OCD) both score highly on measures of compulsivity. However, in individuals with gambling disorder these impairments are apparently limited to poor control over mental activities and ability to control motor behavior-related urges [50].

Regulation of addictive behaviors maybe motivated by either delayed negative consequences or immediate reward: that is, temporal or delay discounting. Reduction in prefrontal cortex control over subcortical processes may culminate in motivations to engage in addictive behavior [51]. Individuals with disordered gambling and substance use disorder (SUD) display rapid temporal discounting of rewards; that is diminished temporal or delay discounting. Therefore, they are more prone to select smaller, earlier rewards than larger ones that come later [52, 53]. Although some data suggest that abstinent individuals with substance use disorders (SUDs) perform better than do individuals with current SUDs, other data suggest no significant differences [52]. A recent study suggests that delay discounting did not differ in individuals with disordered gambling pretreatment and one-year posttreatment [54].

Dopamine has been implicated in learning, motivation, salience attribution, and the processing of rewards and losses (including their anticipation [reward prediction] and the representation of their values) [55]. Dopamine plays a significant role in reward circuits, including projections from the ventral tegmental area to ventral striatum in SUDs [55]. Therefore, it makes immanently good sense for studies on behavioral addictions to focus on investigating dopamine transmission. Dopamine release in the ventral striatum has been positively associated with Iowa Gambling Task performance in healthy control subjects but negatively in individuals with disordered gambling [56]. This indicates that dopamine release probably plays a role in both adaptive and maladaptive decision-making.

Serotonin is implicated in emotions, motivation, decision-making, behavioral control, and inhibition of behavior. All of which in turn play a significant role are vital in addictive behavior. Therefore, it is not surprising that dysregulation of serotonin functioning may mediate behavioral inhibition and impulsivity in disordered gambling [57]. Levels of the serotonin metabolite 5-hydroxyindoleacetic acid (5-HIAA) in cerebrospinal fluid are reduced in disordered gambling [58]. The peripheral marker of serotonin activity, platelet monoamine oxidase is also low in men with disordered gambling [59, 60] providing additional support for serotonergic dysfunction. Furthermore, striatal binding of a ligand with high affinity for the serotonin 1B receptor was associated with problem-gambling severity among individuals with disordered gambling [61]. These findings are consistent with those from challenge studies using meta-chlorophenylpiperazine (m-CPP), a partial agonist with high affinity for the serotonin 1B receptor. These studies observe different biological and behavioral responses in individuals with behavioral or substance addictions relative to those without SUDs/behavioral disorders in response to m-CPP. Other studies indicate dysregulated hypothalamic-pituitary-adrenal axis has been observed in disordered gambling [62]. Noradrenaline may be involved in the peripheral arousal associated with gambling [63, 64].

Data suggest neurocircuitry between behavioral and substance addictions is shared; especially in involving the frontal and striatal regions. Studies using reward-processing and decision-making tasks have identified important contributions from subcortical (e.g., striatum) and frontal cortical areas, particularly the ventromedial prefrontal cortex (vmPFC). Among disordered gamblers, versus healthy controls, both decreased [65] and increased vmPFC activity [66] have been reported during simulated gambling and decision-making tasks. These findings may have been influenced by the specific tasks used, the populations studied, or other factors [67]. Relatively greater activation of other frontal and basal ganglia areas, including the amygdala, during high-risk gambling decision making in the Iowa Gambling Task has been observed among disordered gamblers [66]. While data are relatively limited for other behavioral addictions, several recent cue-induction studies have demonstrated activation of brain regions associated with drug-cue exposure.

The mesolimbic pathway ("reward pathway") from the ventral tegmental area to the nucleus accumbens has been implicated in both substance and behavioral addictions [68]. Relatively decreased ventral striatal activation has been reported in disordered gamblers during monetary reward anticipation [69] and simulated gambling [70]. More recent data using larger samples, however, show smaller amygdala and hippocampal volumes in individuals with disordered gambling, similar to findings in SUDs [71].

Twin studies suggest that genetic factors may contribute more than environmental factors to the overall variance of risk for developing disordered gambling [72]. Data from the Vietnam Era Twin Registry (using men only) estimate the heritability of disordered gambling to be 50–60% [73], a statistic similar to the percentages for SUDs [74].

Pharmacotherapy

Opioid receptor antagonists such as naltrexone currently have the most empirical support. Data suggest naltrexone is effective in reducing the intensity of urges to gamble, gambling thoughts, and gambling behavior especially in individuals reporting higher intensity of gambling urges [75]. The positive effects persist in some cases after naltrexone discontinuation [76]. Dosage may play an important role in ensuring efficacy. Naltrexone in doses of 100–200 mg/day successfully reduced symptoms of hypersexual disorder and compulsive shopping disorder [77]. Nalmefene (40 mg/day) significantly improved disordered gambling [78]. Naltrexone (50 mg/day) was also effective and associated with fewer adverse effects [78]. Stronger urges at treatment onset and a positive family history of alcoholism are associated with better treatment outcome with naltrexone and nalmefene [79].

Although selective serotonin reuptake inhibitors (SSRIs) were one of the first medications that were used to treat disordered gambling, controlled clinical trials assessing SSRIs have demonstrated mixed results for both behavioral and substance addictions. Fluvoxamine and paroxetine were reported to be superior to placebo in several trials [80, 81] but not in others [82, 83]. Efficacy may differ among behavioral addictions. Citalopram, another SSRI, was found effective in reducing hypersexual disorder symptoms among homosexual and bisexual men [84] but, among individuals with Internet addiction disorder, did not reduce the number of hours spent online or improve global functioning [85]. SSRI treatments remain an active area of investigation, and further research is needed to assess the potential clinical utilization of SSRIs for disordered gambling and other behavioral addictions.

Glutamatergic treatments have shown mixed promise in small controlled trials. N-acetyl cysteine has shown preliminary efficacy both as a stand-alone agent [86] and in conjunction with behavioral treatment [87]. Topiramate, however, did not show any differences to placebo in treating disordered gambling [88]. Additionally, the results from these and most other pharmacotherapy trials of behavioral addictions are limited because of the trials' small sample sizes and short-term treatment durations.

Behavioral Treatments

Meta-analyses of psychotherapeutic and behavioral treatment approaches for disordered gambling suggest that they can result in significant improvements. Positive effects can be retained (though to a lesser degree) over follow-ups of up to two years [89].

One approach that has gained empirical support from randomized trials is cognitive behavioral therapy (CBT). This semi-structured, problem-oriented approach focuses, in part, on challenging the irrational thought processes and beliefs that are thought to maintain compulsive behaviors. During therapy, patients learn and then implement skills and strategies to change those patterns and interrupt addictive behaviors [90, 91]. Therapists facilitate the replacement of dysfunctional emotions, behaviors, and cognitive processes through engagement in alternative behaviors and a series of goal-orientated, explicit, systematic procedures. CBT is multifaceted but typically involves keeping a diary of significant events and associated feelings, thoughts, and behaviors; recording cognitions, assumptions, evaluations, and beliefs that may be maladaptive; trying new ways of behaving and reacting (e.g., replacing video-game playing with outdoor activities); and, in the cases of disordered gambling and compulsive shopping, learning techniques to properly manage finances [92]. Such factors are important for initial abstinence but are also essential for relapse prevention. The particular therapeutic techniques that are employed may vary according to the particular type of patient or issue. For example, patients who are having trouble controlling cravings may utilize modules that teach coping strategies specifically for managing cravings. CBT approaches have the strongest evidence base of any of the psychotherapeutic approaches [93], with a meta-analysis of randomized, controlled trials demonstrating improvement in gambling-related variables after treatment and at follow-ups in problem gamblers [89]. In individuals with Internet addiction, CBT has demonstrated efficacy in reducing time spent online, improving social relationships, increasing engagement in offline activities, and increasing the ability to abstain from problematic Internet use.

In addition to psychotherapeutic treatments such as CBT, self-help options are available. Although such options have been found to be beneficial for a range of individuals, they may be especially attractive to those people who do not meet diagnostic criteria for disordered gambling and who find psychotherapeutic intervention too costly or intensive [94]. A recent study suggests that Internet-based programs may help reduce disordered gambling symptoms, including at a three-year follow-up [95]. A popular self-help group based on mutual support is Gambler's Anonymous (GA). Based on the 12-step model of Alcoholics Anonymous, GA stresses commitment to abstinence, which is facilitated by a support network of more experienced group members ("sponsors"). The steps involve admitting loss of control over gambling behavior; recognizing a higher power that can give strength; examining past errors (with the help of a sponsor or experienced member) and making amends; learning to live a new life with a new code of behavior; and helping and carrying the message to other problem gamblers [96]. Interestingly, individuals with (vs. without) a history of GA attendance were more likely to display higher disordered gambling severity, more years of gambling problems, and larger debts at intake to (other) treatment [97]. GA has been shown to have beneficial effects for attendees with varying degrees of gambling severity; [98] however, attrition rates are often high [99]. The benefits of GA may be increased with adjunctive personalized therapy, and these two approaches, when combined, may be mutually beneficial in promoting continuation of treatment [100]. Meta-analyses indicate other self-help interventions (e.g., self-help workbooks and audiotapes) also demonstrate beneficial effects in disordered gambling and are superior to no treatment or placebo. The positive effects, however, are typically not as strong as those of other empirically tested psychotherapeutic approaches [89].

Brief motivational interviewing or enhancement—even as little as a 15-minute telephone consultation—has not only been demonstrated to be effective but in several studies has been shown to be more effective than other lengthier and more intensive approaches [101]. Motivational interventions center on exploring and resolving a patients' ambivalence toward change, with the aim of facilitating intrinsic motivation and self-efficacy through dealing with problem behaviors. Such interventions could provide a cost-effective, resource-conserving approach and could be particularly useful in individuals reluctant to engage in prolonged therapy on account of stigma, shame, or financial concerns.

Although the precise neural mechanisms mediating the effects of behavioral and pharmacological treatments are unclear, an improved understanding of them could provide insight into the mechanisms underlying specific therapies and assist in treatment development and in matching treatments and individuals. Many promising facets of treatment have yet to be examined in the context of behavioral addictions. For example, positive family involvement has been shown to be beneficial in the treatment of SUDs [102] and may be similarly helpful in treating behavioral addictions. Additionally, phenotypic heterogeneity exists within each behavioral addiction, and identifying clinically relevant subgroups remains an important endeavor. Testing specific, well-defined behavioral therapies in randomized, controlled trials is also important in validating treatment approaches. Neurocircuitry relating to specific behavioral therapies has been proposed [103]. The incorporation of pre- and posttreatment neuroimaging assessments into clinical trials represents an important next step for testing these hypotheses.

While much progress has been made in identifying and developing effective pharmacological and behavioral therapies, no existing treatment is completely effective on its own. Combining complementary treatments may help to address weaknesses in either therapy and may thereby catalyze beneficial treatment outcomes. Initial trials using combined approaches have yielded mixed results, with some positive results reported for disordered gambling [87].

Conclusion

Gambling disorder is a significant global public health and economic issue. Gambling as a behavioral disorder is more acceptable to society at large than substance use. The perils of substance use and potential for a disorder are more obvious. The peril of gambling and the potential culmination in a gambling disorder is salient. This makes gambling disorder more likely to be underestimate and therefore more likely evoke relatively greater havoc than substance use disorder.

The DSM V Classification of gambling disorder is a great start to addressing the challenge of a litany of definitions such as pathological gambling, disordered gambling, problem gambling, etc. Under the DSM V definition, future researchers can be on the same page as they seek out the etiology and potential solutions to this problem.

It is apparently however that the etiology is multifactorial and that the solution must be multifactorial. The data suggest promising pharmacological and psychotherapeutic solutions. However, similar to substance use disorders, a significant review of global policy will be necessary for the successful eradication of gambling disorder. Policies should promote responsible engagement in these behaviors and improve treatment access.

References

1. Kessler RC, Hwang I, LaBrie R, Petukhova M, Sampson NA, Winters KC, Shaffer HJ. DSM-IV pathological gambling in the National Comorbidity Survey Replication. Psychol Med. 2008;38:1351–60. https://doi.org/10.1017/S0033291708002900.
2. Petry NM. Should the scope of addictive behaviors be broadened to include pathological gambling? Addiction. 2006;101(Suppl 1):152–60.
3. Leeman RF, Potenza MN. Similarities and differences between pathological gambling and substance use disorders: a focus on impulsivity and compulsivity. Psychopharmacology (Berl). 2012;219:469–90. https://doi.org/10.1007/s00213-011-2550-7.
4. American Psychiatric Association. Diagnostic and statistical manual of mental disorders. 5th edn. Washington, DC: American Psychiatric Association. 2013. https://doi.org/10.1176/appi.books.9780890425596, https://dx.doi.org/10.1176%2Fappi.books.9780890425596. [Google Scholar].
5. Petry NM, Blanco C, Auriacombe M, et al. An overview of and rationale for changes proposed for pathological gambling in DSM-5. J Gambl Stud. 2014;30(2):493–502. https://doi.org/10.1007/s10899-013-9370-0. [PMC free article] [PubMed] [CrossRef] [Google Scholar].
6. Petry NM, Blanco C, Auriacombe M, Borges G, Bucholz K, Crowley TJ, Grant BF, Hasin DS, O'Brien C. An overview of and rationale for changes proposed for pathological gambling in DSM-5. J Gambl Stud. 2013. https://doi.org/10.1007/s10899-013-9370-0.

7. Hodgins DC, Stea JN, Grant JE. Gambling disorders. Lancet. 2011;378(9806):1874–84. Miers D. Regulating commercial gambling. Oxford: Oxford University Press; 2004.
8. Wakefield JC. DSM-5: an overview of changes and controversies. Clin Soc Work J. 2013;41(2):139–54.
9. Lesieur HR, Blume SB. The South Oaks Gambling Screen (SOGS): a new instrument for the identification of pathological gamblers. Am J Psychiatry. 1987;144:1184–8. [PubMed] [Google Scholar].
10. Shaffer HJ, Hall MN, Vander BJ. Estimating the prevalence of disordered gambling behavior in the United States and Canada: a research synthesis. Am J Public Health. 1999;89:1369–76. [PMC free article] [PubMed] [Google Scholar].
11. Petry NM, Stinson FS, Grant BF. Comorbidity of DSM-IV pathological gambling and other psychiatric disorders: results from the National Epidemiologic Survey on Alcohol and Related Conditions. J Clin Psychiatry. 2005;66:564–74. [PubMed] [Google Scholar].
12. Lorains FK, Cowlishaw S, Thomas SA. Prevalence of comorbid disorders in problem and pathological gambling: systematic review and meta-analysis of population surveys. Addiction. 2011;106:490–8. [PubMed] [Google Scholar].
13. Blinn-Pike L, Worthy SL, Jonkman JN. Disordered gambling among college students: a meta-analytic synthesis. J Gambl Stud. 2007;23:175–83. [PubMed] [Google Scholar].
14. Gentile DA, Choo H, Liau A, et al. Pathological video game use among youths: a two–year longitudinal study. Pediatrics. 2011;127:e319–29. [PubMed] [Google Scholar].
15. Ko CH, Yen JY, Chen SH, Yang MJ, Lin HC, Yen CF. Proposed diagnostic criteria and the screening and diagnostic tool of Internet addiction in college students. Compr Psychiatry. 2009;50:378–84. [PubMed] [Google Scholar].
16. Young KS. Internet addiction: symptoms, evaluation and treatment. In: Vande Creek L, Jackson T, editors. Innovations in clinical practice: a source book. Sarasota: Professional Resource; 1999. p. 19–31. [Google Scholar].
17. Yau YHC, Crowley MJ, Mayes LC, Potenza MN. Are Internet use and video-game-playing addictive behaviors? Biological, clinical and public health implications for youths and adults. Minerva Psichiatr. 2012;53:153–70. [PMC free article] [PubMed] [Google Scholar].
18. Williams RJ, Volberg RA, Stevens RMG. The population prevalence of problem gambling: methodological influences, standardized rates, jurisdictional differences, and worldwide trends. Lethbridge: University of Lethbridge. Northampton: Gemini Research; 2012. Prepared for the Ontario Problem Gambling Research Centre and the Ontario Ministry of Health and Long Term Care.
19. Williams RJ, West BL, Simpson R.I. Prevention of problem gambling: a comprehensive review of the evidence and identified best practices. Report prepared for the Ontario Problem Gambling Research Centre and The Ontario Ministry of Health and Long Term Care, 2012. Retrieved from https://www.uleth.ca/dspace/handle/10133/3121.
20. Browne M, Bellringer M, Greer N, Kolandai-Matchett K, Rawat V, Langham E, et al. Permit but discourage: regulating excessive consumption. New York: Oxford University Press, Inc.; 2017, preprint.
21. Calado F, Griffiths MD. Problem gambling worldwide: an update and systematic review of empirical research (2000–2015). J Behav Addict. 2016;5(4):592–613.
22. Storer J, Abbott M, Stubbs J. Access or adaptation? A meta-analysis of surveys of problem gambling prevalence in Australia and New Zealand with respect to concentration of electronic gaming machines. Int Gambling Stud. 2009;9(3):225–44. https://doi.org/10.1080/14459790903257981. The data team, (2017). The world's biggest gamblers, The Economist. 9 February 2017. Retrieved from http://www.economist.com/blogs/graphicdetail/2017/02/daily-chart-4.
23. Abbott M. Beyond Reno: a critical commentary on Hancock and Smith [Advance online publication]. Int J Ment Heal Addict. 2017. https://doi.org/10.1007/s11469-017-9794-3.
24. Abbott M, Stone CA, Billi R, Yeung K. Gambling and problem gambling in Victoria, Australia: changes over 5 years. J Gambl Stud. 2016;32(1):47–78.
25. Williams RJ, Hann RG, Schopflocher D, West B, McLaughlin P, White N, et al. Quinte longitudinal study of gambling and problem gambling. Report prepared for the Ontario Problem Gambling Research Centre. Guelph, Ontario. February 20, 2015. 2015. Available from: https://www.uleth.ca/dspace/handle/10133/3641.
26. Romild U, Volberg R, Abbott M. The Swedish longitudinal gambling study (Swelogs): design and methods of the epidemiological (EP-) track. Int J Methods Psychiatr Res. 2014;23(3):372–86. 8.
27. Rash CJ, Weinstock J, Van Patten R. A review of gambling disorder and substance use disorders. Subst Abuse Rehabil. 2016;7:3–13. https://doi.org/10.2147/SAR.S83460. [PMC free article] [PubMed] [CrossRef] [Google Scholar] F1000 Recommendation.
28. Felsher JR, Derevensky JL, Gupta R. Young adults with gambling problems: the impact of childhood maltreatment. Int J Mental Health Addict. 2010;8:545–56.
29. 77. Nastally BL, Dixon MR. Adolescent gambling: current trends in treatment and future directions. Int J Adolesc Med Health. 2010;22(1):95–111. [PubMed] [Google Scholar].
30. 78. Zhai ZW, Yip SW, Steinberg MA, et al. Relationships between perceived family gambling and peer gambling and adolescent problem gambling and binge-drinking. J Gambl Stud. 2017;33(4):1169–

85. https://doi.org/10.1007/s10899-017-9670-x. [PMC free article] [PubMed] [CrossRef] [Google Scholar] F1000 Recommendation.
31. Dowling NA, Shandley KA, Oldenhof E, et al. The intergenerational transmission of at-risk/problem gambling: the moderating role of parenting practices. Am J Addict. 2017;26(7):707–12. https://doi.org/10.1111/ajad.12599. [PubMed] [CrossRef] [Google Scholar] F1000 Recommendation.
32. Dowling NA, Merkouris SS, Greenwood CJ, et al. Early risk and protective factors for problem gambling: a systematic review and meta-analysis of longitudinal studies. Clin Psychol Rev. 2017;51:109–24. https://doi.org/10.1016/j.cpr.2016.10.008. [PubMed] [CrossRef] [Google Scholar] F1000 Recommendation.
33. Subramaniam M, Wang P, Soh P, et al. Prevalence and determinants of gambling disorder among older adults: a systematic review. Addict Behav. 2015;41:199–209. https://doi.org/10.1016/j.addbeh.2014.10.007. [PubMed] [CrossRef] [Google Scholar].
34. Sauvaget A, Jiménez-Murcia S, Fernández-Aranda F, et al. Unexpected online gambling disorder in late-life: a case report. Front Psychol. 2015;6:655. https://doi.org/10.3389/fpsyg.2015.00655. [PMC free article] [PubMed] [CrossRef] [Google Scholar].
35. Steward T, Mestre-Bach G, Fernández-Aranda F, et al. Delay discounting and impulsivity traits in young and older gambling disorder patients. Addict Behav. 2017;71:96–103. https://doi.org/10.1016/j.addbeh.2017.03.001. [PubMed] [CrossRef] [Google Scholar].
36. Estevez A, Herrero-Fernández D, Sarabia I, et al. The impulsivity and sensation-seeking mediators of the psychological consequences of pathological gambling in adolescence. J Gambl Stud. 2015;31(1):91–103. https://doi.org/10.1007/s10899-013-9419-0. [PubMed] [CrossRef] [Google Scholar].
37. Rodda SN, Lubman DI, Iyer R, et al. Subtyping based on readiness and confidence: the identification of help-seeking profiles for gamblers accessing web-based counselling. Addiction. 2015;110(3):494–501. https://doi.org/10.1111/add.12796. [PubMed] [CrossRef] [Google Scholar].
38. Jiménez-Murcia S, Granero R, Fernández-Aranda F, et al. Predictors of outcome among pathological gamblers receiving cognitive behavioral group therapy. Eur Addict Res. 2015;21(4):169–78. https://doi.org/10.1159/000369528. [PubMed] [CrossRef] [Google Scholar.
39. Petry NM, Kiluk BD. Suicidal ideation and suicide attempts in treatment-seeking pathological gamblers. J Nerv Ment Dis. 2002;190(7):462–9. [PMC free article] [PubMed] [Google Scholar].
40. Battersby M, Tolchard B, Scurrah M, et al. Suicide ideation and behaviour in people with pathological gambling attending a treatment service. Int J Ment Health Addiction. 2006;4:233–46. https://doi.org/10.1007/s11469-006-9022-z. [CrossRef] [Google Scholar].
41. Slutske WS. Natural recovery and treatment-seeking in pathological gambling: results of two U.S. national surveys. Am J Psychiatry. 2006;163(2):297–302. https://doi.org/10.1176/appi.ajp.163.2.297. [PubMed] [CrossRef] [Google Scholar].
42. Nautiyal KM, Okuda M, Hen R, et al. Gambling disorder: an integrative review of animal and human studies. Ann N Y Acad Sci. 2017;1394(1):106–27. https://doi.org/10.1111/nyas.13356. [PMC free article] [PubMed] [CrossRef] [Google Scholar] F1000 Recommendation.
43. Abbott MW, Romild U, Volberg RA. Gambling and problem gambling in Sweden: changes between 1998 and 2009. J Gambl Stud. 2014;30(4), 985–99. Australian Government Productivity Commission (2010). Gambling: Productivity Commission Inquiry Report. Report no. 50. Canberra, Australia: Productivity Commission. Retrieved from www.pc.gov.au/projects/inquiry/gambling%2D%2D-2009/report.
44. Hancock L, Smith G. Critiquing the Reno model I-IV international influence on regulators and governments (2004–2015): the distorted reality of "responsible gambling" [Advance online publication]. Int J Ment Heal Addict. 2017. https://doi.org/10.1007/s11469-017-9746-y.
45. Browne M, Langham E, Rawat V, Greer N, Li E, Rose J, et al. Assessing gambling related harm in victoria: a public health perspective. Melbourne, Australia: Victorian Responsible Gambling Foundation; 2016. Retrieved from https://www.responsiblegambling.vic.gov.au. el-Guebaly N, Casey DM, Currie SR, Hodgins DC, Schopflocher DP, Smith GJ, Williams RJ. The Leisure, Lifestyle, & Lifecycle Project (LLLP): a longitudinal study of gambling in Alberta. Final Report for the Alberta Gambling Research Institute. 2015. Retrieved from http://prism.ucalgary.ca/handle/1880/50377.
46. Abbott M. Gambling and gambling harm in New Zealand: a 28-year case study. Int J Mental Health Addict [Advance online publication]. 2017. https://doi.org/10.1007/s11469-017-9767-6.
47. Yau YH, Potenza MN. Gambling disorder and other behavioral addictions: recognition and treatment. Harv Rev Psychiatry. 2015;23(2):134–46. https://doi.org/10.1097/HRP.0000000000000051.
48. Menchon JM, Mestre-Bach G, Steward T, Fernández-Aranda F, Jiménez-Murcia S. An overview of gambling disorder: from treatment approaches to risk factors. F1000Research. 2018;7:434. https://doi.org/10.12688/f1000research.12784.1.
49. Tavares H, Zilberman ML, Hodgins DC, El-Guebaly N. Comparison of craving between pathological gamblers and alcoholics. Alcohol Clin Exp Res. 2005;29:1427–31. [PubMed] [Google Scholar].
50. Odlaug BL, Chamberlain SR, Grant JE. Motor inhibition and cognitive flexibility in pathologic

skin picking. Prog Neuropsychopharmacol Biol Psychiatry. 2010;34:208–11. [PubMed] [Google Scholar].
51. Everitt BJ, Robbins TW. Neural systems of reinforcement for drug addiction: from actions to habits to compulsion. Nat Neurosci. 2005;8:1481–9. [PubMed] [Google Scholar].
52. Reynolds B. A review of delay-discounting research with humans: relations to drug use and gambling. Behav Pharmacol. 2006;17:651–67. [PubMed] [Google Scholar].
53. Mitchell MR. MNP addictions and personality traits: impulsivity and related constructs. Curr Behav Neurosci Rep. 2014;1:1–12. [PMC free article] [PubMed] [Google Scholar].
54. Petry NM. Discounting of probabilistic rewards is associated with gambling abstinence in treatment-seeking pathological gamblers. J Abnorm Psychol. 2012;121:151–9. [PMC free article] [PubMed] [Google Scholar].
55. Koob GF, Volkow ND. Neurocircuitry of addiction. Neuropsychopharmacology. 2010;35:217–38. [PMC free article] [PubMed] [Google Scholar].
56. Linnet J, Moller A, Peterson E, Gjedde A, Doudet D. Inverse association between dopaminergic neurotransmission and Iowa Gambling Task performance in pathological gamblers and healthy controls. Scand J Psychol. 2011;52:28–34. [PubMed] [Google Scholar].
57. Linnet J, Møller A, Peterson E, Gjedde A, Doudet D. Dopamine release in ventral striatum during Iowa Gambling Task performance is associated with increased excitement levels in pathological gambling. Addiction. 2011;106:383–90. [PubMed] [Google Scholar].
58. Nordin C, Eklundh T. Altered CSF 5–HIAA disposition in pathological male gamblers. CNS Spectr. 1999;4:25–33. [PubMed] [Google Scholar].
59. de Castro IP, Ibanez A, Saiz–Ruiz J, Fernandez–Piqueras J. Concurrent positive association between pathological gambling and functional DNA polymorphisms at the MAO-A and the 5-HT transporter genes. Mol Psychiatry. 2002;7:927–8. [PubMed] [Google Scholar].
60. Ibanez A, Perez de Castro I, Fernandez–Piqueras J, Blanco C, Saiz–Ruiz J. Pathological gambling and DNA polymorphic markers at MAO-A and MAO-B genes. Mol Psychiatry. 2000;5:105–9. [PubMed] [Google Scholar].
61. Potenza MN, Walderhaug E, Henry S, et al. Serotonin 1B receptor imaging in pathological gambling. World J Biol Psychiatry. 2013;14:139–45. [PMC free article] [PubMed] [Google Scholar].
62. Meyer G, Schwertfeger J, Exton MS, et al. Neuroendocrine response to casino gambling in problem gamblers. Psychoneuroendocrinology. 2004;29:1272–80. [PubMed] [Google Scholar].
63. Pallanti S, Bernardi S, Allen A, et al. Noradrenergic function in pathological gambling: blunted growth hormone response to clonidine. J Psychopharmacol. 2010;24:847–53. [PubMed] [Google Scholar].
64. Elman I, Becerra L, Tschibelu E, Yamamoto R, George E, Borsook D. Yohimbine-induced amygdala activation in pathological gamblers: a pilot study. PLoS One. 2012;7:e31118. [PMC free article] [PubMed] [Google Scholar].
65. Tanabe J, Thompson L, Claus E, Dalwani M, Hutchison K, Banich MT. Prefrontal cortex activity is reduced in gambling and nongambling substance users during decision-making. Hum Brain Mapp. 2007;28:1276–86. [PMC free article] [PubMed] [Google Scholar].
66. Power Y, Goodyear B, Crockford D. Neural correlates of pathological gamblers preference for immediate rewards during the Iowa gambling task: an fMRI study. J Gambl Stud. 2011:1–14. [PubMed] [Google Scholar].
67. 108. Leyton M, Vezina P. On cue: striatal ups and downs in addictions. Biol Psychiatry. 2012;72:e21–e2. [PMC free article] [PubMed] [Google Scholar].
68. Hommer DW, Bjork JM, Gilman JM. Imaging brain response to reward in addictive disorders. Ann N Y Acad Sci. 2011;1216:50–61. [PubMed] [Google Scholar].
69. 100. Choi J-S, Shin Y-C, Jung WH, et al. Altered brain activity during reward anticipation in pathological gambling and obsessive-compulsive disorder. PLoS One. 2012;7:e45938. [PMC free article] [PubMed] [Google Scholar].
70. Reuter J, Raedler T, Rose M, Hand I, Glascher J, Buchel C. Pathological gambling is linked to reduced activation of the mesolimbic reward system. Nat Neurosci. 2005;8:147–8. [PubMed] [Google Scholar].
71. Rahman AS, Xu J, Potenza MN. Hippocampal and amygdalar volumetric differences in pathological gambling: a preliminary study of the associations with the behavioral inhibition system. Neuropsychopharmacology. 2014;39:738–45. [PMC free article] [PubMed] [Google Scholar].
72. Blanco C, Myers J, Kendler KS. Gambling, disordered gambling and their association with major depression and substance use: a Web-based cohort and twin-sibling study. Psychol Med. 2012;42:497–508. [PMC free article] [PubMed] [Google Scholar].
73. Shah KR, Eisen SA, Xian H, Potenza MN. Genetic studies of pathological gambling: a review of methodology and analyses of data from the Vietnam Era Twin Registry. J Gambl Stud. 2005;21:179–203. [PubMed] [Google Scholar].
74. Kreek MJ, Nielsen DA, Butelman ER, LaForge KS. Genetic influences on impulsivity, risk taking, stress responsivity and vulnerability to drug abuse and addiction. Nat Neurosci. 2005;8:1450–7. [PubMed] [Google Scholar].
75. Grant JE, Kim SW, Hartman BK. A double-blind, placebo-controlled study of the opiate antagonist

naltrexone in the treatment of pathological gambling urges. J Clin Psychiatry. 2008;69:783–9. [PubMed] [Google Scholar].
76. Dannon PN, Lowengrub K, Musin E, Gonopolsky Y, Kotler M. 12-month follow-up study of drug treatment in pathological gamblers: a primary outcome study. J Clin Psychopharmacol. 2007;27:620–4. [PubMed] [Google Scholar].
77. Grant JE. Three cases of compulsive buying treated with naltrexone. Int J Psychiatry Clin Pract. 2003;7:223–5. [Google Scholar].
78. Grant JE, Potenza MN, Hollander E, et al. Multicenter investigation of the opioid antagonist nalmefene in the treatment of pathological gambling. Am J Psychiatry. 2006;163:303–12. [PubMed] [Google Scholar].
79. Grant JE, Kim SW, Hollander E, Potenza MN. Predicting response to opiate antagonists and placebo in the treatment of pathological gambling. Psychopharmacology (Berl). 2008;200:521–7. [PMC free article] [PubMed] [Google Scholar].
80. Hollander E, DeCaria CM, Finkell JN, Begaz T, Wong CM, Cartwright C. A randomized double-blind fluvoxamine/placebo crossover trial in pathologic gambling. Biol Psychiatry. 2000;47:813–7. [PubMed] [Google Scholar].
81. Kim SW, Grant JE, Adson DE, Shin YC, Zaninelli R. A double-blind placebo-controlled study of the efficacy and safety of paroxetine in the treatment of pathological gambling. J Clin Psychiatry. 2002;63:501–7. [PubMed] [Google Scholar].
82. Blanco C, Petkova E, Ibanez A, Saiz-Ruiz J. A pilot placebo-controlled study of fluvoxamine for pathological gambling. Ann Clin Psychiatry. 2002;14:9–15. [PubMed] [Google Scholar].
83. Grant JE, Kim SW, Potenza MN, et al. Paroxetine treatment of pathological gambling: a multi-centre randomized controlled trial. Int Clin Psychopharmacol. 2003;18:243–9. [PubMed] [Google Scholar].
84. Wainberg ML, Muench F, Morgenstern J, et al. A double-blind study of citalopram versus placebo in the treatment of compulsive sexual behaviors in gay and bisexual men. J Clin Psychiatry. 2006;67:1968–73. [PubMed] [Google Scholar].
85. Dell'Osso B, Hadley S, Allen A, Baker B, Chaplin WF, Hollander E. Escitalopram in the treatment of impulsive-compulsive internet usage disorder: an open-label trial followed by a double-blind discontinuation phase. J Clin Psychiatry. 2008;69:452–6. [PubMed] [Google Scholar].
86. Grant JE, Kim SW, Odlaug BL. N-acetyl cysteine, a glutamate–modulating agent, in the treatment of pathological gambling: a pilot study. Biol Psychiatry. 2007;62:652–7. [PubMed] [Google Scholar].
87. Grant JE, Odlaug BL, Chamberlain SR, et al. A randomized, placebo-controlled trial of N-acetylcysteine plus imaginal desensitization for nicotine-dependent pathological gamblers. J Clin Psychiatry. 2014;75:39–45. [PubMed] [Google Scholar].
88. Berlin HA, Braun A, Simeon D, et al. A double-blind, placebo-controlled trial of topiramate for pathological gambling. World J Biol Psychiatry. 2013;14:121–8. [PubMed] [Google Scholar].
89. Pallesen S, Mitsem M, Kvale G, Johnsen BH, Molde H. Outcome of psychological treatments of pathological gambling: a review and meta-analysis. Addiction. 2005;100:1412–22. [PubMed] [Google Scholar].
90. Tolin DF. Is cognitive-behavioral therapy more effective than other therapies?: a meta-analytic review. Clin Psychol Rev. 2010;30:710–20. [PubMed] [Google Scholar].
91. Petry NM, Ammerman Y, Bohl J, et al. Cognitive-behavioral therapy for pathological gamblers. J Consult Clin Psychol. 2006;74:555–67. [PubMed] [Google Scholar].
92. Petry NM. Pathological gambling: etiology, comorbidity, and treatment. Washington, DC: American Psychological Association; 2005. [PubMed] [Google Scholar].
93. Cowlishaw S, Merkouris S, Dowling N, Anderson C, Jackson A, Thomas S. Psychological therapies for pathological and problem gambling. Cochrane Database Syst Rev. 2012;11:CD008937. [PubMed] [Google Scholar].
94. Raylu N, Oei TP, Loo J. The current status and future direction of self-help treatments for problem gamblers. Clin Psychol Rev. 2008;28:1372–85. [PubMed] [Google Scholar].
95. Carlbring P, Degerman N, Jonsson J, Andersson G. Internet-based treatment of pathological gambling with a three-year follow-up. Cogn Behav Ther. 2012;41:321–34. [PMC free article] [PubMed] [Google Scholar].
96. Gamblers anonymous: recovery program. 2013. http://www.gamblersanonymous.org/ga/content/recovery-program.
97. Petry NM. Patterns and correlates of Gamblers Anonymous attendance in pathological gamblers seeking professional treatment. Addict Behav. 2003;28:1049–62. [PubMed] [Google Scholar].
98. Petry NM. Gamblers anonymous and cognitive-behavioral therapies for pathological gamblers. J Gambl Stud. 2005;21:27–33. [PubMed] [Google Scholar].
99. Brewer JA, Grant JE, Potenza MN. The treatment of pathologic gambling. Addict Disord Their Treat. 2008;7:1–13. [Google Scholar].
100. Grant JE, Odlaug BL. National Center for Responsible Gaming. What clinicians need to know about gambling disorders, vol. 7. Washington, DC: NCRG; 2012. Psychosocial interventions for gambling disorders; pp. 38–52. Increasing the odds: a series dedicated to understanding gambling disor-

ders. At http://www.ncrg.org/resources/monographs. [Google Scholar].

101. Hodgins DC, Currie S, el-Guebaly N, Peden N. Brief motivational treatment for problem gambling: a 24-month follow-up. Psychol Addict Behav. 2004;18:293. [PubMed] [Google Scholar].
102. Copello AG, Velleman RD, Templeton LJ. Family interventions in the treatment of alcohol and drug problems. Drug Alcohol Rev. 2005;24:369–85. [PubMed] [Google Scholar].
103. Potenza MN, Balodis IM, Franco CA, et al. Neurobiological considerations in understanding behavioral treatments for pathological gambling. Psychol Addict Behav. 2013;27:380–92. [PMC free article] [PubMed] [Google Scholar].

Part III

Mechanisms, Race and Gender

Neurobiological Process of Addiction

9

Khai Tran, Sasidhar Gunturu, and Panagiota Korenis

The current approach to understanding addiction is by utilizing the "disease model." Addiction is viewed as a chronic, relapsing disease of the brain where multiple neurological pathways involved are permanently changed leading to not only worsening prognosis but also the development of many other psychiatric illnesses [1]. Experimental research that focuses on the neurobiological functions of the brain has provided a deeper understanding of addiction and its corresponding treatment. Substance use alters the axonal network in the brain that is considered the "reward pathway."

K. Tran
BronxCare Health System, Icahn School of Medicine, New York, NY, USA
e-mail: ktran@bronxcare.org

S. Gunturu
BronxCare Health System, Icahn School of Medicine, New York, NY, USA

Columbia University, New York, NY, USA
e-mail: sguntur1@bronxcare.org

P. Korenis (✉)
BronxCare Health System, Icahn School of Medicine, New York, NY, USA

Albert Einstein College of Medicine, St. George's University School of Medicine, West Indies, Grenada
e-mail: pkorenis@bronxcare.org

Overview in Addiction-Related Brain Regions

The anatomical regions involved in addictions are areas involved in the reward pathway, a complex neuronal arrangement when stimulated provides a pleasurable feeling that leads to the reinforcement of behaviors. Altering this system leads to the development of addictive, tolerance, and withdrawal behaviors [2].

- *Ventral tegmental area (VTA):* A collection of cell bodies located in the floor of the midbrain projecting their axons to numerous areas of the brain. These cell bodies are the origin of the dopaminergic pathway in the brain. It is the starting point of the mesocorticolimbic system that regulates pleasure and pain feelings.
- *Nucleus accumbens (NA):* This area lies in the basal forebrain serving as the relay station for many neurological functions, but most importantly, it processes rewarding stimuli leading to reinforcing behaviors. Its operation is controlled mainly by two essential neurotransmitters: dopamine for desire and serotonin for inhibition.
- *Prefrontal cortex (PFC):* Perhaps the most essential area in complex cognitive behaviors, planning, decision-making, and moderating behaviors. The basic function of this area is to moderate and project behaviors according to

E. Akerele (ed.), *Substance and Non-Substance Related Addictions*,
https://doi.org/10.1007/978-3-030-84834-7_9

internal thoughts and goals. It is a significant relay in the reward pathway and modulated by dopamine.

- *Amygdala:* Small clusters of neurons located deep in the temporal lobe. It is a part of the limbic system. Its primary role is to process memory and emotional responses. It is also modulated by dopamine and plays an active part in reward circuit. It imparts attachment or aversion affective discolorations to perceptions.
- *Hippocampus:* Located in the medial temporal lobe, it is another component of the limbic system that plays an essential role in the consolidation of memory. In addiction, it preserves the pleasant memories associated with substance use and contributes to recidivism. It is regulated by a number of neurotransmitters including dopamine, cannabinoid, and opiate.
- *Locus coeruleus (LC):* The alarm center of the brain located in the posterior pons, it is part of the reticular activating system that responds to stress and panic. This is the primary site in the brain for norepinephrine production. When activated by a lack of drug stimulation, this area is the driving force behind drug-seeking behaviors. It is involved in withdrawal and tolerance pathways.

Neurotransmitter Involved in Addiction

The major neurotransmitters that are directly stimulated by substances are opioid, cannabinoids, and gamma-aminobutyric acid (GABA) [3]. Different substances stimulate the receptors resulting in the direct release of this neurotransmitter. Dopamine, norepinephrine, and serotonin are the neurotransmitters that are responsible for the feedback and reinforcing behaviors that result in substance dependence. Dopamine acts on receptors D1 and D2 and is directly involved in the regulation of pleasure, mood, euphoria, and motor function. It is the most important neurotransmitter in the brain reward circuitry. Serotonin acts on 5HT1, 5HT2, and 5HT3; it is responsible for mood, impulsivity, anxiety, sleep, and cognition [4]. Norepinephrine releases from LC to act on G-coupled protein alpha and beta receptors to stimulate or decrease the level of arousal. Cannabinoids whether from intrinsic or extrinsic sources acts on CB1 and CB2 receptors to control pain, appetite, and memory [5]. Opioid peptides such as endorphins and enkephalins act on pain receptors kappa, mu, and delta to mediate pain. Lastly, GABA is the main inhibitory neurotransmitter in the central nervous system with the primary role to suppress the neuronal activity in the nervous system. Alteration to the level and balance of these neurotransmitters results in intoxication, withdrawal of substances, and the development of tolerance.

Reward Pathway in Addiction: Concept and Physiology

The mesocorticolimbic pathway in the brain also known as the brain-reward circuitry is the dopaminergic pathway in the brain that leads to behavioral enforcement via a positive feedback system [6]. Organisms tend to engage in behaviors that result in rewards or pleasurable feelings; the pleasure provides positive reinforcement so that a particular behavior is repeated. The reward system is activated by two types of drives: the natural rewarding stimulus such as food, water, sex, and nurture; or the artificial rewarding stimulus such as drugs and alcohol [7]. Regardless what the stimulus source is, the neurological process is the same.

When stimulated, the dopaminergic neurons in the VTA release dopamine to stimulate the nucleus accumbens. The influx of dopamine in NA activates the GABAergic medium spiny neurons in the NA to release GABA into the limbic system as well as the prefrontal cortex [8]. Activation of the mesolimbic system that results in a perception of reward leads to the initiation of learned reward-seeking behaviors (Fig. 9.1). This reward-seeking behavior is considered incentive salience which is a cognitive process in which an individual is motivated to seek out a rewarding stimulus in which the driving force is not for survival but rather "desire" attributes.

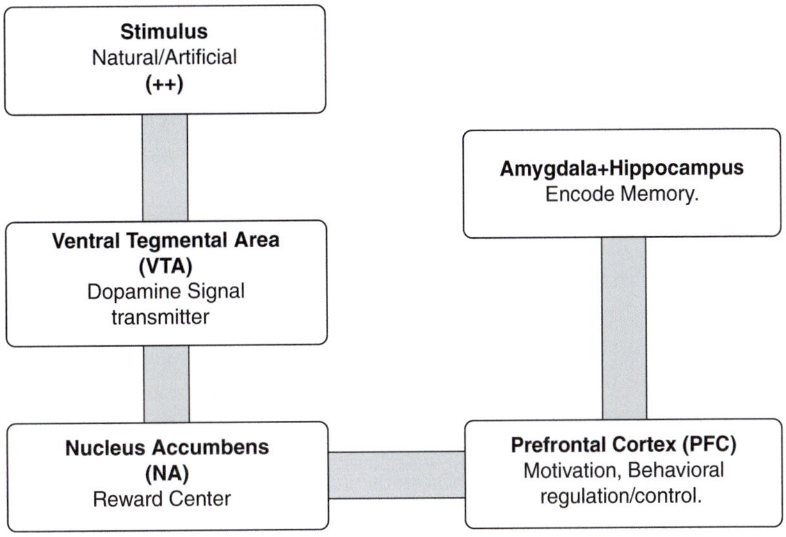

Fig. 9.1 Reward pathway [6]

Substances and Respective Proposed Neurobiological Pathway

Recreational substances act on the reward pathway via two different mechanisms of action: a direct and an indirect pathway. Substances such as cocaine utilize the direct pathway. Cocaine binds to the dopamine transporter DAT [8]. By inactivating the transporter, extracellular dopamine cannot reuptake back into the presynaptic neuron, leading to an accumulation of dopamine in the synaptic cleft. Other substances such as alcohol and heroin inactivate the inhibitory GABAergic neurons that project into the VTA, leading to increased release of dopamine from the VTA. Alcohol also binds to NMDA and endorphins to activate a second messenger system and has serotonergic effects in the reward system [9]. Heroin is converted to morphine in the brain and binds to opiate receptors. This has two effects: first, opiate receptors located within the reward pathway become activated and lead to pleasurable feelings, and second, opiate receptors also decrease GABA release, leading to an increased release of dopamine. Nicotine on the other hand stimulates the dopamine release via cholinergic neurons that are projected into the VTA (Table 9.1).

Table 9.1 Drug mechanism of action summary [1]

Substance	Mechanism of action
Cocaine	Blocks the function of DAT by binding to DAT and slowing transport
Heroin	Binds to opioid receptors that inhibit GABAergic neurons that project to dopaminergic neurons in the VTA
Nicotine	Activates cholinergic neurons that project to dopaminergic neurons in the VTA
Alcohol	Inhibits GABAergic neurons that project to dopaminergic neurons in the VTA

Tolerance and Withdrawal: Concept and Physiology

Adaptation or tolerance is the phenomenon in which after frequent and repeated use, the same amount of substance can no longer produce the same effect felt by the user as the original dose. This is caused by repeated stimulation of neurons. The higher the frequency of use, the faster tolerance is produce. Recurrent use of drugs causes the repeated activation of neuron. This leads to the chemical adaptation of neurons and results in decreased intensity of cellular response to the drug via downregulation of expressed receptors [10]. The desired effect of drug decreases; consequently, the user has to utilize a large dose to achieve a similar effect.

Withdrawal is a substance-specific syndrome which happens when there is an abrupt cessation of the drug. The syndrome is characterized by the disturbance of the autonomic nervous system. With chronic substance use, the homeostatic system had been reconditioned to a new state of balance, so with the abrupt withdrawal, the homeostasis is disrupted, resulting in the activation of acute stress response. Corticotrophin-releasing factor (CRF) is released by the paraventricular nucleus of the hypothalamus that mediates the affective and somatic symptoms of drug withdrawal [11]. CRF acts on three main systems, the amygdale, the medulla oblongata, and the pituitary gland.

The Development of Addiction

The use of recreational drugs results in neurological activation of positive feedback system; by coupling the perception of expected reward (pleasurable feeling, euphoria) with the activation of the dopaminergic system, this association is resistant to extinction and reinforce the behaviors [12]. Through repeated use, the number of receptors in the central nervous system (CNS) gradually increases to accommodate for the continual presence of drug abuse. With the constant neuronal activation, the number of receptors and neurotransmitter released gradually decrease through depletion and feedback inhibition. This leads to the tolerance phenomenon where the reinforcing properties of the substance are decreased. The user's increased need for drug to maintain the new homeostatic state therefore increased, thus begins the substance dependence.

References

1. http://www.karg.cbi.pku.edu.cn/brain-info regions of addiction.
2. http://www.pubs.niaaa.nih.gov/publications/arh312/119-136.
3. http://www.drugabuse.gov/publications/teaching-packets/neurobiology-drug-addiction/section-iii-action-heroin-morphine/5-rats-self-administer-heroin.
4. Parsons. et al. J Pharmacol Exp Ther. 1995;274.
5. Ikemoto S. Brain reward circuitry beyond the mesolimbic dopamine system: a neurobiological theory. Neurosci Biobehav Rev. 2010;35(2):129–50.
6. Berridge KC, Kringelbach ML. Pleasure systems in the brain. Neuron. 2015;86(3):646–64.
7. Olsen CM. Natural rewards, neuroplasticity, and non-drug addictions. Neuropharmacology. 2011;61(7):1109–22.
8. Adinoff B. Neurobiologic processes in drug reward and addiction. Harv Rev Psychiatry. 2004;12(6):305–20.
9. Berridge KC, Kringelbach ML. Neuroscience of affect: brain mechanisms of pleasure and displeasure. Curr Opin Neurobiol. 2013;23(3):294–303.
10. Schultz W. Neuronal reward and decision signals: from theories to data. Physiol Rev. 2015;95(3):853–95.
11. Berridge KC. From prediction error to incentive salience: mesolimbic computation of reward motivation. Eur J Neurosci. 2012;35(7):1124–43.
12. Substance Abuse and Mental Health Services Administration (US); Office of the Surgeon General (US). Facing addiction in America: The surgeon general's report on alcohol, drugs, and health. 2016.

The Genetics of Substance Abuse

10

Olawale Ojo

Introduction

Man has been fascinated by mechanisms of transmission of genetic material through generations. The works of Aristotle, Hippocrates, Epicurus, and *Charaka Samhita* reference the contribution of genetic material from male and female. Indeed, mankind has been able to harness this knowledge in several ways: the genetic cultivation of date palms was practiced in ancient Egypt, while the ancient Jewish writings, including the *Bible* and Babylonian Talmud, describe in detail Mendelian genetics in the transmission of hemophilia.

The discovery of deoxyribonucleic acid (DNA) and ribonucleic acid (RNA) affirms the transfer of genetic material from parents to offspring. Further advances suggest that the environment modifies genes and genetic materials. Having candidate genes does not translate to having a disease or disorder. Genes may not be fully express phenotypically or maybe "turned on and off" by environmental influences. It may be harder for people with genes to quit or may have more severe withdrawal effects.

Addictions are complex and multifactorial in nature, usually occurring in the context of heritability and exposure of the addiction. Different factors exert influences across and individual's lifetime and at different stages of the disorder. These factors include intrinsic factors such as sex, age, age of first use, and family history. Important extrinsic factors include peer influences and socioeconomic status. The nature of the addictive agent such as pharmacokinetics and the mode of use or administration [1]. Other factors such as penetrance, phenocopies, variable expressivity, gene-environment interactions, genetic heterogeneity, polygenicity, and epistasis are also confounders in genetic research [2]. Addiction research for candidate genes is unlikely to yield a single addiction gene. Genes may not be phenotypically expressed; however, the role of genetics cannot be over emphasized in the search for the etiology of substance use disorders. The discovery of new genes opens the potential development of medication which targets and modifies such genes. An understanding of genetics also informs on likely effective medications based on individual's genetic profile further the role of pharmacogenomics.

Gene Structure and Expression in Humans

The body is made of three types of cell lines: the gametes, somatic, and stem cells. The cell's life cycle is divided into cell dividing phase called mitosis and interphase when the cells are not dividing. Somatic and stem cells divide by mitosis, while stem cells divide by meiosis. Genetic information is stored in the DNA is a complex

O. Ojo (✉)
Interfaith Medical Center, Brooklyn, NY, USA

E. Akerele (ed.), *Substance and Non-Substance Related Addictions*,
https://doi.org/10.1007/978-3-030-84834-7_10

structure comprising two helical strands of polymers of nucleotides. Information coding portions of the DNA are called exons. Exons are interspersed by noncoding sequences called introns. The DNA is read by DNA polymerase to produce messenger ribonucleic acid (mRNA) in a process called transcription. Transcription is initiated by a promoter sequence on the coding sequence. mRNA which still contains exons and introns is modified and spliced to remove introns. The exons of the mRNA are translated to protein with the help of transfer RNA (tRNA) and ribosomes.

Posttranslational changes and modification further refines the protein – several molecules may be added or removed for some proteins to become fully functional. Crossing over and independent assortment during meiosis prophase 1 and metaphase 1 ensure genetic diversity and variability. The environment also plays a role and may alter gene expression [3].

Inheritance of Addictions

Much of our knowledge about the heritability of substance abuse comes from family, adoption, and twins' studies. Studies suggest addictions are among the most heritable of psychiatric disorders with heritability range from 0.39 for hallucinogens to 0.72 for cocaine [4]. More addictive substance tends to be more heritable and less heritable. The genetic effect of addiction tends to be more influential as age increases [5].

Heritability also depends on the stage of use – heritability of initiation is generally lower than for abuse [6, 7]. It may seem counterintuitive that substance use is hereditary, putting into consideration the need for initial exposure to the substance; however, some individuals are more susceptible to developing use disorder after exposure to an addictive agent [8].

Candidate Gene Search

The complexity of addiction makes it difficult to examine candidate genes and replicate the results. Genes of biological relevance are examined for single nucleotide polymorphism (SNP) which may be associated with targeted disorders. The difference in the frequency of a genetic variant is examined between control and case groups [9]. Candidate gene search has the potential for false positives which are susceptible to type 1 error.

Alcohol- related genes The most widely studied genes are variants of genes that code for alcohol dehydrogenase (ADH) and aldehyde dehydrogenase (ALDH) which play an important role in the metabolism of alcohol. ADH oxidizes ethanol to acetaldehyde which is then acetate by ALDH (disulfiram acts by inhibiting ALDH, thereby increasing acetaldehyde). Polymorphisms in the genes (ADH1B and ALDH2) influence the consumption and are protective against alcoholism [10]. The His48Arg locus (rs1229984) on the ADH1B gene increases the activity of ADH. His48/His48 homozygotes oxidize alcohol 100 times faster than Arg48/Arg48 homozygotes. The ALDH2 Glu487Lys locus (rs671) inactivates the ALDH 2. Increase in ADH1B or decrease in ALDH2 activity causes the accumulation of acetaldehyde. With the consumption of alcohol, acetaldehyde accumulation releases histamine and causes flushing, headaches, palpitations, and flushing of the skin [2]. His48 and Lys487 occurring commonly in Asian population protect against alcoholism but are implicated in gastrointestinal cancers [11]. ADH1C genes polymorphisms are common in non-Asian populations [2, 12]. Serotonergic variant are also being researched; however, the association with alcoholism is weak [12, 13].

Nicotine Genetic variations in nicotinic acetylcholine receptor cluster (CHRNA5/CHRNA3-CHRNB4) on chromosome 15 have associations with tobacco consumption and increased risk of smoking–related diseases and death. These genes code for α5-α3-β4 subunits. Neuronal nicotinic receptors in the neurons are ligand-gated channels which are pentamers of combinations of α and β subunits. Nicotine-medicated dopamine release is responsible for the stimulation of the reward pathway and substance dependence [14].

Cannabis Variants of cannabinoid receptor 1 and 2 genes (CNR1 and CNR2) are related to a general vulnerability to substances use disorder (nicotine and alcohol, respectively) and not specifically to cannabis dependence. Missense mutation (C385A) of FAAH gene is associated with risk for substance dependence in Caucasian and African-American, but not in Japanese or other Asians [15].

Cocaine The genes involved in cocaine addiction include DRD2/ANKK149 [16], NCAM1 and TTC12, CALCYON [17], dopamine beta-hydroxylase (DBH), and catechol-O-methyltransferase (COMT) [18]. The CHRNA5/CHRNA3-CHRNB4 cluster offers protection from cocaine addiction (although it increases the risk of nicotine dependence) [14].

Opiates OPRM1, which codes for the mu-opioid receptor, is the most frequently studied candidate gene for opioid dependence with mixed results [19].

Pathological gambling Polymorphisms in the promoter region of dopamine receptor 1 (DRD1) may be responsible for decreased impulse control and increased vulnerability to addictive behaviors [20, 21].

Pavlovian-Conditioned Learning and Place Preference

Monoamine genes Catechol-O-methyltransferase (COMT) is responsible for the breakdown of dopamine and norepinephrine in the prefrontal cortex. The substitution of valine for methionine (Val158Met) is a common single nucleotide polymorphism that influences the stability of the COMT enzyme [22]. The Val158 allele was found to be in excess among methamphetamine, nicotine, and polysubstance addicts [23, 24], while late-onset alcoholics have the Met158 allele [25]. Serotonin also plays a role in the regulation of mood and impulse control. Variation (variable number tandem repeats) in the promoter region HTTLPR of the serotonin transporter gene SLC6A4 regulates the synaptic levels of serotonin [2]. The L-allele increases the transcription of the transporter protein, while the S-allele is associated with low transcriptional efficiency. The low transcription of HTTLPR genotypes is associated with alcoholism, depression, and suicidality [26, 27].

Genome-Wide Association Studies

Candidate gene studies are often difficult to replicate and are cost-intensive. Genome-wide association studies (GWAS) are to identify common genotypic variants (minor allele frequency MAF > 5%) on a large scale. Single nucleotide polymorphisms are linked with the interested disorder using a large study sample. Affected individuals (cases) are often compared to unaffected individual (control). As many as five million SNPs may be tested at the same time. To account for the effects of large sample size, multiple testing and the possibility of false positives, the effective P value of 0.05, the genome-wide significance threshold is usually set at approximately 10^{-8} [2].

The most widely studied GWAS is for CHRNA5CHRNA3-CHRNB4 gene cluster on chromosome 15q25 which codes for α5, α3, and β4 subunits of nicotinic receptors. Functional missense polymorphism, rs16969968 (substitution of aspartic acid, Asp with asparagine, Asn) at codon 398 of CHRNA5, is associated with nicotine addiction. Asn398 allele is also correlated with heavy smoking [28], "pleasurable buzz" with smoking [29], and increased occurrence of smoking-related disease among smokers [30–32]. Asn398 allele exhibit an altered response to nicotine agonist. Asn398 predicts the strengths of the connection between the anterior cingulate and the ventral striatum, increasing the reward associated with smoking. Functional polymorphisms of cytochrome P450, family 2, subfamily A, and polypeptide 6 (CYP2A6) have been linked with the number of cigarettes smoked a day. (CYP2A6 enzyme is responsible for 70% of initial nicotine metabolism by converting nicotine to continue.) Polymorphism in the dopamine β-hydroxylase (DBH) gene has been associated with smoking cessation [33].

GWAS of alcohol addiction has not yielded much result. The most promising lead is the variant rs6943555 in autism susceptibility candidate 2 gene (AUTS2), which has been studied in alcoholic mice and found postmortem in humans [34].

Rare and Common Variants

Candidate gene studies and genome-wide associations focus solely on common alleles which have small to moderate effect on susceptibility to a common disorder [2]. However, rare variants may have a strong influence on and may be responsible for more severe forms of the disorder. These are variants may be sporadic or of recent origin [2]. An example is a rare variant of HTR2B gene located on chromosome 2 (2q36.3-q37.1) that is linked to severe alcoholism, extreme impulsivity, aggression, and antisocial personality disorder. The HTR2B gene codes for serotonin 2B receptor. This variant, Q20* stop codon, was studied in the Finnish population. Genetic sequences of individuals who committed violent-premeditated crimes were done. These individuals were often intoxicated with alcohol, suggesting that alcohol influences the stop codon [35].

Summary

The social and economic impact of addiction is very high. Genetic and environmental influences contribute to the vulnerability to substance use disorders which pose a wide range of challenges. The goal of genetic research in addiction is to understand the etiology of the disorders and improve the treatment alternative to individuals who are suffering from addiction despite the traditional approach. By studying heritability, candidate genes, and genome-wide studies, we are able to better predict which individuals may develop addiction. Current research is still in infancy, but promising genes have been identified.

References

1. Agrawal A, Verweij KJH, Gillespie NA, Heath AC, Lessov-Schlaggar CN, Martin NG, et al. The genetics of addiction—a translational perspective. Transl Psychiatry. 2012;2:e140.
2. Ducci F, Goldman D. Genetic approaches to addiction: genes and alcohol. Addiction. 2008;103(9):1414–28.
3. Watson JD, Baker TA, Bell SP, Gann A, Levine M, Losick R. Molecular biology of the gene. 5th ed. San Francisco: Benjamin Cummings; 2003.
4. Goldman D, Oroszi G, Ducci F. The genetics of addictions: uncovering the genes. Nat Rev Genet. 2005;6(7):521–32.
5. Kendler KS, Schmitt E, Aggen SH, Prescott CA. Genetic and environmental influences on alcohol, caffeine, cannabis, and nicotine use from early adolescence to middle adulthood. Arch Gen Psychiatry. 2008;65(6):674–82.
6. Li MD, Cheng R, Ma JZ, Swan GE. A meta-analysis of estimated genetic and environmental effects on smoking behavior in male and female adult twins. Addiction. 2003;98:23–31.
7. Kendler KS, Karkowski LM, Neale MC, Prescott CA. Illicit psychoactive substance use, heavy use, abuse, and dependence in a US population-based sample of male twins. Arch Gen Psychiatry. 2000;57:261–9.
8. Bevilacqua L, Goldman D. Genes and addictions. Clin Pharmacol Ther. 2009;85(4):359–61.
9. Sullivan PF, Eaves LJ, Kendler KS, Neale MC. Genetic case–control association studies in neuropsychiatry. Arch Gen Psychiatry. 2001;58:1015–24.
10. Edenberg HJ. The genetics of alcohol metabolism: role of alcohol dehydrogenase and aldehyde dehydrogenase variants. Alcohol Res Health. 2007;30(1):5–13.
11. Brooks PJ, Goldman D, Li TK. Alleles of alcohol and acetaldehyde metabolism genes modulate susceptibility to oesophageal cancer from alcohol consumption. Hum Genomics. 2009;2009(3):2.
12. Dick DM, Bierut LJ. The genetics of alcohol dependence. Curr Psychiatry Rep. 2006;8(2):151–7.
13. McHugh RK, Hofmann SG, Asnaani A, Sawyer AT, Otto MW. The serotonin transporter gene and risk for alcohol dependence: a meta-analytic review. Drug Alcohol Depend. 2010;108(1):1–6.
14. Bierut LJ, Stitzel JA, Wang JC, Hinrichs AL, Grucza RA, Xuei X, et al. Variants in nicotinic receptors and risk for nicotine dependence. Am J Psychiatry. 2008;165(9):1163–71.
15. Agrawal A, Lynskey MT. Candidate genes for cannabis use disorders: findings, challenges and directions. Addiction. 2009;104(4):518–32.
16. Gelernter J, Yu Y, Weiss R, Brady K, Panhuysen C, Yang BZ, et al. Haplotype spanning TTC12 and ANKK1, flanked by the DRD2 and NCAM1 loci, is strongly associated to nicotine dependence in two distinct American populations. Hum Mol Genet. 2006;15:3498–507.

17. Luo X, Kranzler H, Lappalainen J, Rosenheck R, Charney D, Zuo L, et al. CALCYON gene variation, schizophrenia, and cocaine dependence. Am J Med Genet B Neuropsychiatr Genet. 2004;125B(1):25–30.
18. Ittiwut R, Listman JB, Ittiwut C, Cubells JF, Weiss RD, Brady K, et al. Association between polymorphisms in catechol-O-methyltransferase (COMT) and cocaine-induced paranoia in European-American and African-American populations. Am J Med Genet B Neuropsychiatr Genet. 2011;156B(6):651–60.
19. Glatt SJ, Bousman C, Wang RS, Murthy KK, Rana BK, Lasky-Su JA, et al. Evaluation of OPRM1 variants in heroin dependence by family-based association testing and meta-analysis. Drug Alcohol Depend. 2007;90(2–3):159–65.
20. da Silva Lobo DS, Vallada HP, Knight J, Martins SS, Tavares H, Gentil V, et al. Dopamine genes and pathological gambling in discordant sib-pairs. J Gambl Stud. 2007;23(4):421–33.
21. Lobo DS, Souza RP, Tong RP, Casey DM, Hodgins DC, Smith GJ, et al. Association of functional variants in the dopamine D2-like receptors with risk for gambling behaviour in healthy Caucasian subjects. Biol Psychol. 2010;85(1):33–7.
22. Lachman HM, Papolos DF, Saito T, Yu YM, Szumlanski CL, Weinshilboum RM. Human catechol-O-methyltransferase pharmacogenetics: description of a functional polymorphism and its potential application to neuropsychiatric disorders. Pharmacogenetics. 1996;6(3):243–50.
23. Tammimäki AE, Männistö PT. Are genetic variants of COMT associated with addiction? Pharmacogenet Genomics. 2010;20(12):717–41.
24. Vandenbergh DJ, Rodriguez LA, Miller IT, Uhl GR, Lachman HM. High-activity catechol-O-methyltransferase allele is more prevalent in polysubstance abusers. Am J Med Genet. 1997;74(4):439–42.
25. Tiihonen J, Hallikainen T, Lachman H, Saito T, Volavka J, Kauhanen J, et al. Association between the functional variant of the catechol-O-methyltransferase (COMT) gene and type 1 alcoholism. Mol Psychiatry. 1999;4(3):286–9.
26. Barr CS, Newman TK, Becker ML, Parker CC, Champoux M, Lesch KP, et al. The utility of the non-human primate model for studying gene by environment interactions in behavioral research. Genes Brain Behav. 2003;2(6):336–40.
27. Caspi A, Sugden K, Moffitt TE, Taylor A, Craig IW, Harrington H, et al. Influence of life stress on depression: moderation by a polymorphism in the 5-HTT gene. Science. 2003;301(5631):386–9.
28. Bierut LJ, Madden PA, Breslau N, Johnson EO, Hatsukami D, Pomerleau OF, et al. Novel genes identified in a high-density genome wide association study for nicotine dependence. Hum Mol Genet. 2007;16(1):24–35.
29. Sherva R, Wilhelmsen K, Pomerleau CS, Chasse SA, Rice JP, Snedecor SM, et al. Association of a single nucleotide polymorphism in neuronal acetylcholine receptor subunit alpha 5 (CHRNA5) with smoking status and with 'pleasurable buzz' during early experimentation with smoking. Addiction. 2008;103(9):1544–52.
30. Amos CI, Wu X, Broderick P, Gorlov IP, Gu J, Eisen T, et al. Genome-wide association scan of tag SNPs identifies a susceptibility locus for lung cancer at 15q25.1. Nat Genet. 2008;4(5):616–22.
31. Hung RJ, McKay JD, Gaborieau V, et al. A susceptibility locus for lung cancer maps to nicotinic acetylcholine receptor subunit genes on 15q25. Nature. 2008;452(7187):633–7.
32. Timofeeva MN, McKay JD, Smith GD, et al. Genetic polymorphisms in 15q25 and 19q13 loci, cotinine levels, and risk of lung cancer in EPIC. Cancer Epidemiol Biomark Prev. 2011;20(10):2250–61.
33. Thorgeirsson TE, Gudbjartsson DF, Surakka I, Vink JM, Amin N, Geller F, et al. Sequence variants at CHRNB3-CHRNA6 and CYP2A6 affect smoking behavior. Nat Genet. 2010;42:448–53.
34. Schumann G, Coin LJ, Lourdusamy A, Charoen P, Berger KH, Stacey D, et al. Genome-wide association and genetic functional studies identify autism susceptibility candidate 2 gene (AUTS2) in the regulation of alcohol consumption. Proc Natl Acad Sci U S A. 2011;108:7119–24.
35. Bevilacqua L, Doly S, Kaprio J, Yuan Q, Tikkanen R, Paunio T, et al. A population-specific HTR2B stop codon predisposes to severe impulsivity. Nature. 2010;468(7327):1061–6.

11 Drug Abuse and Race

Evaristo Akerele

Introduction

Substance use disorder is a significant public health issue. One modality of addressing this challenge is to assess the impact on racial/ethnic groups. These data may be useful in improving the general well-being of the population. It is of paramount importance to clarify the definitions of race and ethnicity in order to obtain useful data. According to the Interagency Committee's recommendations, the minimum categories for data on race and ethnicity or Federal statistics and program administrative reporting are defined as follows [7]:

- American Indian or Alaska Native—a person having origins in any of the original peoples of North and South America (including Central America) who maintains cultural identification through tribal affiliations or community recognition.
- Asian or Pacific Islander—a person having origins in any of the original peoples of the Far East, Southeast Asia, the Indian subcontinent, or the Pacific Islands. These areas include, for example, China, India, Japan, Korea, the Philippine Islands, Hawaii, and Samoa.
- Black or African American—a person having origins in any of the Black racial groups of Africa.
- Hispanic—a person of Mexican, Puerto Rican, Cuban, Central or South American, or other Spanish culture or origin, regardless of race.
- White—a person having origins in any of the original peoples of Europe, North Africa, or the Middle East.

The recommended changes for data collection also include an emphasis on data quality. The committee recommended that when race and ethnicity data are collected separately, ethnicity data should be collected first. In addition, the minimum designations for ethnicity and race are as follows:

- Ethnicity
  - Hispanic origin
  - Not of Hispanic origin

- Race
  - American Indian or Alaska Native
  - Asian or Pacific Islander
  - Black or African American
  - White

E. Akerele (✉)
Department of Psychiatry, New Jersey Medical School, Rutgers University, Newark, NJ, USA

E. Akerele (ed.), *Substance and Non-Substance Related Addictions*,
https://doi.org/10.1007/978-3-030-84834-7_11

In addition, persons are allowed but are not required to report more than one race. A minimum of one additional racial category, designated "more than one race," has been recommended to report the aggregate number of multiple race responses. This classification system allows for the collection of data on special subgroups, such as "Hispanic and one or more races" and "more than one race."

In sections that follow the relationship between race and the use of these substances explored.

Racial/Ethnic Differences [5]

The racial/ethnic comparisons made here are only for students who identify as being members of one race/ethnicity only. Although the Monitoring the Future (MTF) design did not include an oversampling of any racial/ethnic minority groups, the large overall sample sizes at each grade level do produce fair numbers of African American and Hispanic respondents, and the size of these populations has increased in recent decades. Furthermore, these findings combined data from two adjacent years to augment the sample sizes on which estimates for these two minority groups (as well as Whites) are based and, thus, increase the reliability of the estimates. The sampling error of differences among groups is likely to be larger than would be true for other demographic and background variables such as gender or college plans because African Americans and Hispanics are more likely to be clustered by neighborhood, and therefore by school. The data discussed here refer to the 2-year combined (i.e., 2017–2018) prevalence estimates for lifetime, annual, 30-day, and selected daily use for the three racial/ethnic groups at all three grade levels. *For a number of years,* 12th grade African American students *reported lifetime, annual, 30-day, and daily prevalence levels for nearly all drugs that were lower—sometimes dramatically so—than those for White or Hispanic 12th graders.* Recent data tell a different story, with levels of drug use among African Americans more similar to the other groups. This narrowing of the gap between African Americans and other racial/ethnic groups is also seen in eighth and tenth grades. This suggests that this narrowing in 12th grade is probably not due primarily to differential dropout rates. Whites have the lowest levels of annual marijuana use in eighth grade, at 7.5% compared to 10.7% and 12.4% for African American and Hispanic students, respectively. In tenth and 12th grades, the annual marijuana use differs little by race/ethnicity. These data may suggest that minority students are getting more comfortable reporting marijuana use.

These categories are broad. The Hispanic category encompasses people with various Latin American, Caribbean, and European origins. These are not addressed here due to small sample sizes. Furthermore, small numbers of cases present challenges in the detailed analysis of students who indicate membership in the other racial/ethnic groups, as well as those who indicate membership in multiple racial/ethnic groups and the many specific combinations these students comprise. More complete treatments of racial/ethnic differences, as well as interactions with other demographic characteristics, are addressed elsewhere [1–4, 6, 8, 10, 11]

- The use of some drugs is less common among African American teens relative to White teens. These include nicotine vaping, marijuana vaping, use of hallucinogens, and nonmedical use of sedatives (barbiturates), tranquilizers, and narcotics other than heroin. Other drugs less commonly used by among African American teens did not show much difference in 2018 among eighth graders. However they still are less commonly used in the upper grades. These include LSD, MDMA (ecstasy, Molly), cocaine (in recent years), cocaine other than crack, and nonmedical use of amphetamines and Vicodin. (African American levels of Vicodin use are actually highest in the eighth grade, but lowest in tenth and 12th grades.)
- **For 12th grade**, White students *have the highest lifetime and annual prevalence levels*

among the three major racial/ethnic groups for many substances, including marijuana, LSD, hallucinogens other than LSD, MDMA (ecstasy, Molly), and nonmedical use of narcotics other than heroin, amphetamines, and tranquilizers. They also have the lowest lifetime and annual prevalence of alcohol use and being drunk. Not all of these findings are replicated at lower grade levels.

- **For ALL Three grades**, Hispanics in 2018 had the highest annual prevalence at all three grade levels for synthetic marijuana, cocaine, crack, and cocaine other than crack. It bears repeating that Hispanics have a considerably higher dropout rate than Whites or African Americans, based on the Census Bureau statistics, which should tend to diminish any such differences by 12th grade, yet there remain sizeable differences even in the upper grades.
- **For Eighth grade**—before most dropping out occurs—Hispanics had the highest levels of use of almost all substances, whereas by the 12th grade, Whites have the highest levels of use of most. Certainly, the considerably higher dropout rate among Hispanics could help explain this shift, and it may be the most plausible explanation. Another explanation worth considering is that Hispanics may tend to start using drugs at a younger age, but Whites overtake them at older ages. These explanations are not mutually exclusive, of course, and to some degree both explanations may hold true.
- **For Cigarettes**, White students have by far the highest prevalence of daily cigarette smoking, while African American and Hispanic students are now fairly close to each other among all three grades, for example, 12th grade Whites have a 5.0% daily smoking prevalence; Hispanics, 1.8%; and African Americans, 2.0%.
- The thirty-day prevalence of smokeless tobacco use is highest among White students in all three grades.
- African American students have the lowest 30-day prevalence for alcohol use in all three grades. They also have the lowest prevalence for self-reports of having been drunk. A more extensive discussion of possible explanations (including the possibility of differential validity of reporting) can be found in Wallace et al. [9] for the prior 30 days. The differences are largest at 12th grade, with 23% of Whites reporting having been drunk, 13% of Hispanics, and 10% of African Americans.
- Recent binge drinking (having five or more drinks in a row during the prior 2 weeks) is also lowest among African Americans in all three grades; in 12th grade, their level of use is 7.4% versus 19% for Whites and 12% for Hispanics. The corresponding prevalence levels for the tenth grade are 3.9% for African Americans versus 10.5% for Whites and 10.8% for Hispanics. In the eighth grade, Hispanics have the highest prevalence at 5.2% compared to 2.9% for Whites and 2.6% for African Americans.
- In ADHD treatment related to student race/ethnicity. In general, White students are considerably more likely to have used prescription ADHD drugs at each grade than African American or Hispanic students. The current use of either subclass of drugs (stimulant or non-stimulant) is also substantially higher among White students than among African American or Hispanic students in all three grades, with the exception that these differences are somewhat smaller for non-stimulant drugs in grades 10 and 12. In all three grades, African Americans and Hispanics have lifetime levels of use that are close to each other. However, in the eighth grade, Hispanics have a somewhat lower level than African Americans in the current use of each class of drugs and of any ADHD drug, while in tenth and 12th grade, there is little difference in their use. As to why White students are more likely to be treated with ADHD drugs than African American and Hispanic students, it again may well be due to White families being more likely to get access to, or being able to afford, professional assessment and treatment.
- Levels of past year use for diet pills are highest for Whites. In 2018, levels of past year use were about two times as high for Whites as compared to Hispanics, at 4.4% and 1.9%,

respectively. Racial/ethnic differences have diminished in recent years as overall prevalence has declined.

- Levels of past year use of stay-awake pills are about twice as high for Whites as they are for African Americans, at 2.2% and 1.1%, respectively, with Hispanic levels closer to Whites at 1.8%. Differences in these groups were larger in the past years when overall prevalence was higher. The use of stay-awake pills has not varied consistently by any of the other subgroup categories.
- In all grades Whites have the lowest levels of medical marijuana use, although overall use levels are low. In tenth and 12th grades, the differences are the largest, with use levels among Whites less than half of those among Hispanics and African Americans.

Review of Data from the National Survey of Drug Use and Health 2018

There is no significant change in alcohol use initiation rate among African American youths since 2015. There is a decline in alcohol use disorder among African American youth and young adults during 2015–2018. Among African Americans aged 12+, there are significant decreases in prescription opioid misuse initiation, misuse, and use disorders during 2015–2018. A majority of African Americans continue to obtain drugs from friends/relatives and from healthcare provider/prescriber, underscoring the need for ongoing education of practitioners, appropriate pain management, and partnership with states to monitor opioid prescribing. There are significant decreases in prescription opioid misuse among African American youth and young adults. There are no significant changes in heroin initiation, heroin use, and heroin use disorder among African Americans during 2015–2018. Marijuana use disorder increased in 2018 to 2.2% relative to 2017 in the 12- to 17-year-olds and 18- to 25-year-olds to 6.9% in African Americans with a slight decrease in the 26-year-old and above age group. There are no significant changes in marijuana use disorder among African Americans across all age groups. The lifetime use of cocaine in 2018 for individuals over 26 years old; White 19.6%, African American 10.6%, and Hispanic 13.1%. The lifetime use of marijuana in individuals over 26 years old in 2018 were as follows: Whites 14.1%, African American 14.8%, and Hispanic 9.7%.

Conclusions and Future Directions

The data suggest that both in high school, ages 12–17, ages 18–25, and age 26 or over African Americans had the lowest drug use or drug use disorder. African American were not at the top in any of these categories. There a few clear differences: a) Whites are more likely to use drugs in later grades of high school, choice of drug is race/ethnicity dependent, c) dropout rates seem to correlate negatively with drug use in the later part of high school. However, despite the lower rates of drug use, African Americans are least likely to obtain treatment for substance use disorder. This maybe in part, due to early dropout being more likely to culminate in lower socioeconomic status.

There are a number of additional factors such as outreach challenges, and cultural factors. Substance Abuse and Mental Health Services Administration (SAMSHA) has made significant efforts to improve the challenges with substance use disorder in African Americans. These include: (a) establishment of Provider Clinical Support System (PCSS)-universities to embed data waiver training in pre-graduate education for physicians, nurse practitioners, and physician assistants; (b) expansion of training and technical assistance on opioids issues in rural America through supplements to USDA Cooperative Extension programs; (c) re-establishment of the Drug Abuse Warning Network (DAWN); (d) expansion of the Suicide Prevention Lifeline network; and (e) public-targeted messaging based on areas of concern identified in National Survey of Drug Use and Health (NSDUH): marijuana, methamphetamine, and suicide prevention. Future efforts must include putting in place modalities to address the cultural stigma that may be a barrier to presentation for treatment. Clearly more needs to done to obtain significant change the ability or desire to seek treatment. The stigma and ability to reenter the workforce maybe more significant for African Americans. As a result there may be a greater reluctance to openly seek treatment. Other barriers such as lower socioeconomic standards that result in financial challenges need to be addressed. This can be done by providing free access to treatment irrespective of ability to pay. Finally, there is a need to ensure that outreach to African Americans is enhanced through a variety of modalities that include but are not limited to the following:

(1) Diversity of treatment programs to ensure all adequate representation of all groups; (2) Culturally trained and sensitive outreach workers and staff embedded in African American communities who have earned the trust of the community; (3) Significant grants to community clinics to study the challenges faced in these communities such as access to good schools, job opportunities, and appropriate job training.

Another possibility may be that the low treatment rate among African Americans is primarily gender or age specific, for example, men and the elderly. Targeted interventions to increase the participation of these groups in treatment could be developed. Treatment facilities also need to pay special attention to ensure all cultural group needs are addressed. More work is necessary to identify factors within each racial/ethnic group that increase the risk of susceptibility to drug use. The ultimate goal should then be to eradicate the negative impact of such factors.

References

1. Bachman JG, O'Malley PM, Johnston LD, Schulenberg JE. Impacts of parental education on substance use: differences among white, African-American, and Hispanic students in 8th, 10th, and 12th grades (1999–2008) (monitoring the future occasional paper no. 70). Ann Arbor: Institute for Social Research; 2010. Available: http://www.monitoringthefuture.org/.
2. Bachman JG, O'Malley PM, Johnston LD, Schulenberg JE, Wallace JM. Racial/ethnic differences in the relationship between parental education and substance use among U.S. 8th-, 10th-, and 12th-grade students: findings from the monitoring the future project. J Stud Alcohol Drugs. 2011;72(2):279–85. https://doi.org/10.15288/jsad.2011.72.279.
3. Bachman JG, Wallace JM Jr, O'Malley PM, Johnston LD, Kurth CL, Neighbors HW. Racial/ethnic differences in smoking, drinking, and illicit drug use among American high school seniors, 1976-89. Am J Public Health. 1991;81(3):372–7. https://doi.org/10.2105/ajph.81.3.372.
4. Delva J, Wallace JM Jr, O'Malley PM, Bachman JG, Johnston LD, Schulenberg JE. The epidemiology of alcohol, marijuana, and cocaine use among Mexican American, Puerto Rican, Cuban American, and other Latin American eighth-grade students in the United States: 1991-2002. Am J Public Health. 2005;95(4):696–702. https://doi.org/10.2105/AJPH.2003.037051.
5. Miech RA, Johnston LD, O'Malley PM, Bachman JG, Schulenberg JE, Patrick ME. Monitoring the future national survey results on drug use, 1975–2019: volume I, secondary school students. Ann Arbor: Institute for Social Research, The University of Michigan; 2020. Available at http://monitoringthefuture.org/pubs.html#monographs.
6. Miech R, Terry-McElrath YM, O'Malley PM, Johnston LD. Increasing marijuana use for black adolescents in the United States: a test of competing explanations. Addict Behav. 2019;93:59–64. https://doi.org/10.1016/j.addbeh.2019.01.016.
7. NIDA. (2003, September 1). Drug use among racial/ethnic minorities. Retrieved from https://archives.drugabuse.gov/publications/drug-use-among-racialethnic-minorities on 2020, October 21.
8. Terry-McElrath YM, Patrick ME. U.S. adolescent alcohol use by race/ethnicity: consumption and perceived need to reduce/stop use. J Ethn Subst Abus. 2020;19(1):3–27. https://doi.org/10.1080/15332640.2018.1433094.
9. Wallace JM Jr, Bachman JG, O'Malley PM, & Johnston LD. Racial/ethnic differences in adolescent drug use: exploring possible explanations. In G. Botvin et al. (Eds), Drug abuse prevention with multiethnic youth. National Criminal Justice Reference Service. 1995. pp. 59–80. https://www.ncjrs.gov/App/Publications/abstract.aspx?ID=159985.
10. Wallace JM Jr, Bachman JG, O'Malley PM, Johnston LD, Schulenberg JE, Cooper SM. Tobacco, alcohol, and illicit drug use: racial and ethnic differences among U.S. high school seniors, 1976-2000. Public Health Rep. 2002;117(Suppl 1):S67–75.
11. Wallace JM Jr, Vaughn MG, Bachman JG, O'Malley PM, Johnston LD, Schulenberg JE. Race/ethnicity, socioeconomic factors, and smoking among early adolescent girls in the United States. Drug Alcohol Depend. 2009;104(Suppl 1):S42–9. https://doi.org/10.1016/j.drugalcdep.2009.06.007.

12 Women and Substance Use Disorders

Tolulope Olupona and Olaniyi Olayinka

Introduction

Substance Use in Women

Substance use continues to affect American women at alarming rates. In 2016, according to the National Survey of Drug Use and Health, 19.5 million females (or 15.4%) ages 18 or older have used illicit drugs in the past year [1].

Substance use in women affects various physiological aspects of women's life including menstrual cycle, pregnancy, fertility, breastfeeding, and menopause. Women use substances for various reasons including use to cope with emotions, weight regulation, reduce anxiety, reduce stress, rewards for celebration, and socialization tool. Women's substance use behavior also differs from men [2–4]. Studies have shown that women often use a smaller amount of substances before getting addicted [2]. They also respond differently to substances including having more drug cravings and are more likely to relapse from treatment [5]. Sex hormones also make women more sensitive to the effects of substances. Women who use substances are more likely to have been victims of emotional or sexual trauma and are more likely to have experienced Posttraumatic Stress Disorder [4].

T. Olupona (✉)
Psychiatry Residency Training Program, Interfaith Medical Center, Brooklyn, NY, USA
e-mail: tolupona@interfaithmedical.org

O. Olayinka
Department of Psychiatry and Behavioral Sciences, Brooklyn, NY, USA

Alcohol Use Disorder

Alcohol use is increasing among women in the United States, although the use appears to be diminishing in men. A recent study suggested that women may be drinking as much as men [6]. Rates of alcohol-related visits to hospital increased by 50% between 2006 and 2014 [7]. Death rates from alcohol-related cirrhosis increased by 57% for women between the ages of 45 and 64 and 18% for women between the ages of 25 and 44 according to the CDC between 2000 and 2015 [8]. Researchers are studying why women are drinking more, and several factors are being considered including increasing marketing of alcohol including wines and spirits to women. Marketing of alcohol emphasizes the pleasurable aspects of alcohol. Increasingly, social media, TV, and entertainment industry's portrayal of alcohol as necessary aspects of "fun" socialization may also be increasing the social acceptability of problematic drinking behavior. Also, women's participation in the workforce and pressures to succeed both at work and at home maybe leading more women to use alcohol to manage stress. Women may also be drinking more to reduce anxiety and using alcohol as rewards.

E. Akerele (ed.), *Substance and Non-Substance Related Addictions*,
https://doi.org/10.1007/978-3-030-84834-7_12

There are physiological differences in how alcohol affects men and women [9]. Compared to men, women become more intoxicated after drinking half as much as men. They also metabolize alcohol differently and develop cirrhosis of the liver more rapidly. They also have a greater risk of dying from alcohol-related injury. Alcohol increases the risk of high blood pressure, bone fractures, and injuries in women. Excessive alcohol use in women increases psychiatric problems including depression, posttraumatic stress disorders, eating disorders, and suicidality [10]. Alcohol use also increases the risk of breast cancer [11].

Several studies have looked at the effects of alcohol consumptions on breast cancer. Studies have found an increased risk of breast cancer with increasing alcohol intake. A meta-analysis of 53 studies, which included over 58,000 women, showed that women who drank more than 45 grams of alcohol showed the risk of developing breast cancer 1.5 times than those who did not consume alcohol [12]. The risk of breast cancer was also usage dependent; for every 10 grams of alcohol consumed, researchers observed a small increase in the risk of breast cancer. Alcohol use can also have damaging effects during pregnancy. Alcohol use during pregnancy can lead to fetal alcohol syndrome, causing brain damage and subsequent developmental issues [13]. Alcohol abstinence during pregnancy can prevent the development of fetal alcohol syndrome.

Tobacco Use Disorder

In 2016, 13.5% of women in the United States smoked, compared to 17.5% of men [14]. Smoking rates appear to be reducing in women from high-income countries and is increasing in women from low- to middle-income countries. The smoking rate between men and women continues to close. Increase smoking among women is leading to an increase rate of smoking-related health issues. Smoking is directly responsible for 80% of lung cancer death annually. In the United States, in 2014, smoking led to 70,700 lung and bronchus cancer deaths [15]. Smoking also increases the risk of various cancers including oral cancer, esophageal cancer, laryngeal cancer, and pharyngeal cancer. Smoking also increased the risk of cervical cancer in women. Women who smoke and who are on oral contraceptives also have a higher rate of blood clots, heart attacks, and strokes. Female smokers are 22 times more likely to die from Chronic Obstructive Pulmonary Disease. Despite the negative health effects of smoking, women continue to smoke at an alarming rate which is likely related to friendly marketing of cigarette smoking to women.

Nicotine has many serious effects on women's life cycle including serious effects during pregnancy and effects on fertility. Smoking can also lead to low birth weight, premature rupture of membranes, placenta previa, miscarriage, and neonatal death. Neonates of mothers who smoke also have nicotine in their bloodstream. Smoking also leads to more difficulty conceiving than in mothers who do not smoke. Smoking also increases the risk of pelvic inflammatory diseases and leads to an earlier onset of menopause.

Opioid Use Disorder

There is scientific evidence suggesting the current epidemic of opioid overdose and related deaths disproportionately affecting women. A review of health data from 1997 to 2005 found higher use of opioids among older women compared to men [15]. In a 2011 study of 892 opioid-dependent individuals, women reported significantly higher cravings (assessed using the visual analog scale) compared to male participants [5]. Women using heroin are more likely to also be misusing prescription drugs, increasing the risk for opioid overdose and subsequently death. Other factors related to opioid use in this subgroup include a higher report of pain and childhood trauma.

In Hemsing and colleague's review of prescription opioid misuse among women, the authors found positive history of physical or psychological trauma, younger or older age, pregnancy, or being a first nations, lesbian, bisexual or transgendered woman were associated with opioid misuse [16]. Opioid use during pregnancy poses the double risk of harming both the mother and the unborn child. Neonatal abstinence syndrome, characterized by drug withdrawal symptoms, is particularly common in newborns exposed to opioids in utero [17, 18]. Additionally, affected neonates may develop life-threatening seizures.

Opioid misuse may also impact psychosocial functioning in women. Those who develop opioid use disorder often spend time trying to obtain opioids and are likely to neglect child care. These may lead to physical or emotional harm to a child and ultimately separation of such a child from the family. Therefore, early identification and treatment of women with opioid use disorder are crucial in preserving maternal and child health while fostering family cohesion.

Cocaine Use Disorder

The prevalence of cocaine use among women has been estimated to be steady since 2009. The 2017 National Survey on Drug Use and Health study reported approximately two million women aged 12 years or older used cocaine in the past year [19]. Recreational cocaine use is associated with significant morbidity and mortality among women. As a potent psychostimulant, acute and chronic cocaine use has been linked to cardiovascular, neurologic, psychiatric, behavioral, and respiratory adverse events among others. These effects include acute myocardial infarction, extreme paranoia, and cocaine-induced psychosis. Recent studies suggest the highest prevalence of cocaine use is among women of childbearing age. An estimated 750,000 pregnant women use cocaine annually, with the highest cocaine-exposure rates reported among those aged 18–25 years [20]. Hence, obstetric complications of cocaine use, which include fetal effects, are not uncommon [21]. In 2005, a study of over 700 infants exposed to cocaine in utero found low birth weight and infectious disease correlated positively with maternal cocaine exposure [22].

Studies investigating sex differences in the use of psychostimulants such as cocaine found that women, compared to men, progress faster from initial exposure to dependence and have higher relapse rates [2, 3]. It is posited these factors may contribute to the increased risk for drug overdose and death in women. Cocaine is a highly addictive and potentially dangerous drug. Its nonmedical use under any circumstance should be discouraged.

Cannabis Use Disorder

The prevalence of cannabis use among women continues to rise [23]. This is in tandem with changing government policies regarding medical and recreational use of cannabis. Of note, the pattern of cannabis use among men now approximates that of women. A recent analysis of the National Epidemiologic Survey on Alcohol and Related Conditions data reveals an increase in the past year prevalence of cannabis use among US adults from 2.5% in 2001–2002 to 6.9% in 2012–2013 [24]. Some studies suggest no significant differences in the pattern of cannabis use among pregnant compared to non-pregnant women. For instance, a nationally representative study found among approximately 18,000 cannabis users about 16% of pregnant participants reported daily cannabis use, compared to 13% of nonpregnant participants [25]. The rising prevalence of cannabis use, however, has public health ramifications on women's health, given some of its negative effects both on maternal and fetal health [23]. In a meta-analysis of 24 eligible studies relating the maternal cannabis exposure and fetal outcomes, Gunn and colleagues found active cannabis use increased the odds of anemia in pregnant women by approximately 36%. The study also reported an increased odds of low birth weight and admission to a neonatal intensive care unit among infants exposed to cannabis in utero compared with nonexposed infants [26].

Another general health concern regards cannabis exposure during adolescence as this has been associated with the development of psychosis in genetically susceptible individuals [27, 28].

While there is a growing literature on the clinical benefits of cannabis (e.g., in treating intractable seizures and pain and improving appetite in HIV and cancer patients), its negative health consequences are real and should be considered when developing policies regulating the availability and use of marijuana.

Conclusion

New studies have emerged showing the rising prevalence of substance use among women and its impact on women's health and society. The effort to establish evidence-based and cost-effective interventions for opioid and tobacco use is particularly crucial as current data shows their increased use among women globally. Novel approaches to evaluate the impact of marijuana legalization on women's health should also be encouraged.

References

1. Center for Behavioral Health Statistics and Quality. Results from the 2016 National Survey on drug use and health: detailed tables. Rockville: Substance Abuse and Mental Health Services Administration; 2017. https://www.samhsa.gov/data/sites/default/files/NSDUH-DetTabs-2016/NSDUH-DetTabs-2016.pdf. Retrieved 26 Jan 2019.
2. Greenfield SF, Back SE, Lawson K, Brady KT. Substance abuse in women. Psychiatr Clin. 2010;33(2):339–55.
3. Becker JB, McClellan ML, Reed BG. Sex differences, gender and addiction. J Neurosci Res. 2017;95(1–2):136–47.
4. Cormier RA, Dell CA, Poole N. Women and substance abuse problems. BMC Womens Health. 2004;4(1):S8.
5. Back SE, Payne RL, Wahlquist AH, Carter RE, Stroud Z, Haynes L, et al. Comparative profiles of men and women with opioid dependence: results from a national multisite effectiveness trial. Am J Drug Alcohol Abuse. 2011;37(5):313–23.
6. Nyaronga D, Greenfield TK, McDaniel PA. Drinking context and drinking problems among Black, White, and Hispanic men and women in the 1984, 1995, and 2005 US National Alcohol Surveys. J Stud Alcohol Drugs. 2009;70(1):16–26.
7. White AM, Slater ME, Ng G, Hingson R, Breslow R. Trends in alcohol-related emergency department visits in the United States: results from the Nationwide emergency department sample, 2006 to 2014. Alcohol Clin Exp Res. 2018;42(2):352–9.
8. QuickStats: death rates for chronic liver disease and cirrhosis, by sex and age group — national vital statistics system, United States, 2000 and 2015. MMWR Morb Mortal Wkly Rep. 2017;66:1031. https://doi.org/10.15585/mmwr.mm6638a9.
9. Glenn SW, Parsons OA, Stevens L. Effects of alcohol abuse and familial alcoholism on physical health in men and women. Health Psychol. 1989;8(3):325.
10. Nolen-Hoeksema S. Gender differences in risk factors and consequences for alcohol use and problems. Clin Psychol Rev. 2004;24(8):981–1010.
11. Collaborative Group on Hormonal Factors in Breast Cancer. Alcohol, tobacco and breast cancer–collaborative reanalysis of individual data from 53 epidemiological studies, including 58 515 women with breast cancer and 95 067 women without the disease. Br J Cancer. 2002;87(11):1234.
12. Alcohol's Effects on the Body | National Institute on Alcohol Abuse and Alcoholism (NIAAA). 2019. Niaaa.nih.gov. Retrieved 1 Feb 2019 from https://www.niaaa.nih.gov/alcohol-health/alcohols-effects-body.
13. Popova S, Lange S, Probst C, Gmel G, Rehm J. Estimation of national, regional, and global prevalence of alcohol use during pregnancy and fetal alcohol syndrome: a systematic review and meta-analysis. Lancet Glob Health. 2017;5(3):e290–9.
14. CDC - Fact Sheet - Adult Cigarette Smoking in the United States - Smoking & Tobacco Use. 2019. Smoking and tobacco use. Retrieved 1 Feb 2019 from https://www.cdc.gov/tobacco/data_statistics/fact_sheets/adult_data/cig_smoking/index.htm.
15. Campbell CI, et al. Age and gender trends in long-term opioid analgesic use for noncancer pain. Am J Public Health. 2010;100(12):2541–7. https://doi.org/10.2105/AJPH.2009.180646.
16. Hemsing N, Greaves L, Poole N, Schmidt R. Misuse of prescription opioid medication among women: a scoping review. Pain Res Manag. 2016;2016:1754195.
17. Reddy UM, Davis JM, Ren Z, Greene MF, Opioid Use in Pregnancy, Neonatal Abstinence Syndrome, and Childhood Outcomes Workshop Invited Speakers. Opioid use in pregnancy, neonatal abstinence syndrome, and childhood outcomes: executive summary of a joint workshop by the Eunice Kennedy Shriver National Institute of Child Health and Human Development, American College of Obstetricians and Gynecologists, American Academy of Pediatrics, Society for Maternal-Fetal Medicine, Centers for Disease Control and Prevention, and the March of Dimes Foundation. Obstetr Gynecol. 2017;130(1):10–28.
18. Kocherlakota P. Neonatal abstinence syndrome. Pediatrics. 2014;134(2):e547–61. https://doi.org/10.1542/peds.2013-3524.
19. Center for Behavioral Health Statistics and Quality. 2017 National Survey on drug use and health: detailed

tables. Rockville: Substance Abuse and Mental Health Services Administration; 2018. Retrieved 31 Jan 2019.
20. NIDA. 2016. Cocaine. Retrieved from https://www.drugabuse.gov/publications/research-reports/cocaine on 2019, January 31.
21. McHugh RK, Wigderson S, Greenfield SF. Epidemiology of substance use in reproductive-age women. Obstet Gynecol Clin N Am. 2014;41(2):177–89.
22. Bauer CR, Langer JC, Shankaran S, et al. Acute neonatal effects of cocaine exposure during pregnancy. Arch Pediatr Adolesc Med. 2005;159(9):824–34. https://doi.org/10.1001/archpedi.159.9.824.
23. Mark K, Terplan M. Cannabis and pregnancy: maternal child health implications during a period of drug policy liberalization. Prev Med. 2017;104:46–9.
24. Hasin DS, Saha TD, Kerridge BT, et al. Prevalence of marijuana use disorders in the United States between 2001-2002 and 2012-2013. JAMA Psychiat. 2015;72(12):1235–42. https://doi.org/10.1001/jamapsychiatry.2015.1858.
25. Ko JY, Farr SL, Tong VT, Creanga AA, Callaghan WM. Prevalence and patterns of marijuana use among pregnant and nonpregnant women of reproductive age. Am J Obstet Gynecol. 2015;213(2):201–e1.
26. Gunn JKL, Rosales CB, Center KE, et al. Prenatal exposure to cannabis and maternal and child health outcomes: a systematic review and meta-analysis. BMJ Open. 2016;6:e009986. https://doi.org/10.1136/bmjopen-2015-009986.
27. Hall W, Degenhardt L. Cannabis use and the risk of developing a psychotic disorder. World Psychiatry. 2008;7(2):68–71.
28. Malone DT, Hill MN, Rubino T. Adolescent cannabis use and psychosis: epidemiology and neurodevelopmental models. Br J Pharmacol. 2010;160(3):511–22.

Part IV

Key Drugs of Abuse

13 Cannabinoids: The Case for Legal Regulation That Permits Recreational Adult Use

Tiesha T. Gregory, Kate O'Malley, Christopher Medina-Kirchner, Marc Grifell Guàrdia, and Carl L. Hart

Introduction

Currently, in the United States, there are few issues that animate the public discourse as much as cannabinoids and policies regulating their use. Discussions range from whether marijuana should be used medically to whether it should be legally available to adults seeking to alter their consciousness. Other hotly contested issues range from whether the enforcement of existing laws that regulate cannabis is conducted in a racially discriminatory manner to whether current draconian policies jeopardize the health of cannabinoid users seeking psychoactive alternatives in an effort to circumvent restrictive laws. The current chapter explores these and other pertinent cannabis-related issues. The chapter begins with a brief overview of cannabinoids and concludes with specific policy recommendations.

Cannabinoids These chemicals are generally defined as molecules that bind to cannabinoid receptors. They modify and regulate the activity of these receptors. Some are endogenously produced (endocannabinoids), whereas others are plant-derived (phytocannabinoids) or synthesized (synthetic cannabinoids). From a chemical structural perspective, cannabinoids are diverse. For example, many synthetic cannabinoids do not share structural commonality with the plant-derived cannabinoid Δ^9-tetrahydrocannabinol (THC), the major psychoactive component in marijuana.[1]

Medical Marijuana

Cannabis is still listed on Schedule I under the Federal Controlled Substance Act. This designa-

[1] For simplicity sake, we use the terms cannabis and marijuana interchangably throughout the chapter.

T. T. Gregory · C. Medina-Kirchner
Department of Psychology, Columbia University, New York, NY, USA
e-mail: ttg2110@columbia.edu; cmk2206@columbia.edu

K. O'Malley
Department of Psychological Sciences, Swinburne University, Hawthorn, VIC, Australia
e-mail: kate.omalley@columbia.edu

M. G. Guàrdia
Department of Psychology, Columbia University, New York, NY, USA

Department of Psychiatry and Legal Medicine, Universitat Autònoma de Barcelona, Cerdanyola del Vallés and IMIM (Hospital del Mar Medical Research Institute), Bellaterra, Spain

C. L. Hart (✉)
Department of Psychology, Columbia University, New York, NY, USA

Division on Substance Abuse, New York State Psychiatric Institute and Department of Psychiatry, Columbia University Irving Medical Center, Vagelos College of Physicians and Surgeons, New York, NY, USA
e-mail: clh42@columbia.edu

E. Akerele (ed.), *Substance and Non-Substance Related Addictions*,
https://doi.org/10.1007/978-3-030-84834-7_13

tion denotes that cannabis has "no currently accepted medical use, a lack of accepted safety for use under medical supervision, and a high potential for abuse." In short, cannabis itself is banned in the United States. Theoretically, this is true: Federal law forbids the use of cannabis as a medical treatment. But in practice, this issue is not so simple. Since 1978, the US Federal government has supplied (and still does) cannabis to a selective group of patients through the Compassionate Investigational New Drug program. The number of patients in the program was always small, about 15; the number of patients registered in 1992 when enrollment of new patients was discontinued. Today, there are only three patients enrolled.

Despite being categorized as a Schedule I drug, cannabis-related medical usefulness has been documented in the scientific literature. Dozens of scientists—myself (CH) included—have been engaged in such research for decades. That is how we know, for example, that the drug stimulates appetite in HIV-positive patients (e.g., [23]) and that cannabis is useful in the treatment of neuropathic pain, chronic pain, and spasticity due to multiple sclerosis [31]. While we recognize that the number of ailments for which cannabis has been demonstrated to mitigate seems to increase each year, we are cognizant and suspicious of exaggerated claims promoting the substance as a cure for everything from heartache to cancer.

Nevertheless, it is incumbent upon scientists to acknowledge cannabis-related potential medical utility. Citizens in multiple US states certainly have. Cannabis-related therapeutic benefits have compelled many throughout the country to vote to legalize medical marijuana at the state level. Since 2010, for example, the number of states that allow patients to take the drug for specific medical conditions has jumped from 16 to 33—a figure that is expected to climb steadily with each successive election season. And yet Federal law still technically forbids the use of medical marijuana. The inconsistency of Federal laws with these other programs and initiatives, and with the increasing number of studies demonstrating the medical usefulness of the substance, makes marijuana's Schedule I status seem like medical and/or governmental hypocrisy, undermining peoples' trust in the relevant Federal agencies.

Cannabis-based medications Perhaps as some acknowledgment of the perceived hypocrisy, the US Food and Drug Agency has approved one cannabis-derived and three cannabis-related medications. Epidiolex, which contains cannabidiol (CBD)—a cannabinoid found in the cannabis plant, is indicated to treat seizures associated with Lennox-Gastaut syndrome or Dravet syndrome in patients 2 years of age and older. The FDA also has approved Marinol and Syndros for the treatment of conditions such as anorexia associated with weight loss in AIDS patients and chemotherapy-induced nausea. Marinol and Syndros include the active ingredient dronabinol, which is synthetic Δ^9-tetrahydrocannabinol (THC), the most psychoactive component of cannabis. Finally, Cesamet has been approved for the treatment of nausea and vomiting associated with cancer chemotherapy in patients who have failed to respond adequately to other standard antiemetic treatments. Cesamet contains the active ingredient nabilone, which is a synthetic cannabinoid similar to THC.

Adult Recreational Cannabis Use

Another factor that potentially erodes public trust in governmental agencies and media outlets is the distorted claims made about the effects produced by the *drogue du jour*. Public statements regarding the recreational use of cannabis have been outstanding in this regard. For example, there has been a resurgence of media coverage drawing a causal link between cannabis use and psychosis. Popular press headlines blare, for example, "Higher than ever: New study links strong weed to psychosis" [38]. The implication is, of course, that cannabis smoking leads to psychotic disorders. This reasoning ignores the fact that such conclusions are based on data from correlational studies (e.g., [13]), which are insufficient to determine a cause-effect relationship. Even worse, some observers assert that the drug causes people to behave violently (e.g., [10]). Given the growing popularity of such claims, we felt that it is important to address two questions specifically: Does cannabis cause psychotic disorders such as schizophrenia, and do associated symptoms like paranoia lead to violent crimes?

To be clear, we find these assertions to be misinformed and even reckless.

It is true that people diagnosed with psychosis are more likely to report current or prior use of cannabis than people without psychosis [6]. The easy conclusion to draw from that is that cannabis use caused an increased risk of psychosis, and it is that easy answer that some—especially those seeking to sell newspapers, books, and sensational movies—have seized upon. However, this ignores the evidence that psychotic behavior is also associated with higher rates of tobacco use [43] and with the use of stimulants [42]. Do all these things "cause" psychosis, or is there another, more likely answer? One of the most important things science professors try to impart to undergraduate students is the distinction between correlation (two things are statistically associated) and causation (one thing causes another). For example, the wearing of light clothing is more likely during the same months as higher sales of ice cream, but we do not believe that either causes the other.

Psychosis In our extensive 2016 review of the cannabis-psychosis literature [34], we concluded that those individuals who are susceptible to developing psychosis (which usually does not appear until around the age of 20) are also susceptible to other forms of problem behavior, including poor school performance, lying, stealing, and early and heavy use of various substances. Many of these behaviors appear earlier in development, but the fact that one thing occurs before another also is not proof of causation. Actually, this is one of the standard logical fallacies taught in logic classes, post hoc *ergo propter hoc*, which means "after this, therefore because of this." It is also worth noting that tenfold increases in cannabis use in the United Kingdom from the 1970s to the 2000s were not associated with an increase in rates of psychosis over this same period; further evidence that changes in cannabis use in the general population are unlikely to contribute to changes in psychosis [19].

Violence Evidence from research tells us that aggression and violence are highly unlikely outcomes of cannabis use. Based on our own laboratory research, during which we have given thousands of doses of cannabis to people—carefully studying their brain, behavioral, cognitive, and social responses—we have never seen a research participant become violent or aggressive while under the influence of the drug (see, [25–27, 29, 33]), as have been alleged. The main effects of smoking cannabis are contentment, relaxation, sedation, euphoria, and increased hunger. Still, very high THC concentrations can cause mild paranoia, visual, and/or auditory distortions, but even these effects are rare and usually seen only in very inexperienced users. It is possible that the rarely experienced, temporary paranoid state seen in some cannabis users has fueled notions that cannabis *causes* a permanent psychotic disorder. But it is paramount to distinguish between these two concepts. The temporary effects of a drug should not be confused with the drug-induced permanent alterations.

Reefer madness: before and now There is a broader point that needs to be made—one that speaks to the recklessness of the "cannabis causes violence" claim. In the 1930s, numerous media reports in the Unites States exaggerated the connection between cannabis use by Black people and violent crimes. During Congressional hearings concerning the regulation of the drug, Harry J. Anslinger, commissioner of the US Bureau of Narcotics, repeated such claims and declared, "Marijuana is the most violence-causing drug in the history of mankind." Anslinger's fabricated testimony was used to justify racial discrimination and to facilitate passage of the Marijuana Tax Act in 1937, which essentially banned the drug. As we see, the reefer madness rhetoric of the past has not just evaporated; it continued and has evolved, reinventing itself perhaps even more powerfully today.

In the United States, there have been several recent cases during which police officers cited the fictitious dangers posed by cannabis to justify their deadly actions. Michael Brown of Ferguson, MO, in 2014; Philando Castile of St. Paul, MN, in 2016; and Keith Lamont Scott, of Charlotte, North Carolina, in 2016, were all killed by police who used some version of this bogus defense.

Ramarley Graham of New York, New York, in 2012; Trayvon Martin of Sanford, FL, in 2012; Rumain Brisbon of Phoenix, AZ, in 2014; and Sandra Bland of Prairie View, Texas, in 2015, all also had their lives cut short as a result of an interaction with law enforcement (or a proxy) initiated under the pretense of cannabis use suspicion.

Racial discrimination in arrests In the Unites States, Black people are four times more likely to be arrested for cannabis possession than their White counterparts [15], despite the fact that both groups use and sell cannabis at similar rates [50]. This, by the way, is the definition of racial discrimination: an action(s) that results in disproportionate unjust or unfair treatment of persons from a specific racial group [30]. Note that malicious intent of the perpetrator is not required. What is required is that the treatment be unjust or unfair and that such injustice is disproportionately experienced by at least one racial group.

Even worse, the racial discrimination that occurs with cannabis arrests continues to go on despite the fact that the possession of the drug had been decriminalized in many US cities. Take Baltimore, for example, where Black people represent about 60% of the population and about as many cannabis users. Decriminalization took effect there in October of 2014. Yet, between 2015 and 2017, Baltimore police arrested 1514 individuals for weed possession; 1450 were Black people [40]. That's 96%. Similar numbers have been reported for cities like Brooklyn, Chicago, Manhattan, and Philadelphia.

Table 13.1 States where adult recreational marijuana use is legal

State	Year passed
Alaska	2014
Arizona	2020
California	2016
Colorado	2012
Connecticutt	2021
Illinois	2020
Maine	2016
Massachusetts	2016
Michigan	2018
Montana	2020
Nevada	2016
New Jersey	2020
New Mexico	2021
New York	2021
Oregon	2014
Virginia	2021
Vermont	2018
Washington	2012

Citizens calling for legalization The fact that cannabis is the most widely used banned substance—25 million US citizens use it monthly—makes it difficult to justify the above injustices [50]. In addition, the momentum for legalizing adult recreational cannabis use has steadily increased since 2000. According to the most recent Gallup Poll, more than 60% of Americans say that cannabis should be legalized [39]. This figure marks the highest support for legalization over nearly half a century. Correspondingly, a growing number of states have legalized recreational use of marijuana via ballot initiatives. As of June 2019, ten states allow adults to purchase and consume the drug recreationally (Table 13.1).

In 2013, Uruguay became the first country in the world to legalize the recreational use of cannabis, and in 2018, Canada became the second.

Synthetic Cannabinoids

Despite the above legal developments, it is important to emphasize that recreational cannabis use is still prohibited by the US federal law and by state law in a majority of jurisdictions, not to mention cannabis prohibition that continues around the globe. As a result, some have sought psychoactive alternatives that produce cannabis-like effects, namely, synthetic cannabinoids. Typically, these substances are not yet banned, and many are not detected by traditional urine drug screens.

Synthetic cannabinoids are the fastest-growing and largest group of new psychoactive substances (NPS), with hundreds of these compounds now developed [16]. Initially, these drugs were synthesized by scientists such as John W. Huffman (JWH) and others for the purpose of studying the endocannabinoid system. Huffman's research, for example, sought to better understand how cannabinoids could be used in medicine. Since then, the number of clandestine laboratories producing synthetic cannabinoids for recreational use has proliferated. This has prompted several governments around the world to act. Most have acted predictably by prohibiting these drugs with little, if any, consideration for the fact that restrictive policies will hamper medical research using synthetic cannabinoids. Even less attention has been focused on how these policies could adversely impact the health of adults who use cannabinoids to alter their consciousness and/or behavior.

Recreational use and subsequent banning of these compounds in the United States is emblematic of a larger drug policy problem that extends beyond synthetic cannabinoids and well beyond North America. Thus, we believe the synthetic cannabinoid-marijuana story in the United States is instructive for anyone interested in formulating drug policies that respect individuals' civil liberties and enhance public health and safety.

Recreational Appeal of Synthetic Cannabinoids

Starting around the mid-2000s, when synthetic cannabinoids were legally available, reports began surfacing about the growing consumption of products containing these drugs, including JWH-018, JWH-073, and CP 47,497. Like THC, many of these drugs stimulate cannabinoid receptors in the brain. Although the pharmacological effects of synthetic cannabinoids can vary widely, some, when inhaled, engender psychoactive effects similar to those produced by smoked marijuana, including euphoria and relaxation (e.g., [11, 20, 21]). Indeed, synthetic cannabinoids are sometimes referred to as synthetic marijuana. Not surprisingly, responses obtained from survey questionnaires indicate that most users report that they consume synthetic cannabinoids primarily because of the pleasurable effects produced by these drugs (e.g., [51]). Given that the recreational use of marijuana was legally prohibited throughout the United States until 2014, the year when the use by adults was legalized in only two states (Colorado and Washington), it is not difficult to see the appeal of synthetic cannabinoids for those seeking a legal alterative to marijuana use.

At the time, synthetic cannabinoid-containing products were legal and widely available. They were sold in "head shops," convenience stores, and through the Internet to anyone seeking a "marijuana-like high." These products were marketed as natural herbal incense or potpourri under various brand names such as "Spice" or "K2," and they were available to anyone in the know, regardless of age. This, combined with the fact that most synthetic cannabinoids were not detected by standard urine drug tests, further enhanced their appeal among specific individuals, especially those under the age of 21 years and those subjected to random drug screens as a condition of employment, among other reasons (e.g., [21, 51]).

Little Is Known About the Effects of Synthetic Cannabinoids in Humans

Over the past several decades, there have been hundreds of laboratory studies investigating the direct effects of marijuana on human behavior. As a result, our knowledge about marijuana-related effects in humans has increased dramatically. Such knowledge affords us the ability to maximize beneficial effects while minimizing deleterious ones. For example, our research demonstrates that marijuana attenuates performance and mood disruptions during night shift work [33]. Another beneficial effect produced by marijuana is the stimulation of appetite in HIV-positive patients (e.g., [23]), which could be lifesaving for someone suffering from AIDS wasting syndrome.

On the other hand, there is empirical evidence demonstrating marijuana withdrawal symptoms following abrupt discontinuation of heavy, near-daily use of the drug (e.g., [22, 28]). Marijuana withdrawal is not life threatening, but symptoms can be unpleasant and can persist from 4 to 12 days, depending on an individual's level of dependence. Importantly, marijuana withdrawal symptoms can be mitigated with the use of specific medications, including synthetic cannabinoid agonists, oral THC, and nabilone (e.g., [22, 24, 28]). As noted above, both of these medications are also FDA-approved for the treatment of nausea and vomiting associated with cancer chemotherapy. Oral THC is also approved to treat loss of appetite and weight loss in patients with HIV infection. These observations show that there is a large database assessing marijuana-related effects and that the drug has been demonstrated to produce a range of effects, including therapeutic.

And while there is growing evidence in support of the notion that synthetic cannabinoids, such as oral THC and nabilone, are important tools in the medical armamentarium, a comparable database does not exist for other synthetic cannabinoids. In fact, with the exception of the FDA-approved oral synthetic cannabinoids, there are no published laboratory studies assessing the direct effects of these drugs in humans, nor there are data evaluating human response following abrupt discontinuation of the regular use of synthetic cannabinoids in research participants. Consequently, our understanding of the effects produced by the majority of drugs from this class is primarily based on results from in vitro receptor-binding studies, data collected using laboratory animals, survey responses of synthetic cannabinoids users, and anecdotal and case reports.

While information obtained from the above sources can provide some clues about the behavioral effects of synthetic cannabinoids in humans, these data, when used alone, are limited. For instance, there are two types of cannabinoid receptors, designated CB_1 and CB_2. The structures of these two receptors and their anatomical distribution in the body vary considerably. CB_2 receptors are found mainly outside the brain in immune cells, suggesting that cannabinoids may play a role in the modulation of the immune response. CB_1 receptors are found primarily in the brain and are thought to mediate psychoactive effects produced by cannabinoids such as THC. Data from receptor-binding studies have revealed that several synthetic cannabinoids found in products sold for recreational purposes (e.g., JWH-018 and AMB-FUBINACA) have greater affinities for the CB_1 receptor and are more potent agonists than THC [7–9, 37]. But this information alone tells us nothing about the subjective or behavioral effects produced by these drugs in people. In other words, simply knowing a drug's receptor affinity does not provide sufficient information to determine the myriad of potential psychoactive effects produced by that drug.

Still, consistent findings from survey data and case reports show that synthetic cannabinoids, when smoked, are generally well-tolerated and produce overlapping subjective effects with marijuana [21]. In fact, some users have even reported that they smoke these substances to alleviate marijuana withdrawal [20], further suggesting pharmacological specificity between smoked marijuana and synthetic cannabinoids. Of course, this information is largely anecdotal, which raises concern about the veracity of their purported effects in humans. Evidence from rigorously conducted studies are needed to help resolve this issue, but such investigations seem unlikely given recent legislative trends that reflexively prohibit nearly all novel synthetic cannabinoids that act as agonists at CB_1 receptors.

Unintended Consequences of Prohibition

As can be seen in Table 13.2, US authorities began prohibiting synthetic cannabinoids in 2011. Similar legal actions have been taken by many European countries as well, and the number of banned synthetic cannabinoids continues to grow with each successive year. In the United States alone, there are now dozens of compounds on the prohibited list (Table 13.2).

The prohibition of these substances has been far-reaching, precipitating a range of consequences, especially undesired ones. Under the current legal scheme, criminal sanctions can be imposed not only for possessing, manufacturing, distributing, importing, or exporting these substances, but also for the use of these compounds in the pursuit of research or instructional activities. In laymen's terms, this means that there will be virtually no further scientific investigation of banned synthetic cannabinoid drugs. Given that some of these drugs are highly selective for cannabinoid receptors—receptors that are much more abundant than wide-spread opioid receptors (important pain modulators), indicating that they are crucial in modulating many basic human functions—the potential negative impact of the ban on research aimed at better understanding the endocannabinoid system, including the of development of medical treatments, is difficult to understate. In short, our knowledge about these banned substances as well as the endogenous cannabinoid system has been inappropriately truncated by politics and remains limited as a result of implementing less than thoughtful regulatory schemes.

Table 13.2 A list of synthetic cannabinoids and the year they were banned in the United States

Synthetic cannabinoid	Year banned
Cannabicyclohexanol, CP 47,497; JWH-018, JWH-073, and JWH200	2011
AM2201, AM694, JWH-019, JWH-081, JWH-122, JWH-203, JWH-250, JWH-398, SR-18, and SR-19	2012
APINACA, UR-144, and XLR11	2013
5F-PB-22, AB-FUBINACA, ADB-PINACA, and PB-22	2014
AB-CHMINACA, AB-PINACA, and THJ-2201	2015
ADB-CHMINACA	2016
5F-ADB, 5F-AMB, 5F-APINACA, ADB-FUBINACA, AMB-FUBINACA, MDMB-CHMICA, and MDMB-FUBINACA	2017
4-CN-CUMYL-BUTINACA, 5F-AB-PINACA, 5F-CUMYL-P7AICA, 5F-EDMB-PINACA, 5F-MDMB-PICA, FUB-144, FUB-AKB48, **MAB-CHMINACA,** MMB-CHMICA, NM2201, and SGT-25	2018

To put this in practical terms, consider the growing evidence indicating that THC-based cannabinoids modestly enhance the analgesic effects of opioid medications [1, 12, 44, 45–47]. Conceivably, synthetic cannabinoids, with a more favorable receptor-binding profile than THC, could turn out to be even more effective therapeutic tools to enhance opioid-related analgesia. In addition, this approach potentially mitigates some adverse effects of opioids by allowing lower doses of these medications. Relatedly, the observation that the annual number of opioid-related overdose deaths is lower than expected in states that permit the medical use of marijuana is intriguing [5]. Of course, these findings are correlational and a causal relationship between marijuana use and opioid-related deaths has yet to be established. Nonetheless, by reflexively banning synthetic cannabinoids, it precludes our ability to study these compounds as potential therapeutics in dealing with the so-called opioid crisis.

Another unintended consequence of prohibiting specific synthetic cannabinoid drugs is the rapid introduction of slightly modified chemicals to circumvent existing laws. It works like this: Law enforcement detects a new synthetic cannabinoid in the illicit market; it's then banned, followed by a proliferation of new, yet-to-be-banned, usually more potent and potentially dangerous substances introduced as replacements. In 2008, there were only five compounds included on the United Nations Office on Drugs and Crime (UNODC) synthetic cannabinoid list. By the end of 2018, the number had ballooned to nearly 300 [52].

These developments can contribute to considerable health-related harms for individuals who consume products containing newer, unknown synthetic cannabinoids. For example, between 2009 and 2011, if a consumer purchased a product called "K2," it most likely contained JWH-018 as the active ingredient. In 2011, JWH-018 was banned, prompting illicit manufactures to replace the compound with a less known, more potent synthetic cannabinoid or with multiple agents. In light of the fact that products sold as synthetic cannabinoids on the illicit market are frequently poorly labeled, containing a mixture of herbs and aromatic extracts sprayed with unspecified synthetic cannabinoid compounds, consumers who purchased K2 in 2012 (or subsequently) seeking the exact high that they experienced from previously purchased K2 products might be unpleasantly surprised and/or untoward effects.

In a series of experiments aimed at assessing the presence of synthetic cannabinoids in the German market, Beuerle and colleagues have provided empirical support for the above (e.g., [17, 18, 35, 36]). Between 2012 and 2015, these researchers found that (1) the number of new synthetic cannabinoids, with slightly modified chemical structures, dramatically increased; (2) the active ingredient in several products changed frequently; (3) many products contained multiple new synthetic cannabinoids; and (4) the doses contained in these products varied widely, despite having identical package labeling. Others, using forensic analyses, have also reported that many synthetic cannabinoids found in these products are not included on package labeling (e.g., [14, 32, 36]).

Sometimes it is easy to forget that the above is not merely an intellectual exercise. Indeed, overly restrictive drug policies and their unintended consequences frequently have bona fide harmful health effects on the lives of everyday people. A good case in point is the events of July 12, 2016, in New York City. On this day, 33 people in a predominately Black, Brooklyn neighborhood were reported to be stupendously intoxicated after consuming what was referred to as "synthetic marijuana." Some of these individuals temporarily lost consciousness, became debilitated, and disoriented, but fortunately, no one died. Meanwhile, local and national media headlines blared with titles such as "Synthetic marijuana overdose turns dozens into 'zombies' in NYC" [41]. Accompanying stories and videos dramatized the extraordinary potency and ill effects of K2. Each was peppered with sensational quotes like this one from an article in *The New York Times*: "It's like a scene out of a zombie movie, a horrible scene" [48]. The conspicuous moralism dehumanizing users of this class of drug was palpable.

But unfortunately, virtually all of these pieces were devoid of any useful information that would enhance public health and safety. For example, not one article confirmed that a synthetic cannabinoid had indeed been ingested. Not one reported the actual contents contained in the products the victims were alleged to have consumed. Not one mentioned that the observed ill effects could have been caused by other substances or some other factor. This point is particularly important because most of the victims had been observed next to a local methadone clinic, suggesting that some were patients at the clinic. Obviously, the combined effects of the opioid medication with other drugs could have been a contributing factor in the reported adverse effects.

Frustrated by such irresponsible reporting and patent neglect for public health, I (CH) went on a local news program calling for city health officials to retrieve the alleged products and test them in order to determine their constituents (https://www.youtube.com/watch?v=MqqM2QSVjRA). I also called for officials to obtain biological assays (blood, urine) from patients who were transported to the hospital to see if this information corresponded with results from the tested products. In this way, specific possible causes of the problem could have been carefully investigated, and findings could have been widely publicized. Members of the press, the local community, and the broader drug-using community, among others, could have all have been alerted, potentially preventing further harms to unsuspecting users of the agent that turned out to be the culprit. This didn't happen, at least not initially.

Several months passed before the general public was provided with any useful information regarding a potential causal agent in the so-called zombie outbreak. On December 14, 2016, 5 months after sensationalistic zombie stories appeared in the popular press, *The New York Times* published an article identifying a new, more potent synthetic cannabinoid as the culprit [49]. This conclusion was based on findings from an article published in the prestigious *New England Journal of Medicine* about the incident [2]. This group of researchers obtained and tested blood and urine samples from 8 individuals among the 33 who had been reported to have experienced adverse effects of an alleged synthetic cannabinoid. They also tested a sample of the herbal "incense" product "AK-47 24 Karat Gold," which was claimed to be the item responsible for the ill effects. The findings revealed that the synthetic cannabinoid AMB-FUBINACA was identified in all eight individually tested packets of AK-47 24 Karat Gold and that its metabolite was found in the blood of all eight individuals. Importantly, the amount of AMB-FUBINACA contained in individual AK-47 24 Karat Gold packets was not consistent, ranging from 14 to 25 mg/g. In addition, half of the tested patients had other drugs in their system, including an antidepressant, antihistamine, benzodiazepine, and opioid medications.

Back in 2016, AMB-FUBINACA was not yet banned in the United States. So, it is quite likely that manufacturers of synthetic marijuana included it in their products as the active component for this reason. But, it is important to note that AMB-FUBINACA is considerably more potent than THC, meaning far less of this substance is needed to produce psychoactive and other effects, including deleterious. Similarly, AMB-FUBINACA is even more potent than JWH-018—one of the earlier cannabinoids found in "fake" marijuana products.

Incorporating Evidence Into Policy and Practice

Perhaps the most important factor in determining the effects produced by any drug is the amount taken. In general, larger amounts increase the likelihood of harmful effects. This is one of the most basic principles of pharmacology. For this reason, we are concerned that knee-jerk responses to ban any new substances will invariably lead to a burgeoning number of less well-known and potentially more dangerous substances in the illicit market. As can be seen from the Brooklyn example, this approach has been consistently shown to jeopardize the health of people who consume products obtained on the illicit market.

It is naïve to believe that people will not engage in an activity simply because it has been deemed forbidden by a government. Indeed, a mistaken underlying assumption guiding many overly restrictive approaches to drug regulation is that once a drug is banned, then the demand for that drug and its desired effects will dissipate. Nothing could be further from the truth. Since humans have inhabited the earth, they have always sought to alter their consciousness with psychoactive plants and other materials. This is a normal human pursuit. And it continues today with no foreseeable abatement in the near future. Given this reality, it is incumbent upon any responsible government to think cogently about how to balance the natural human desire to alter one's mood with public health and safety.

As we consider this challenge within the context of cannabinoids, it is important to remember that most recreational users of synthetic cannabinoids consume these substances in search of a marijuana-like high and that unfavorable outcomes are rarely associated with the use of marijuana. Furthermore, an outbreak of negative health reactions to synthetic cannabinoids—like that which has been reported in several states, including Connecticut, Illinois, Maryland, and New York—is virtually unheard of in states where marijuana use by adults is legal (Table 13.1). *Thus, our first policy recommendation is the expansion of legalized recreational marijuana.* This would be a simple measure to mitigate many problems related to synthetic cannabinoid use. It would also remove a conspicuous tool—enforcement of restrictive marijuana laws—used to discriminate against Black people. Of course, this can be done by state ballot initiatives. But it would be ideal for the US government to follow the leads of Uruguay and Canada by legalizing the drug at the federal level.

The fact remains that recreational marijuana is still banned in the United States. As such, people will continue to consume alternative substances, including synthetic cannabinoids, seeking the marijuana high. A key drawback is that some products contain dangerous adulterants and/or extremely potent cannabinoids that are not included on the package labeling. The consumption of these products by unwitting consumers can lead to severe adverse consequences, including delirium, cardiotoxicity, seizures, acute kidney injury, hyperthermia, and death (e.g., [3, 4]). *Thus, our second policy recommendation is the implementation of free, anonymous drug safety testing services.* It works like this: drug samples can be submitted for testing in order to determine the constituents contained in that sample. This information can be given to the user, so they can decide whether or not to take a particular drug and how much of it to take. These procedures have been shown to reduce the number of people exposed to harmful effects of unknown drugs (e.g., Measham 2019).

In conclusion, cannabinoids are a hot topic, and their consumption by humans remains steady, despite years of draconian policies designed to eliminate their use but have instead limited personal freedoms and have contributed to racial discrimination, among other negative consequences. Thus, it is imperative that responsible governments take necessary steps to ensure the autonomy, health, and safety of their citizens. Authorities in a growing number of US states, as well as those in the countries of Uruguay and Canada, have implemented cannabis regulatory schemes in line with these goals. We hope others will follow.

Acknowledgments Dr. Grifell's time and contributions to this project were made possible thanks to the Rio Hortega grant (CM18/00168) from Instituto de Salud Carlos III (ISCIII) and Fondo Social Europeo (FSE) and a grant from the Open Society Foundation (OR2018-44135). The authors declare that they have no conflicts of interest.

References

1. Abrams DI, Couey P, Shade SB, Kelly ME, Benowitz NL. Cannabinoid–opioid interaction in chronic pain. Clin Pharmacol Ther. 2011;90(6):844–51. https://doi.org/10.1038/clpt.2011.188.
2. Adams AJ, Banister SD, Irizarry L, Trecki J, Schwartz M, Gerona R. "Zombie" outbreak caused by the synthetic cannabinoid AMB-FUBINACA in New York. N Engl J Med. 2017;376:235–42. https://doi.org/10.1056/NEJMoa1610300.
3. Alipour A, Patel PB, Shabbir Z, Gabrielson S. Review of the many faces of synthetic cannabinoid toxicities. Mental Health Clin. 2019;9(2):93–9. https://doi.org/10.9740/mhc.2019.03.093.
4. Armstrong F, McCurdy MT, Heavner MS. Synthetic cannabinoid-associated multiple organ failure: Case series and literature review. Pharmacotherapy. 2019;39(4):508–13. https://doi.org/10.1002/phar.2241.
5. Bachhuber MA, Saloner B, Cunningham CO, Barry CL. Medical cannabis laws and opioid analgesic overdose mortality in the United States, 1999-2010. JAMA Intern Med. 2014;174(10):1668–73. https://doi.org/10.1001/jamainternmed.2014.4005.
6. Bahorik AL, Newhill CE, Eack SM. Neurocognitive functioning of individuals with schizophrenia: Using and not using drugs. Schizophr Bull. 2014;40(4):856–67. https://doi.org/10.1093/schbul/sbt099.
7. Banister SD, Moir M, Stuart J, Kevin RC, Wood KE, Longworth M, et al. Pharmacology of indole and indazole synthetic cannabinoid designer drugs AB-FUBINACA, ADB-FUBINACA, AB-PINACA, ADB-PINACA, 5F-AB-PINACA, 5F-ADB-PINACA, ADBICA, and 5F-ADBICA. ACS Chem Neurosci. 2015a;6(9):1546–59. https://doi.org/10.1021/acschemneuro.5b00112.
8. Banister SD, Stuart J, Kevin RC, Edington A, Longworth M, Wilkinson SM, et al. Effects of bioisosteric fluorine in synthetic cannabinoid designer drugs JWH-018, AM-2201, UR-144, XLR-11, PB-22, 5F-PB-22, APICA, and STS-135. ACS Chem Neurosci. 2015b;6(8):1445–58. https://doi.org/10.1021/acschemneuro.5b00107.
9. Banister SD, Longworth M, Kevin R, Sachdev S, Santiago M, Stuart J, et al. Pharmacology of valinate and tert-leucinate synthetic cannabinoids 5F-AMBICA, 5F-AMB, 5F-ADB, AMB-FUBINACA, MDMB-FUBINACA, MDMB-

CHMICA, and their analogues. ACS Chem Neurosci. 2016;7(9):1241–54. https://doi.org/10.1021/acschemneuro.6b00137.
10. Berenson A. Tell your children: The truth about marijuana, mental illness, and violence. New York: Free Press; 2019.
11. Cooper ZD, Haney M. Sex-dependent effects of cannabis-induced analgesia. Drug Alcohol Depend. 2016;167:112–20. https://doi.org/10.1016/j.drugalcdep.2016.08.001.
12. Cooper ZD, Bedi G, Ramesh D, Balter R, Comer SD, Haney M. Impact of co-administration of oxycodone and smoked cannabis on analgesia and abuse liability. Neuropsychopharmacology. 2018;43(10):2046. https://doi.org/10.1038/s41386-018-0011-2.
13. Di Forti MD, Quattrone D, Freeman TP, Tripoli G, Gayer-Anderson C, Quigley H, et al. The contribution of cannabis use to variation in the incidence of psychotic disorder across Europe (EU-GEI): a multicentre case-control study. Lancet Psychiatry. 2019;6(5):427–36. https://doi.org/10.1016/S2215-0366(19)30048-3.
14. Dresen S, Ferreirós N, Pütz M, Westphal F, Zimmermann R, Auwärter V. Monitoring of herbal mixtures potentially containing synthetic cannabinoids as psychoactive compounds. J Mass Spectrom. 2010;45(10):1186–94. https://doi.org/10.1002/jms.1811.
15. Edwards E, Bunting W, Garcia L. The war on marijuana in black and white. American Civil Liberties Union report June 2013. 2013. http://www.samhsa.gov/data/sites/default/files/NSDUHresultsPDFWHTML2013/Web/NSDUHresults2013.pdf.
16. EMCDDA. European drug report 2016: Trends and developments. Luxembourg: Publications Office; 2016.
17. Ernst L, Brandhorst K, Papke U, Altrogge A, Zodel S, Langer N, Beuerle T. Identification and quantification of synthetic cannabinoids in 'spice-like' herbal mixtures: Update of the German situation in early 2017. Forensic Sci Int. 2017;277:51–8. https://doi.org/10.1016/j.forsciint.2017.05.019.
18. Ernst L, Langer N, Bockelmann A, Salkhordeh E, Beuerle T. Identification and quantification of synthetic cannabinoids in 'spice-like' herbal mixtures: Update of the German situation in summer 2018. Forensic Sci Int. 2019;294:96–102. https://doi.org/10.1016/j.forsciint.2018.11.001.
19. Gage SH, Zammit S, Hickman M. Stronger evidence is needed before accepting that cannabis plays an important role in the etiology of schizophrenia in the population. F1000 Rep Med. 2013;5:2. https://doi.org/10.3410/M5-2.
20. Gunderson EW, Haughey HM, Ait-Daoud N, Joshi AS, Hart CL. "Spice" and "K2" herbal highs: A case series and systematic review of the clinical effects and biopsychosocial implications of synthetic cannabinoid use in humans. Am J Addict. 2012;21(4):320–6. https://doi.org/10.1111/j.1521-0391.2012.00240.x.
21. Gunderson EW, Haughey HM, Ait-Daoud N, Joshi AS, Hart CL. A survey of synthetic cannabinoid consumption by current cannabis users. Subst Abus. 2014;35(2):184–9. https://doi.org/10.1080/08897077.2013.846288.
22. Haney M. The marijuana withdrawal syndrome: Diagnosis and treatment. Curr Psychiatry Rep. 2005;7(5):360–6. https://doi.org/10.1007/s11920-005-0036-1.
23. Haney M, Gunderson EW, Rabkin J, Hart CL, Vosburg SK, Comer SD, Foltin RW. Dronabinol and marijuana in HIV-positive marijuana smokers: Caloric intake, mood, and sleep. J Acquir Immune Defic Syndr. 2007;45(5):545–54. https://doi.org/10.1097/QAI.0b013e31811ed205.
24. Haney M, Cooper ZD, Bedi G, Vosburg SK, Comer SD, Foltin RW. Nabilone decreases marijuana withdrawal and a laboratory measure of marijuana relapse. Neuropsychopharmacology. 2013;38(8):1557–65. https://doi.org/10.1038/npp.2013.54.
25. Hart CL, van Gorp W, Haney M, Foltin RW, Fischman MW. Effects of acute smoked marijuana on complex cognitive performance. Neuropsychopharmacology. 2001;25(5):757–65. https://doi.org/10.1016/S0893-133X(01)00273-1.
26. Hart CL, Haney M, Ward AS, Fischman MW, Foltin RW. Effects of oral THC maintenance on smoked marijuana self-administration. Drug Alcohol Depend. 2002a;67(3):301–9. https://doi.org/10.1016/S0376-8716(02)00084-4.
27. Hart CL, Ward AS, Haney M, Comer SD, Foltin RW, Fischman MW. Comparison of smoked marijuana and oral delta(9)-tetrahydrocannabinol in humans. Psychopharmacology. 2002b;164(4):407–15. https://doi.org/10.1007/s00213-002-1231-y.
28. Hart CL. Increasing treatment options for cannabis dependence: A review of potential pharmacotherapies. Drug Alcohol Depend. 2005;80(2):147–59. https://doi.org/10.1016/j.drugalcdep.2005.03.027.
29. Hart CL, Ilan AB, Gevins A, Gunderson EW, Role K, Colley J, Foltin RW. Neurophysiological and cognitive effects of smoked marijuana in frequent users. Pharmacol Biochem Behav. 2010;96(3):333–41. https://doi.org/10.1016/j.pbb.2010.06.003.
30. Hart CL, Hart MZ. Opioid crisis: Another mechanism used to perpetuate American racism. Cult Divers Ethn Minor Psychol. 2019;25(1):6–11. https://doi.org/10.1037/cdp0000260.
31. Hill KP. Medical marijuana for treatment of chronic pain and other medical and psychiatric problems: A clinical review. JAMA. 2015;31324:2474–83. https://doi.org/10.1001/jama.2015.6199.
32. Hudson S, Ramsey J. The emergence and analysis of synthetic cannabinoids. Drug Test Anal. 2011;3(7–8):466–78. https://doi.org/10.1002/dta.268.
33. Keith DR, Gunderson EW, Haney M, Foltin RW, Hart CL. Smoked marijuana attenuates performance and mood disruptions during simulated night shift work. Drug Alcohol Depend. 2017;178:534–43. https://doi.org/10.1016/j.drugalcdep.2017.04.036.

34. Ksir C, Hart CL. Cannabis and psychosis: A critical overview of the relationship. Curr Psychiatry Rep. 2016;18:12. https://doi.org/10.1007/s11920-015-0657-y.
35. Langer N, Lindigkeit R, Schiebel H-M, Papke U, Ernst L, Beuerle T. Identification and quantification of synthetic cannabinoids in "spice-like" herbal mixtures: Update of the German situation for the spring of 2016. Forensic Sci Int. 2016;269:31–41. https://doi.org/10.1016/j.forsciint.2016.10.023.
36. Lindigkeit R, Boehme A, Eiserloh I, Luebbecke M, Wiggermann M, Ernst L, Beuerle T. Spice: A never ending story? Forensic Sci Int. 2009;191(1):58–63. https://doi.org/10.1016/j.forsciint.2009.06.008.
37. Longworth M, Banister SD, Mack JBC, Glass M, Connor M, Kassiou M. The 2-alkyl-2H-indazole regioisomers of synthetic cannabinoids AB-CHMINACA, AB-FUBINACA, AB-PINACA, and 5F-AB-PINACA are possible manufacturing impurities with cannabimimetic activities. Forensic Toxicol. 2016;34(2):286–303. https://doi.org/10.1007/s11419-016-0316-y.
38. Maiolo D. Higher than ever: New study links strong weed to psychosis. Summit Daily. 2019. Retrieved from https://www.summitdaily.com/news/higher-than-ever-new-study-links-strong-weed-to-psychosis/.
39. McCarthy J. Two in three Americans now support legalizing marijuana. 2018. Retrieved from Gallup.com website. https://news.gallup.com/poll/243908/two-three-americans-support-legalizing-marijuana.aspx.
40. McLeod E, Friedman A, & Soderberg B. Structural Racism and Cannabis: Black still disproportionately arrested for weed decriminalization. A Baltimore Fishbowl Report, December 2018. 2018. https://baltimorefishbowl.com/stories/structural-racism-and-cannabis-black-baltimoreans-stilldisproportionately-arrested-for-weed-after-decriminalization/.
41. Miller M. Synthetic marijuana overdose turns dozens into "zombies" in NYC. CBS News. 2016. Retrieved from https://www.cbsnews.com/news/synthetic-marijuana-overdose-turn-dozens-into-zombies-in-nyc/.
42. Moran LV, Masters GA, Pingali S, Cohen BM, Liebson E, Rajarethinam RP & Ongur D. Prescription stimulant use is associated with earlier onset of psychosis. Journal of Psychiatric Research, 2015;71:41–47. https://doi.org/10.1016/j.jpsychires.2015.09.012.
43. Mustonen A, Ahokas T, Nordström T, Murray GK, Mäki P, Jääskeläinen E. Niemelä S. Smokin' hot: Adolescent smoking and the risk of psychosis. Acta Psychiatrica Scandinavica, 2018;138(1):5–14. https://doi.org/10.1111/acps.12863.
44. Naef M, Curatolo M, Petersen-Felix S, Arendt-Nielsen L, Zbinden A, Brenneisen R, Naef M, Curatolo M, Petersen-Felix S, Arendt-Nielsen L, Zbinden A, Brenneisen R. The analgesic effect of oral delta-9-tetrahydrocannabinol (THC), morphine, and a THC-morphine combination in healthy subjects under experimental pain conditions. Pain. 2003;105(1):79–88. https://doi.org/10.1016/S0304-3959(03)00163-5.
45. Narang S, Gibson D, Wasan AD, Ross EL, Michna E, Nedeljkovic SS, Jamison RN. Efficacy of dronabinol as an adjuvant treatment for chronic pain patients on opioid therapy. J Pain. 2008;9(3):254–64. https://doi.org/10.1016/j.jpain.2007.10.018.
46. Portenoy RK, Ganae-Motan ED, Allende S, Yanagihara R, Shaiova L, Weinstein S, et al. Nabiximols for opioid-treated cancer patients with poorly-controlled chronic pain: A randomized, placebo-controlled, graded-dose trial. J Pain. 2012;13(5):438–49. https://doi.org/10.1016/j.jpain.2012.01.003.
47. Roberts JD, Gennings C, Shih M. Synergistic affective analgesic interaction between delta-9-tetrahydrocannabinol and morphine. Eur J Pharmacol. 2006;530(1):54–8. https://doi.org/10.1016/j.ejphar.2005.11.036.
48. Rosenberg, E. & Schweber, N. 33 suspected of overdosing on synthetic marijuana in Brooklyn. The New York Times. 2016. Retrieved from https://www.nytimes.com/2016/07/13/nyregion/k2-synthetic-marijuana-overdose-in-brooklyn.html.
49. Santora M. Drug 85 times as potent as marijuana caused a 'zombielike' state in Brooklyn. The New York Times; 2016. Retrieved from https://www.nytimes.com/2016/12/14/nyregion/zombielike-state-was-caused-by-synthetic-marijuana.html
50. Substance Abuse & Mental Health Data Archive (SAMHDA). National survey on drug use and health. 2017. Accessed at https://pdas.samhsa.gov/#/survey/NSDUH-2017-DS0001 on 25 April 2019.
51. Vandrey R, Dunn KE, Fry JA, Girling ER. A survey study to characterize use of Spice products (synthetic cannabinoids). Drug Alcohol Depend. 2012;120(1):238–41. https://doi.org/10.1016/j.drugalcdep.2011.07.011.
52. United Nations Office on Drugs and Crime. World Drug Report 2018. (United Nations publication, Sales No. E.18.XI.9). http://www.unodc.org/unodc/en/data-and-analysis/WDR-2012.html.

Cocaine 14

Eric D. Collins

A Brief History of Cocaine

Like many potentially medicinal, psychoactive compounds derived from plants, naturally occurring cocaine was discovered many centuries ago. Coca leaves, the natural source of cocaine, have been used for over a millennium by the indigenous peoples of the Andean regions of South America in the borderland of the Amazonian basin of Peru, Bolivia, Colombia, Ecuador, and Brazil. Coca leaves are cultivated from one of the two very closely related shrubby plants, *E. coca* (sometimes written *Erythroxylon coca*) and *E. novogranatense*. Each of these species has two varieties, and all coca plants are indigenous to the Andean region of South America.

For centuries, cocaine has been ingested orally and transmucosally by local South American peoples. Its use, as described here, is still common today. For oral (swallowed) use, the leaves of the coca plant are used to make coca tea, which is consumed by drinking, as is done with all teas. For transmucosal use through the buccal mucosa (the lining inside the cheek), the leaf is placed inside the cheek and mixed with alkaline substances such as lime (calcium oxide and/or calcium hydroxide), because alkaline conditions maximize transmucosal absorption of the cocaine molecule. The local term (where cocaine is grown) for such transmucosal use of the coca leaf is *acullico,* though it may also be termed coca "chewing," which is entirely analogous to the "chewing" of tobacco.

The positive effects of coca leaf chewing, *acullico*, and coca tea drinking are straightforward and quite clear, as cocaine ingested in these ways increases energy, improves endurance for hard physical labor, and suppresses appetite, thus enabling people to do strenuous work with fewer breaks for rest or food. In the sixteenth century, these pharmacological effects of cocaine played an important role in the relationship between the indigenous Andean people and the Spanish conquerors, who initially outlawed coca leaf chewing, only to encourage it soon after, when they recognized that the local people they had forced to mine gold and silver worked considerably harder and longer with the coca leaves than without them [13].

The role of cocaine throughout the world began to grow exponentially after the German chemist, Albert Niemann, isolated the drug in 1859. Only 4 years later, another chemist, Angelo Mariani, began marketing a wine, Vin Mariani, that contained cocaine extracted from coca leaves by soaking the leaves in the wine. Vin Mariani and other cocaine-infused wines became very popular during the latter half of the nineteenth century [13]. These alcoholic beverages, as well as the American "soft" drink, Coca-Cola, which

E. D. Collins (✉)
Columbia University Vagelos College of Physicians & Surgeons, New York, NY, USA
e-mail: edc3@cumc.columbia.edu

E. Akerele (ed.), *Substance and Non-Substance Related Addictions*,
https://doi.org/10.1007/978-3-030-84834-7_14

contained cocaine between 1886 and 1903, took advantage of the generally positive pharmacological stimulant effects discussed above (decreased appetite and increased energy and endurance). Interestingly, a decocainized coca leaf extract is still used in Coca-Cola as a flavoring ingredient [28].

In addition, although Niemann had noted the "peculiar numbness" cocaine produced when applied to the tongue [13], its role as a local anesthetic was not formally discovered by the medical profession until 1884, when the German ophthalmologist, Karl Koller, submitted his paper describing the local anesthetic properties of cocaine to an ophthalmological society meeting in Heidelberg.

The year 1884 proved a milestone year, as, only 5 months prior to Koller's presentation, and following a common, recurring pattern observed when highly reinforcing substances are newly described, the world-renowned psychiatrist, Sigmund Freud, gravely underestimated the risk of cocaine addiction, when, in his treatise on cocaine (Über Coca), he stated, "It seems to me noteworthy—and I discovered this in myself and in other observers who were capable of judging such things—that a first dose or even repeated doses of coca produce no compulsive desire to use the stimulant further" ("Classics revisited. Uber Coca. By Sigmund Freud," [3]).

Rather unsurprisingly from today's vantage point, there ensued a massive worldwide increase in cocaine production, facilitated partly by technological advances, as Merck, the leading European manufacturer of cocaine, increased its output of cocaine from less than a pound in 1883 to over 3100 pounds in 1884 and over 158,000 pounds in 1886 [21]. Not to be outdone, the American pharmaceutical company, Parke-Davis, also increased its production of cocaine at the same time. Notably, both Merck and Parke-Davis paid Freud to endorse their cocaine [13].

In the setting of Freud's and others' endorsements of the many benefits of cocaine, a markedly increased demand for cocaine drove the above-noted exponential increase in cocaine production. In the United States, cocaine was available over the counter in various medicines, including tonics and toothache cures, in addition to its inclusion in Coca-Cola, which was initially sold as a patent medication and marketed as a temperance beverage that offered the benefits of cocaine without the problems caused by alcohol.

With the marked increase in the use of cocaine, which Parke-Davis eventually marketed in the late nineteenth century in an injection kit, replete with a syringe and needle, came also the problem of cocaine addiction. By the early twentieth century, cocaine problems in the United States had become quite severe [9]. In his 1910 report to Congress, President Taft described the state of affairs, with respect to cocaine, as follows: "The misuse of cocaine is undoubtedly an American habit, the most threatening of the drug habits that has ever appeared in this Country…." As a result, by 1914, Congress had passed the Harrison Narcotics Tax Act, which prohibited the sale of nonmedical cocaine, prohibited its import, imposed the same penalties for users of cocaine as were in place for users of opium and heroin, and required strict accounting of medical prescriptions for cocaine [13,18].

The twentieth century witnessed episodic epidemics of stimulant use in the United States, occurring roughly every 25–30 years. The use of cocaine, effectively made more scarce and thus more expensive by the Harrison Narcotics Act, gave way to the advent of pharmaceutical amphetamines in the 1930s; amphetamine epidemics returned again in the 1950s/1960s. It is impressive to observe the repeated episodes of "forgetting" of the harms associated with cocaine and other powerful psychostimulants. For example, in 1980, the prevailing medical view was that cocaine use was not a significant problem at all. The *Comprehensive Textbook of Psychiatry* published that year included the following statement, "taken no more than two or three times per week, cocaine creates no serious problems [15]. Moreover, experts held that cocaine only produced relatively minor "psychological addiction," which was thought to be more easily treated than addictions to alcohol, sedatives, and opioids, all of which, unlike cocaine, produced significant physiological addiction" [12].

As has repeatedly occurred when societies markedly underestimate the problems of a powerfully reinforcing substance like cocaine, the stage was thus set in the early 1980s for a resurgence in cocaine use. A dramatic rise in cocaine use in the United States between 1972 and 1985 can be seen in Fig. 14.1. Enterprising chemists had found a way to make cocaine into a smokable form, because cocaine HCl, the crystalline white powder derived from the coca leaf, is mostly destroyed when burned and is therefore not readily smoked. Known commonly as "crack," the new, smokable form of cocaine produced an almost immediate and extremely intense stimulant effect that was much more addicting than coca leaf chewing or intranasal ("snorted") cocaine use, because ingestion of cocaine through the lungs produces very rapid increases in cocaine levels in both the blood and the brain. The resultant cocaine epidemic of the 1980s was both predictable and profound, as it left a significant mark on cities, where huge profits could be made selling the highly addictive, low-cost "crack" rocks that induce a very intense, albeit short-lived, cocaine high. Drug-related crime, connected both to efforts by addicted users to obtain cash and as part of lethal turf battles between rival sellers of cocaine, thus became a staple in most American cities at the time.

Although the use of cocaine, primarily crack, continued at high levels throughout the 1980s, the cocaine epidemic of that decade began to come to an end in 1986 with the death of Len Bias, a very popular and talented college basketball player who died 2 days after the Boston Celtics picked him with the second overall pick in the NBA draft. While Len Bias reportedly did not use crack cocaine, he did use cocaine almost immediately prior to his sudden death, and the national attention of his death focused on the United States' cocaine use problems, including especially the crack cocaine epidemic, brought to the fore the so obviously mistaken notion that cocaine, used in moderation, was not harmful.

Interestingly, although there is a clear consensus that cocaine is a powerfully addicting substance, there has historically been much less concern that ingesting cocaine through coca leaf chewing poses serious health risks. In 1950, the UN commissioned an enquiry into the coca leaf and identified the following harmful effects of chewing coca leaves: It suppresses hunger and thereby produces malnutrition; it produces undesirable intellectual and moral changes in users and hinders the chewer's chances of attaining a higher social standard; and it reduces the economic yield of productive work and contributes to maintenance of a lower socioeconomic status [42]. The same report concluded that coca leaf chewing was not an addiction. More recently, the World Health organization and the UN published a briefing kit [45] that drew the following conclusions: "Use of coca leaves appears to have no negative health effects and has positive thera-

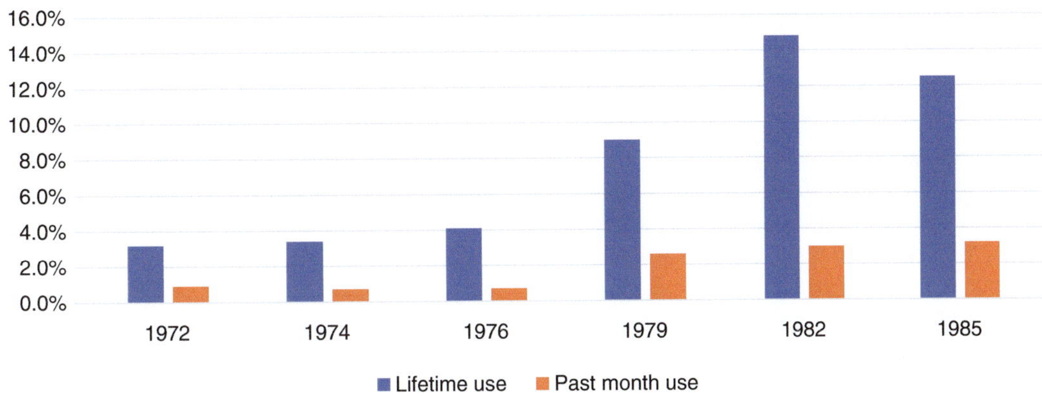

Fig. 14.1 Prevalence of cocaine use by adults ages 18 and older in the United States, 1972–1985. (Data taken from The Epidemiology of Cocaine Use and Abuse [37])

peutic, sacred and social functions for indigenous Andean populations"; and "While it is possible that there are some health problems associated with coca leaf use that are so far unrecognised, this seems unlikely."

Current Global Impact of Cocaine

The world's appetite for illegal drugs, including cocaine, is extremely strong and shows no signs of abating. To put a dollar value on the market for all illegal drugs, in March 2017, the Global Financial Integrity, a nonprofit research and advisory organization in Washington, DC, estimated the retail value of all international crime between $1.6 trillion and $2.2 trillion in 2014. Of this vast sum, drug trafficking constituted the second largest component (behind counterfeiting), bringing in between an estimated $426 and $652 billion, or approximately one-third of the total of all transnational crime. The retail value of the world cocaine trade was estimated between $94 billion and $143 billion (nearly a quarter of the total drug trafficking), second only to the value of the cannabis trade (between $183 billion and $287 billion) and slightly edging out the opiate trade (between $75 and $132 billion). For reference, the global market for amphetamine-type stimulants in 2014 was estimated to be between $74 billion and $90 billion [27].

Besides the market value of world cocaine production, one can also look at other measures of the magnitude of the world's cocaine economy. Other common approaches include measuring the land areas used for cultivating coca plants and tracking the volume of cocaine-related law enforcement seizures. Such data, estimated most recently in 2018, are summarized here.

After peaking in 2000, the area of land on which cocaine was cultivated worldwide declined until 2013, when it turned upward again (see Fig. 14.2). Between 2013 and 2016, the last year for which data are available, the worldwide land area on which coca was cultivated increased 76% to 213,000 hectares. Most of the increase in worldwide cocaine cultivation came from Colombia, where the amount of land cultivating

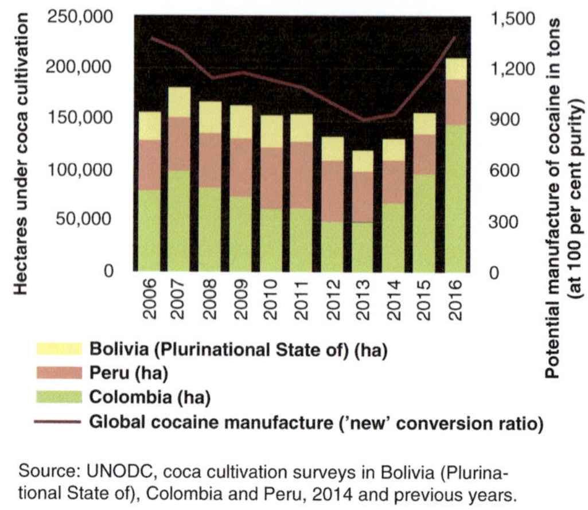

Fig. 14.2 Global coca cultivation and cocaine manufacture, 2006–2016. (Source: United Nations Office on Drugs and Crime. World Drug Report [43])

cocaine tripled between 2013 and 2016. A variety of factors contributed to the marked increase in coca cultivation, including market forces, changed trafficking strategies among producers, suspension of aerial spraying aimed at crop elimination, and reduced interventions aimed at promoting alternative crop production. In 2016, Colombia accounted for 68.5% of the worldwide coca bush cultivation with 146,000 hectares of land used for growing coca species. In 2016, Peru accounted for an additional 21% of worldwide coca cultivation, while Bolivia accounted for an additional 10%. As such, in 2016, these three countries accounted for 99.5% of the world's cocaine production [43].

Figure 14.3 shows global amounts of cocaine (in tons) seized in different parts of the world between 2006 and 2016. Overall, the quantity of cocaine seized worldwide increased 23% from 2015 to 2016 (World Drug Report 2018 (United Nations publication, Sales No. E.18.XI.9)). Between 2013 and 2016, seizures of cocaine hydrochloride increased in Columbia from 167 tons to 378 tons, with seizure of an additional 43 tons of coca paste and cocaine base that year. In 2016, over 90% of the world cocaine seizures occurred in the Americas, with 60% seized in South America (more than half of that in Colombia), 18% seized in the United States, and 11% seized in Central America, the majority in

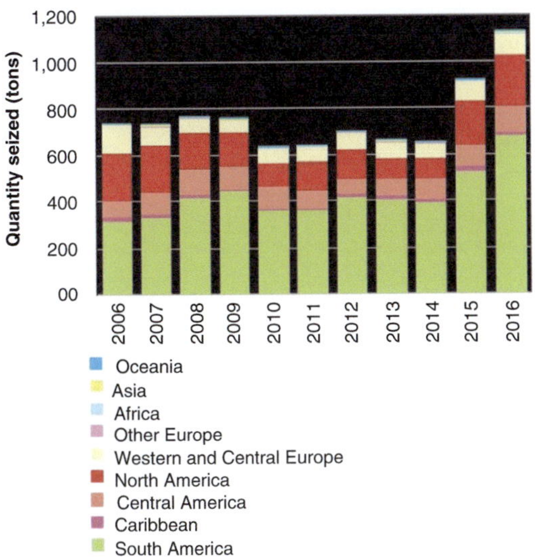

Source: UNODC, responses to the annual report questionaire

Fig. 14.3 Global quantities of cocaine seized by region (and some subregions), 2006–2016 (includes cocaine hydrochloride, coca paste and base, and "crack" cocaine; not adjusted for purity). (Source: United Nations Office on Drugs and Crime. World Drug Report [43])

Panama (note that the majority of Central American cocaine was presumed destined for markets in the United States). An additional 8% of the total global cocaine seizures occurred in Western and Central Europe, with 3% of the global seizures occurring in Belgium and 1% each in Spain and the Netherlands. While the amounts of cocaine seized in the rest of the world are relatively quite small, these regions showed the fastest rates of increase in cocaine seizures and suggest that the world appetite for cocaine remains quite robust. Specifically, from 2015 to 2016, the amounts of cocaine seized in Asia tripled, with a tenfold increase in cocaine seized in South Asia. Africa, the Near East/Mid-East, and Southwest Asia all saw a doubling of the amount of cocaine seized from 2015 to 2016 [43]. More recent data from the United Nations Office on Drugs and Crime [44] show a further increase in worldwide seizures in 2017 to 1275 kg equivalents (up from 652 kg equivalents seized in 2014).

A final measure of the global impact of the cocaine trade comes from estimates of drug-related fatalities. As can readily be seen from Fig. 14.4 [43], while opioid overdose deaths

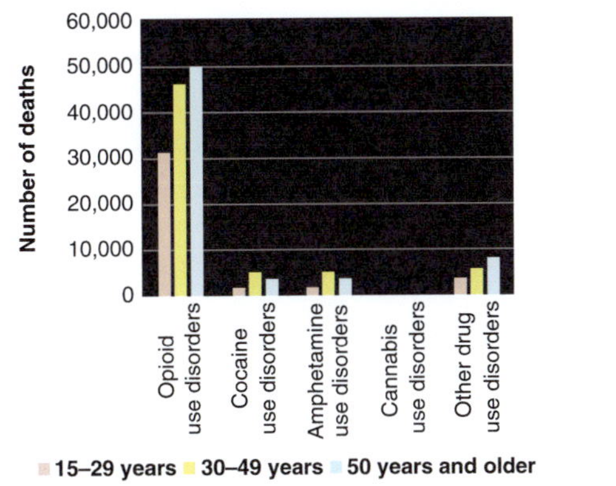

Source: WHO, Global Health Estimates 2015: Deaths by Cause, Age, Sex, by Country and by Region, 2000–2015 (Geneva, 2016)

Fig. 14.4 Deaths resulting from drug use disorders, by main drug categories and age, worldwide, 2015. (Source: United Nations Office on Drugs and Crime. World Drug Report [43])

throughout the world in 2015 dwarfed all other deaths from drug use disorders combined, the deaths from cocaine use disorders worldwide that year were equivalent to those from amphetamine use disorders as well as from the remaining other drug use disorders combined (excluding opioid, cocaine, amphetamine, and cannabis use disorders).

In the United States, the total number of cocaine-related deaths in 2013 was fewer than 5000; that number more than doubled to over 10,000 cocaine-related deaths in the United States in 2016 [43]. From another perspective, the age-adjusted death rate in the United States for all cocaine-involved deaths had peaked in 2006 at approximately 2.5 deaths/100,000 population [22]. This number was surpassed in 2016 and reached over 4 deaths/100,000 population in 2017. While the significant increase in opioid-related deaths during this period, both from synthetic opioids other than methadone and from all opioids, contributed powerfully to this increase (see Fig. 14.5), the age-adjusted rates of cocaine-related deaths in the absence of opioids also increased during the period between 2013 and 2017 [22], suggesting increased cocaine use in the mid-2010s.

The worldwide implications of these significant and very recent increases in cocaine produc-

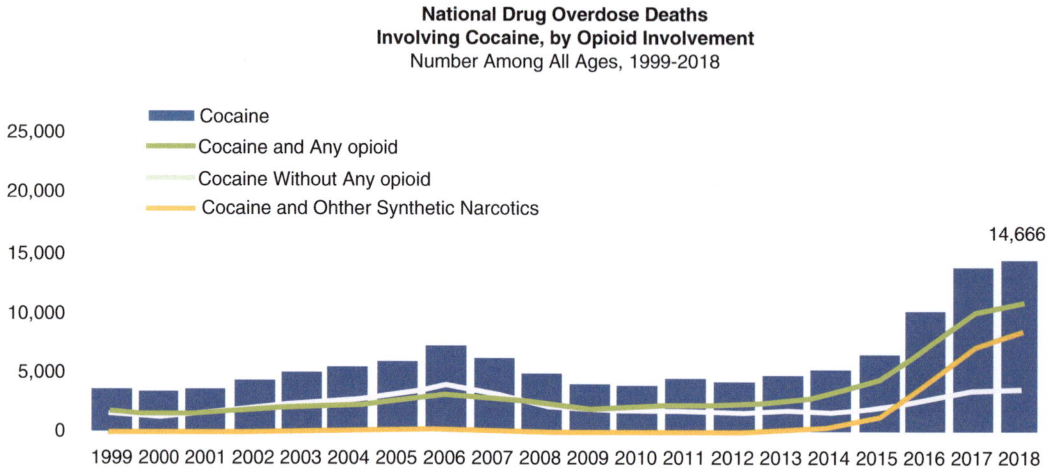

Fig. 14.5 National drug overdose death rates involving cocaine, by opioid involvement. (Source: National Institute on Drug Abuse and CDC Wonder Database [32])

tion and use go well beyond the life-damaging and lethal consequences related directly to cocaine use by individuals. Drug-producing nations, including those that produce coca plants or the opium poppy, are typically poorer nations with higher levels of government corruption, lower adherence to the rule of law, and fewer legal economic opportunities, especially for young people, who are much more commonly involved in the cultivation, harvesting, and manufacture of illegal drugs. The significant power of organized crime in these regions stems from the extremely high profits available for drug traffickers. And high financial flows in the illicit drug economy may undermine democratic processes, fund terrorism, and interfere with the establishment of effective social and governmental institutions in these countries [43].

Epidemiology of Cocaine Use

As shown in Fig. 14.6, cocaine use throughout the world in 2016 was highest in North America, approaching nearly 1.9% of the population, followed by Oceania (Australia, New Zealand, Indonesia, Polynesia, and many small islands in the Southwest Pacific) at almost 1.7%, Western and Central Europe at 1.2%, and South and Central America at 0.8% [43].

In the United States, the prevalence of cocaine use disorder (as distinct from the data above, which only reflect cocaine use) between 2002 and 2018, among individuals aged 12 and older, can be seen in Fig. 14.7 [38]. Overall, from data collected with the National Survey on Drug Use and Health (NSDUH), SAMHSA estimated that, in 2018, about 977,000 people ages 12 and over had a cocaine use disorder. This represents approximately 0.4% of the US population ages 12 and over in 2018. By comparison, that same year, about 526,000 people in the United States had a heroin use disorder, and about 1.7 million had a pain reliever use disorder. While opioid use disorders (taking heroin and prescription pain relievers together) clearly affected a much greater number of people than cocaine use disorder in 2018, for the nearly one million people affected by cocaine use disorder, and for the millions more of their family members, the magnitude of the cocaine problem in the United States is obviously quite significant.

The National Survey on Drug Use and Health [38] also provides insight into the differences in lifetime cocaine use and past year cocaine use, in total and by gender, in the same age groups as shown above (12 and older, 12 to 17, 18 to 25, and 26 or older). The epidemiological data described here are organized neatly in Tables 14.1 and 14.2, taken from the National Survey on

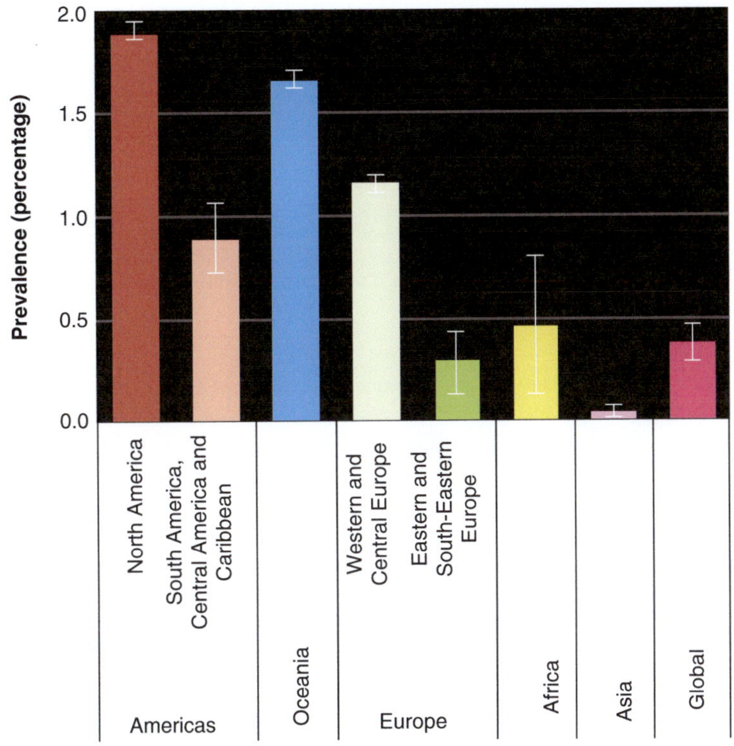

Source: UNODC estimates based on annual reports questionnaire data and other government reports.

Fig. 14.6 Estimated annual prevalence rates of cocaine use among the population aged 15–64 years, 2016. (Source: United Nations Office on Drugs and Crime. World Drug Report [43])

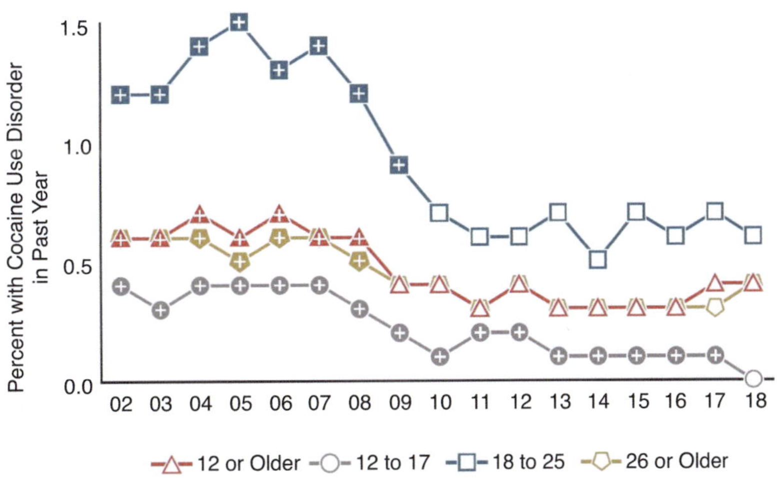

+Difference between this estimate and the 2018 estimate is statistically significant at the .05 level.

Fig. 14.7 Cocaine use disorder in the past year among people aged 12 or older: 2002–2018. +Difference between this estimate and the 2018 estimate is statistically significant at the .05 level. (Source: Key Substance Abuse and Mental Health Indicators in the United States: Results from the 2018 National Survey on Drug Use and Health)

Drug Use and Health [38]. In 2018, approximately 14.7% (more than one in every seven people) of the population aged 12 and over had used cocaine at least once in their lifetime. The proportion of males (18.1%) aged 12 and over with lifetime use of cocaine was considerably higher than that of females (11.5%) aged 12 and over with lifetime use of cocaine. In comparison,

Table 14.1 Cocaine use in lifetime among persons aged 12 or older, by age group and demographic characteristics: percentages, 2017 and 2018

Demographic characteristics	Aged 12+ (2017)	Aged 12+ (2018)	Aged 12-17 (2017)	Aged 12-17 (2018)	Aged 18+ (2017)	Aged 18+ (2018)	Aged 18-25 (2017)	Aged 18-25 (2018)	Aged 26+ (2017)	Aged 26+ (2018)
Total	14.9	14.7	0.7	0.7	16.3	16.1	12.0	11.4	17.0	16.8
Gender										
Male	18.8	18.1	0.6	0.6	20.8	19.9	14.2	12.9	21.9	21.1
Female	11.2	11.5	0.8	0.8	12.2	12.5	9.8	9.9	12.6	12.9

Source: 2018 National Survey on Drug Use and Health, Substance Abuse and Mental Health Services Administration [38]

Table 14.2 Cocaine use in past year among persons aged 12 or older, by age group and demographic characteristics: percentages, 2017 and 2018

Demographic characteristics	Aged 12+ (2017)	Aged 12+ (2018)	Aged 12-17 (2017)	Aged 12-17 (2018)	Aged 18+ (2017)	Aged 18+ (2018)	Aged 18-25 (2017)	Aged 18-25 (2018)	Aged 26+ (2017)	Aged 26+ (2018)
Total	2.2	2.0	0.5	0.4	2.4	2.2	6.2	5.8	1.7	1.6
Gender										
Male	3.0[a]	2.6	0.5	0.4	3.3[a]	2.9	7.5	6.8	2.6	2.2
Female	1.4	1.5	0.5	0.5	1.5	1.5	4.9	4.7	1.0	1.1

Source: 2018 National Survey on Drug Use and Health, Substance Abuse and Mental Health Services Administration [38]

past year cocaine use among individuals 12 and over was 2% of the population in 2018, with 2.6% of males and 1.5% of females reporting cocaine use in the prior year. The 18- to 25-year-old age group showed the highest rates for both lifetime (11.4%) and past year (1.6%) cocaine use. In that young adult age group, 12.9% of males and 9.9% of females reported lifetime cocaine use, while 6.8% of males and 4.7% of females reported past year cocaine use.

Pharmacology

Cocaine enhances the actions of dopamine, norepinephrine, and serotonin through reuptake blockade of these neurotransmitters. This neurobiology of cocaine action makes it more similar to methylphenidate than to amphetamines. Cocaine can be used orally (by swallowing, though this is rare), by the transmucosal route (across the buccal mucosa, which is uncommon in the United States), by intranasal (snorted) means (far more common in the United States), by smoking, or intravenously. Its effects appear within 15 seconds for smoked or intravenous use and within 90 seconds for intranasal use. The offset of effects, however, is comparatively quite rapid—about 15–30 minutes, often with rebound dysphoric mood. The profile of acute cocaine effects typically includes increased mood, energy, confidence, and libido, with decreased appetite and diminution of fatigue.

The pattern of addictive use of cocaine is commonly in a binge-and-rest pattern. Cocaine binges commonly last 48–72 hours, sometimes longer, during which time users may not eat or sleep at all. Following a binge, the "crash" can last a few days, much of which is spent sleeping. Depressed mood, loss of pleasure, irritability, low energy, and poor concentration are common after the post-binge "crash," and relapse is common during this period (certainly in part to treat the unpleasant mood state accompanying the cocaine "crash"). Physiological effects of cocaine include elevated vital signs (including core temperature). After only modest initial cocaine use, further use does not produce additional elevations in vital signs or subjective effects, even while plasma levels rise. Continued use will raise the risk of seizures (though seizures with cocaine use are relatively rare, absent use of overdose amounts or another risk for seizures). Interestingly, and importantly, cocaine can be used medicinally for its local anesthetic properties, and it has sometimes been the local anesthetic of choice for otolaryngology procedures, in which there are often concerns about the potential for significant blood loss, because unlike other local anesthetics, cocaine has intrinsic vasoconstrictor effects.

It is worth reviewing and expanding on some of the variables that made the development of crack cocaine in the 1980s so devastating. First, cocaine hydrochloride, which is crystalline, is virtually completely destroyed, rather than volatilized, when burned. By removing the hydrochloride moiety using simple kitchen chemistry, cocaine as "free base" can be heated without destroying it, making it possible for individuals to ingest the molecule by smoking. Further, very small amounts, often in doses costing \$3 to \$5 or less, could produce extremely intense, but very brief, highs, which many users want to experience again, often within 5 minutes. Anything that could be sold for even small amounts became worth stealing, and the profit in the business for drug dealers became tremendous. This is analogous to the high profit that can be earned by selling shots (45 mL) of hard liquor for \$5/shot compared with selling the entire bottle of 750 mL for \$25.

The potential serious physical effects of cocaine are many and include myocardial infarction, arrhythmias, stroke, seizures, and death. A host of different, unique medical complications accompany each route of administration. For example, because of its vasoconstricting effects, regular use of intranasal cocaine causes necrosis of nasal septal tissue, which ultimately leads to a perforated nasal septum in regular users of intranasal cocaine.

The relatively common, severe psychological complications of cocaine addiction, especially when severe, include paranoid ideas, progressing to delusions (primarily present while a person is under the influence, although sensitization is common, so that less and less cocaine is required to trigger paranoid delusions). The psychosis accompanying regular, heavy cocaine use may appear schizophreniform, manic, or toxic (i.e., delirium). Individuals using cocaine regularly may also hallucinate or develop manic symptoms without psychosis. Repetitive behaviors (stereotypies), including pacing, bruxism, and skin picking may also occur. Depression, often profound, may also develop, particularly, as noted previously, after a cocaine binge. There is also a range of sexual side effects of cocaine abuse, including loss of libido, impotence, priapism, and orgasmic failure.

Diagnosis

The diagnosis of a cocaine use disorder should be made using the *Diagnostic and Statistical Manual of Mental Disorders*, Fifth Edition (DSM-5). Cocaine use disorders are classified in the DSM-5 with other stimulants, including, most notably, amphetamine-type stimulants. The criteria for stimulant use disorders in the DSM-5 are as follows [1]:

A pattern of amphetamine-type substance, cocaine, or other stimulant use leading to clinically significant impairment or distress, as manifested by at least two of the following, occurring within a 12-month period:

1. The stimulant is often taken in larger amounts or over a longer period than was intended.
2. There is a persistent desire or unsuccessful efforts to cut down or control stimulant use.
3. A great deal of time is spent in activities necessary to obtain the stimulant, use the stimulant, or recover from its effects.
4. Craving, or a strong desire or urge to use the stimulant.
5. Recurrent stimulant use resulting in a failure to fulfill major role obligations at work, school, or home.
6. Continued stimulant use despite having persistent or recurrent social or interpersonal problems caused or exacerbated by the effects of the stimulant.
7. Important social, occupational, or recreational activities are given up or reduced because of stimulant use.

8. Recurrent stimulant use in situations in which it is physically hazardous.
9. Stimulant use is continued despite knowledge of having a persistent or recurrent physical or psychological problem that is likely to have been caused or exacerbated by the stimulant.
10. Tolerance, as defined by either of the following:
    (a) A need for markedly increased amounts of the stimulant to achieve intoxication or desired effect
    (b) A markedly diminished effect with continued use of the same amount of the stimulant

    Note: This criterion is not considered to be met for those taking stimulant medications solely under appropriate medical supervision, such as medications for attention-deficit/hyperactivity disorder or narcolepsy.
11. Withdrawal, as manifested by either of the following:
    (a) The characteristic withdrawal syndrome for the stimulant (refer to Criteria A and B of the criteria set for stimulant withdrawal, p. 569)
    (b) The stimulant (or a closely related substance) is taken to relieve or avoid withdrawal symptoms.

    Note: "This criterion is not considered to be met for those taking stimulant medications solely under appropriate medical supervision, such as medications for attention-deficit/hyperactivity disorder or narcolepsy."

It is important to recognize that the DSM-5 diagnostic criteria given above do not include laboratory test results in order to make the diagnosis of a cocaine use disorder (or any substance use disorder). As a behavioral disorder, the condition is diagnosed based on behavior: the use of cocaine in a destructive (i.e., impairing and/or distressing) pattern. Nonetheless, because some individuals choose to lie about their use of substances (i.e., "undeclared substance use"), laboratory drug toxicology testing could theoretically be used to identify occult (unreported) cocaine use. It would, however, arguably be both impractical and unnecessarily expensive and of questionable yield to urine test everyone entering primary care for use of cocaine and other drugs (see section on Screening for Cocaine Use Disorder). In addition, regular drug toxicology testing would likely and dangerously dissuade some individuals from seeking primary care altogether, as some substance users want very much to avoid having their substance use known by anyone.

The information collected in the usual course of clinical care in addiction treatment settings will usually be geared quite specifically toward determining whether each person evaluated meets criteria for substance use disorders generally and for cocaine use disorder specifically. In other clinical settings, particularly in primary care, the typical course of clinical history-taking may not always produce enough information to make the diagnosis of a substance use disorder, particularly related to use disorders for illicit substances. The usual approach is to utilize a screening procedure (questionnaire), followed by a significantly more detailed discussion exploring substance use for individuals who screen positive for a possible substance use disorder.

Screening for Cocaine Use Disorder

Ideally, screening for diseases works best for common illnesses (else it would be too expensive to screen everyone), for which identification of the illness earlier in the natural history of the disease can lead to simpler, more effective treatment than if the illness were detected later, when it has produced greater morbidity and mortality and potentially could no longer be as effectively treated [36]. As noted above, while urine toxicology effectively detects recent cocaine use, it does not reliably identify cocaine use disorder (the illness), because the majority of people with recent cocaine use do not have a cocaine use disorder [36].

Therefore, the best screening tests for substance use disorders, including cocaine use disorder, are interview-based questionnaires that inquire more about the consequences of substance use than about quantity, frequency, and duration of use. An early screening instrument, the Drug Abuse Screening Test, or DAST [39], while demonstrating good sensitivity and specificity, is relatively long, with 28 questions, making it rather inefficient. Over the years, the instrument has been shortened to a questionnaire with 20 items and 1 with 10 items; recently, a 2-item version, the DAST-2 [41] has demonstrated excellent sensitivity and specificity in a primary care setting [41]. The two questions on the DAST-2 are "How many days in the past 12 months have you used drugs other than alcohol?" (with a positive screen set at 7 days), and "How many days in the past 12 months have you used drugs more than you meant to?" (with a positive screen cutoff set at 2 days). Given the good sensitivity and specificity of this two-item screener, it would be most appropriate to include this instrument routinely as a screening procedure in primary care settings.

Toxicology Testing for Cocaine

A detailed discussion of different laboratory toxicology testing technologies is beyond the scope of this chapter, but a brief discussion of the most common testing processes is in order. The most commonly used samples for detection of cocaine use are urine and oral fluid (saliva). Hair testing has gained in popularity in recent years and is being used more frequently in some settings. Plasma/serum are used infrequently for the detection of cocaine metabolites, because the detection window for cocaine metabolites in the blood is much shorter than it is in urine, and drawing blood is far more invasive than the collection of oral fluid, with similar windows of detection.

The most commonly used and oldest method to detect cocaine use is urine toxicology testing, both because of the relative convenience of urine collection and because the kidneys concentrate the urine, which makes possible the detection of substances in urine for a longer period of time compared with the blood. Cocaine itself has a relatively short serum half-life, on the order of 50 minutes [14]. Cocaine metabolites, specifically the inactive metabolites benzoyl ecgonine and ecgonine methyl ester [20], have considerably longer half-lives and are detectable in urine for a wide range of times, depending on many variables, including the magnitude and chronicity of dosing, as well as the technology used for detection. Jufer et al. [20] observed differential elimination kinetics following chronic administration of cocaine and estimated the terminal elimination half-life of benzoyl ecgonine and ecgonine methyl ester ranging between 14 and 52 hours. Recently, some investigators have found that, using a highly sensitive cutoff of 5 ng/mL, benzoyl ecgonine can be detected in urine after chronic cocaine administration for between 17 and 22 days [30].

An alternative to urine testing is oral fluid (saliva) testing, which has the obvious advantage of much greater ease of observed collection, with a much lower likelihood of adulteration. The two main disadvantages to oral fluid testing are the shorter window of detection for cocaine metabolites, as the half-life of benzoyl ecgonine in saliva (and plasma) have been estimated to be approximately 6 hours, and the possibility that antisialogogues (compounds that reduce saliva production) could be used to dry the mouth, reducing markedly the amount of oral fluid that could be collected and therefore making it easier to produce a falsely negative sample. As noted above, blood testing is used quite infrequently for the detection of cocaine metabolites, because it is both more invasive and has a shorter window of drug detection than urine testing. It has the advantage that it cannot readily be diluted or adulterated, unless the phlebotomist serves as a confederate to the patient, which would likely occur only very rarely.

In recent years, hair analysis has been used more frequently in clinical, workplace, and forensic settings to detect illicit substance use, including cocaine use [16]. Compared with urine testing, hair testing for substance use has the following advantages: relatively noninvasive collection, a very much longer window of detection of drug use (about 1 month/half inch of hair), a markedly lower risk of dilution/adulteration, and easy sample preservation at ambient temperature [23]. There remain controversies about the best analytical methods as well as about the possible external contamination of hair, ethnic/racial bias in drug/metabolite incorporation into hair, and deterioration/distortion of the results due to the use of cosmetics and other hair treatments that can interfere with drug detection [23].

Treatment of Cocaine Use Disorder

The treatment of cocaine use disorder, a behavioral illness, is primarily behavioral. Unlike some other substance use disorders, specifically opioid, nicotine and alcohol use disorders, and despite decades of dedicated research efforts, there are, as yet, no FDA-approved medications for cocaine use disorder. A variety of psychosocial interventions, including contingency management techniques as well as motivation enhancement and cognitive behavioral therapy (CBT)-based relapse prevention psychotherapies, have shown efficacy in helping people stop using cocaine. In this section, we review briefly the main research findings for pharmacotherapy and for psychosocial interventions for cocaine use disorder.

Pharmacotherapy of Cocaine Use Disorder

Dozens of medications, mostly alone, some in combination, have been tested for their potential to treat cocaine use disorder. While a comprehensive review of medication trials for cocaine use disorder is beyond the scope of this chapter, this section will highlight some of the more historically important or promising research aimed at finding medications to help individuals achieve and maintain sobriety from cocaine.

One innovative approach to finding medications for cocaine use disorders grew out of decades of behavioral pharmacology research, originally with laboratory animals. Specifically, in laboratories that allow human beings the opportunity to choose between using cocaine or earning money, a number of groups have investigated whether medications can alter the behavioral effects of cocaine, including both self-administration of cocaine and self-report of cocaine effects. A good example of this type of research [10] demonstrated an interesting dissociation between cocaine self-administration, on which desipramine maintenance had no effect, and subjective effects, on which desipramine maintenance had some significant effects, including decreased arousal and vigor, increased anger, anxiety, confusion, and decreased ratings of "I want cocaine" (despite no change in actual choice to use cocaine while on desipramine maintenance vs. placebo maintenance). In another set of studies using the same human laboratory model of cocaine self-administration and subjective effects, the cognitive enhancer, memantine, enhanced some subjective effects of cocaine without altering cocaine self-administration [4, 5].

Notwithstanding the laboratory model described above, the primary focus in this brief review of possible medications for cocaine use disorder will be on randomized, placebo-controlled clinical trials. Many early efforts to find medications for cocaine use disorder focused on antidepressants of multiple classes, including SSRIs, SNRIs, TCAs, and others [34]. In multiple randomized controlled trials (RCTs) of antidepressants, the overall conclusion is that antidepressants do not separate meaningfully from placebo on treatment outcomes for individuals with cocaine use disorders [2, 34].

Given the well-known, albeit secondary, pharmacological effect of disulfiram to inhibit dopamine beta-hydroxylase, thereby reducing the breakdown of dopamine, a number of studies have been conducted, investigating whether disulfiram might reduce cocaine use among individuals with cocaine use disorders [2, 33]. The findings of all the disulfiram studies taken together show heterogeneous results, making it impossible to draw meaningful conclusions regarding the effects of disulfiram on cocaine use disorder [2]. There was evidence in some of the RCTs that disulfiram significantly worsened treatment retention compared to placebo.

Multiple RCTs have investigated anticonvulsants, muscle relaxants, psychostimulants, antipsychotics, dopamine agonists, as well as buspirone, acamprosate, varenicline, naltrexone, and buprenorphine for cocaine use disorder. Chan and colleagues conducted a systematic review and meta-analysis of randomized clinical trials and prior systematic reviews of potential pharmacotherapies for cocaine use disorder. From more than 50 papers they identified that met their inclusion criteria, the authors [2] found the following: there was low strength of evidence favoring psychostimulants over placebo for abstinence rates (but for no other treatment outcomes), low strength of evidence favoring topiramate over placebo, again only for the outcome of cocaine abstinence, and moderate strength of evidence that antipsychotics improve study retention with no demonstrated effects on other treatment outcomes.

One of the more potentially promising pharmacotherapeutic approaches to cocaine use disorder has combined the use of topiramate in combination with mixed amphetamine salts. A recent RCT [25] investigated extended release mixed amphetamine salts up to 60 mg daily combined with topiramate up to 100 mg twice daily. The combination treatment demonstrated a significant difference from placebo on the proportion of individuals able to achieve three consecutive weeks of abstinence, as confirmed by urine toxicology. This study extends previous similar work favoring the combined treatment over placebo on the likelihood of achieving three consecutive weeks of abstinence, particularly for individuals with a higher baseline frequency of cocaine use [26].

More broadly, a very recent systematic review and meta-analysis of psychostimulant medications for psychostimulant use disorders [40] included 38 randomized placebo-controlled trials of prescription stimulant medications for stimulant use disorders. The authors concluded that treatment with prescription amphetamines in "robust doses" can promote illicit stimulant abstinence in individuals with cocaine use disorders (but not with prescription psychostimulant use disorders). The authors concluded that a moderate quality of evidence supported this finding that higher doses of prescription amphetamines promote sustained abstinence in people with cocaine use disorder. In addition, they found that such "agonist maintenance" treatment was particularly effective in promoting abstinence among individuals with both cocaine and opioid use disorders when the opioid users were enrolled in an opioid treatment program, such as a methadone maintenance program.

In addition, recently, ketamine, which in the form of one of its enantiomers, esketamine, FDA-approved in 2019 for the treatment of depression, was investigated recently for its potential to modulate cocaine use in 55 individuals with cocaine use disorder [8]. All participants were treated using a 5-week mindfulness-based relapse prevention treatment protocol, and, during a 5-day inpatient study induction, a subanesthetic dose of ketamine or midazolam (as an active control) was given in a single, 40-minute, continuous, intravenous infusion. Notably, 48.2% of the ketamine-treated subjects compared with only 10.7% of the midazolam-treated subjects were cocaine abstinent during the final 2 weeks of the trial. In addition, ketamine-treated study participants were 53% less likely to drop out of the study and had 58.1% lower craving scores throughout the study. This study, which builds on earlier promising work with ketamine for cocaine use disorder [6, 7], requires replication, but it points toward what so far appears to be one of the more promising advances to date in the pharmacotherapy of cocaine use disorder.

No discussion of pharmacotherapy of cocaine use disorder would be complete without mentioning the potential promise of vaccine therapy for the condition. The most common approach to cocaine use disorder vaccines involves sequestering the cocaine molecule in antibodies, thus preventing the large, conjugated antibody-cocaine complex from crossing the blood-brain barrier [19]. One candidate vaccine (TA-CD) has stimulated the production of antibodies to the cocaine molecule and successfully reduced positive subjective effects of cocaine in a human laboratory model in which individuals were allowed to smoke cocaine and rate the effects of the cocaine

[17]. Unfortunately, when studied in phase III randomized controlled trial, the TA-CD vaccine did not reduce cocaine use [24], probably because the vaccine produced highly variable levels of antibodies and because cocaine use among those who achieved the highest cocaine antibody levels appeared to increase, as individuals with high antibody levels may have attempted to overwhelm and override the blocking effect of the antibodies. At this point, unfortunately, immunotherapy for cocaine use disorder has not yet fulfilled its potential promise, though novel approaches combining an anti-cocaine vaccine with induction of a cocaine hydrolase by gene transfer may yet revive the prospects for anti-cocaine vaccine therapy [11].

Psychotherapy/Psychosocial Treatments for Cocaine Use Disorder

As noted above, because no medications have yet proven beneficial in the treatment of cocaine use disorder, the only available treatments with some demonstrated benefit for the condition are psychosocial interventions. Various psychosocial interventions have been developed for substance use disorders, and many of these have demonstrated efficacy in the treatment of cocaine use disorder. Most of these psychotherapeutic treatments involve concepts and approaches derived from cognitive behavioral therapy (CBT)-based treatments.

The main psychosocial interventions that have shown benefit for cocaine use disorder include the following: cognitive behavioral therapy, relapse prevention/coping skill therapy, contingency management, and 12-step facilitation. This section will very briefly describe each of these interventions, with a brief summary of available evidence for the intervention.

Like cognitive-behavioral therapy for mood and anxiety disorders, CBT for cocaine use disorder is a structured, usually manual-guided and time-limited treatment intervention that focuses on thoughts and feelings related to drug use and aims to teach new behaviors, through role-playing and practice, that will reduce the likelihood of substance use. The basic idea is that people learn to use substances, through modeling, as well as through both classical and operant conditioning. The two main elements of CBT are a functional analysis, in which thoughts and feelings before and after drug use are identified, and skills training, in which a person learns (or relearns) healthier skills or habits. A typical course of CBT might be 8 to 12 1-hour-long sessions, with homework assigned between sessions to allow the patient to practice both the identification of thoughts and feelings surrounding drug use and new skills [35]. As described in more detail below, CBT approaches for substance use disorders have demonstrated benefits, some of which seem to continue to develop for up to a year after a 12-week course of treatment.

Several different specific CBT-derived treatments have been developed for substance use disorders, including cocaine use disorder. These include relapse-prevention/coping skill training, contingency management, and motivation enhancement therapy. The main focus in relapse prevention/coping skill training is to reduce the likelihood of relapse by teaching individuals to prepare for and better cope with high-risk situations. The goals for this treatment include reducing substance craving and building skills, including the identification and practice of alternative behaviors to substance use [29].

Contingency management (CM) interventions are behavioral and based on operant conditioning. The central idea is to reward abstinence through provision of reinforcers for drug-free urine tests. The alternative reinforcers offered have included money, prizes, vouchers to cover the costs of patient-selected, positive alternative activities, and/or clinic or treatment setting privileges. Another CBT-derived approach is the community reinforcement approach, which focuses on environmental factors that strongly influence problem drug-use behavior. Aspects of treatment addressed include skill training, vocational counseling, provision of employment opportunities, improved relationships, and cultivation of new activities and drug-free social networks [29]. Finally, motivation enhancement therapy (MET), also termed motivational interviewing (MI), aims to encourage individuals to express and strengthen their personal motivation for behavior change.

A number of other psychosocial interventions have been studied for cocaine use disorder. Among these are the 12-step facilitation, which draws strongly on the 12 steps of alcoholics anonymous (AA) and similar 12-step self-help groups, with an emphasis on 3 main principles: acceptance that the individual has a chronic disease over which one is powerless unless one becomes abstinent; surrender to a higher power, with participation in the fellowship and support of other people with addiction; and active involvement in 12-step meetings [31]. There have also been studies of a few other psychosocial interventions for cocaine use disorder, including psychodynamic psychotherapy, focused on intrapsychic conflicts and maladaptive defenses related to them, and interpersonal psychotherapy (IPT), based on the view that psychiatric disorders derive from dysfunctional interpersonal relationships.

A recent, comprehensive Cochrane review of psychosocial interventions for stimulant use disorders [29] examined the available well-conducted trials of the above psychotherapies for stimulant use disorders. The review included 27 studies of contingency management, 19 studies of cognitive behavioral therapy (CBT), 5 studies of motivation enhancement therapy, 4 studies of 12-step facilitation, 3 studies of interpersonal psychotherapy, and 1 study of psychodynamic psychotherapy. Taken together, the authors found that, when compared to no intervention at all, there was high-quality evidence that these interventions increased the longest period of continuous abstinence, moderate quality evidence that these interventions reduced dropout rates, and low-quality evidence that they increased continuous abstinence at the end of the treatment. They also found that, when psychosocial interventions were combined or added on, the most studied and also potentially the most promising psychosocial approach was contingency management. The review, however, could not distinguish which psychosocial intervention was most effective.

Conclusions

Cocaine is a local anesthetic with powerfully reinforcing stimulant properties and a relatively high potential to produce addiction. The economic value of transnational crime attributed to cocaine approaches $150 billion annually and represents close to a quarter of the world drug trade. The global impact of the huge and potentially growing market for cocaine has implications for the well-being of individuals throughout the world, including the citizens of the poorer countries where coca plants are grown. In these countries, government corruption and the exploitation of vulnerable young people recruited into the drug trade are powerful factors that contribute to the likely long-term maintenance of drug supply cultures. In addition, while the use of cocaine has historically ebbed and flowed with changes in societal views of the dangers associated with it, the recent increases in cocaine-associated drug overdose fatalities may be the harbinger of a shift in the United States away from opioid use and toward increased cocaine use.

As is true with all addictions, the treatment for cocaine use disorder can and does help some individuals achieve and maintain long-term cocaine abstinence. Thus far, the only proven treatments for cocaine use disorder are psychotherapies, primarily those derived from cognitive behavioral treatment approaches. While the search for medications to treat cocaine use disorder has been long and mostly quite frustrating with no FDA-approved medications to treat the illness, cocaine pharmacotherapy research should continue, as there have been some potentially promising results, both with high-dose prescription amphetamines as a kind of "agonist therapy" for cocaine use disorder and with ketamine. Despite the frustrations, many remain hopeful that we are on the threshold of being able to impact the course of cocaine addiction through the use of medications and/or other biological treatments.

Future Directions

While it is extremely difficult to predict the future, it seems quite safe to anticipate that, in all likelihood, cocaine use disorder will never be eradicated. In that regard, the American "War on Drugs" must be recognized as a complex political act that fails to comprehend the science of drug reinforcement and the inevitable human desire to ingest substances that increase dopamine transmission in the brain reward centers. Thus, the pharmacology of cocaine is too powerful, the world appetite for it too large, and the availability of effective treatments for cocaine use disorder too meager to make eliminating cocaine use a realistic possibility. Nevertheless, there is room for optimism, as research continues to explore combining effective psychotherapies with medications, including possibly vaccines, that together may synergistically reduce cocaine use, even after a person develops cocaine addiction. In addition, we may witness increased efforts to bring more people into contact with treatment providers in harm reduction settings, where individuals with cocaine addiction, who might otherwise have no desire yet to achieve abstinence or even to change much about their drug using behavior, may seek some forms of help to mitigate the deleterious consequences of their substance use. These contacts with treatment-oriented professionals and/or peers may increase the likelihood that some individuals will subsequently seek treatment. Also, there is reason to hope that the future may bring productive, non-stigmatizing shifts in societal attitudes toward individuals with addiction illnesses, as the terrible toll of the current opioid use epidemic has increased discussion and understanding of addiction as the biological, treatable illness, it is rather than as a moral failing or character flaw. Finally, we may hope to see societal shifts away from cocaine (and other drug) use as a result of the growing understanding that the choice to use drugs is not simply an individual choice with no other victims. It is, ultimately, a choice with significant implications both for the loved ones of those using cocaine and for worldwide social justice.

References

1. American Psychiatric Association. Diagnostic and statistical manual of mental disorders. 5th ed. Arlington: American Psychiatric Association; 2013.
2. Chan B, Kondo K, Freeman M, Ayers C, Montgomery J, Kansagara D. Pharmacotherapy for cocaine use disorder-a systematic review and meta-analysis. J Gen Intern Med. 2019;34(12):2858–73. https://doi.org/10.1007/s11606-019-05074-8.
3. Freud S. Classics revisited. Uber Coca. J Subst abuse treat. 1984;1(3):206–17. Retrieved from https://www.ncbi.nlm.nih.gov/pubmed/6399323
4. Collins ED, Vosberg SK, Ward AS, Haney M, Foltin RW. The effects of acute pretreatment with high-dose memantine on the cardiovascular and behavioral effects of cocaine in humans. Exp Clin Psychopharmacol. 2007;15(3):228–37. https://doi.org/10.1037/1064-1297.15.3.228.
5. Collins ED, Ward AS, McDowell DM, Foltin RW, Fischman MW. The effects of memantine on the subjective, reinforcing and cardiovascular effects of cocaine in humans. Behav Pharmacol. 1998;9(7):587–98. https://doi.org/10.1097/00008877-199811000-00014.
6. Dakwar E, Hart CL, Levin FR, Nunes EV, Foltin RW. Cocaine self-administration disrupted by the N-methyl-D-aspartate receptor antagonist ketamine: a randomized, crossover trial. Mol Psychiatry. 2017;22(1):76–81. https://doi.org/10.1038/mp.2016.39.
7. Dakwar E, Levin F, Foltin RW, Nunes EV, Hart CL. The effects of subanesthetic ketamine infusions on motivation to quit and cue-induced craving in cocaine-dependent research volunteers. Biol Psychiatry. 2014;76(1):40–6. https://doi.org/10.1016/j.biopsych.2013.08.009.
8. Dakwar E, Nunes EV, Hart CL, Foltin RW, Mathew SJ, Carpenter KM, et al. A single ketamine infusion combined with mindfulness-based behavioral modification to treat cocaine dependence: a randomized clinical trial. Am J Psychiatry. 2019;176(11):923–30. https://doi.org/10.1176/appi.ajp.2019.18101123.
9. Das G. Cocaine abuse in North America: a milestone in history. J Clin Pharmacol. 1993;33(4):296–310. https://doi.org/10.1002/j.1552-4604.1993.tb04661.x.
10. Fischman MW, Foltin RW, Nestadt G, Pearlson GD. Effects of desipramine maintenance on cocaine self-administration by humans. J Pharmacol Exp Ther. 1990;253(2):760–70. Retrieved from https://www.ncbi.nlm.nih.gov/pubmed/2338656.
11. Gao Y, Geng L, Orson F, Kinsey B, Kosten TR, Shen X, Brimijoin S. Effects of anti-cocaine vaccine and viral gene transfer of cocaine hydrolase in mice on cocaine toxicity including motor strength and liver damage. Chem Biol Interact. 2013;203(1):208–11. https://doi.org/10.1016/j.cbi.2012.08.006.
12. Gawin FH, Kleber HD. Evolving conceptualizations of cocaine dependence. Yale J Biol Med.

1988;61(2):123–36. Retrieved from https://www.ncbi.nlm.nih.gov/pubmed/3043925.
13. Goldstein RA, DesLauriers C, Burda AM. Cocaine: history, social implications, and toxicity--a review. Dis Mon. 2009;55(1):6–38. https://doi.org/10.1016/j.disamonth.2008.10.002.
14. Goodman & Gilman's. The pharmacological basis of therapeutics. 12th ed. New York: McGraw-Hill; 2011.
15. Grinspoon L, Bakalar J. Drug dependence: non-narcotic agents. In: Comprehensive textbook of psychiatry. 3rd ed. Baltimore: Williams and Wilkins; 1980.
16. Gryczynski J, Schwartz RP, Mitchell SG, O'Grady KE, Ondersma SJ. Hair drug testing results and self-reported drug use among primary care patients with moderate-risk illicit drug use. Drug Alcohol Depend. 2014;141:44–50. https://doi.org/10.1016/j.drugalcdep.2014.05.001.
17. Haney M, Gunderson EW, Jiang H, Collins ED, Foltin RW. Cocaine-specific antibodies blunt the subjective effects of smoked cocaine in humans. Biol Psychiatry. 2010;67(1):59–65. https://doi.org/10.1016/j.biopsych.2009.08.031.
18. Harrison Narcotics Tax Act. 1914. Retrieved from http://www.druglibrary.org/schaffer/history/e1910/harrisonact.htm
19. Heekin RD, Shorter D, Kosten TR. Current status and future prospects for the development of substance abuse vaccines. Expert Rev Vaccines. 2017;16(11):1067–77. https://doi.org/10.1080/14760584.2017.1378577.
20. Jufer RA, Wstadik A, Walsh SL, Levine BS, Cone EJ. Elimination of cocaine and metabolites in plasma, saliva, and urine following repeated oral administration to human volunteers. J Anal Toxicol. 2000;24(7):467–77. https://doi.org/10.1093/jat/24.7.467.
21. Karch SB. Cocaine: history, use, abuse. J R Soc Med. 1999;92(8):393–7. https://doi.org/10.1177/014107689909200803.
22. Kariisa M, Scholl L, Wilson N, Seth P, Hoots B. Drug overdose deaths involving cocaine and psychostimulants with abuse potential - United States, 2003-2017. MMWR Morb Mortal Wkly Rep. 2019;68(17):388–95. https://doi.org/10.15585/mmwr.mm6817a3.
23. Kintz P. Hair analysis in forensic toxicology: an updated review with a special focus on pitfalls. Curr Pharm Des. 2017;23(36):5480–6. https://doi.org/10.2174/1381612823666170929155628.
24. Kosten TR, Domingo CB, Shorter D, Orson F, Green C, Somoza E, et al. Vaccine for cocaine dependence: a randomized double-blind placebo-controlled efficacy trial. Drug Alcohol Depend. 2014;140:42–7. https://doi.org/10.1016/j.drugalcdep.2014.04.003.
25. Levin FR, Mariani JJ, Pavlicova M, Choi CJ, Mahony AL, Brooks DJ, et al. Extended release mixed amphetamine salts and topiramate for cocaine dependence: A randomized clinical replication trial with frequent users. Drug Alcohol Depend. 2019:107700. https://doi.org/10.1016/j.drugalcdep.2019.107700.
26. Mariani JJ, Pavlicova M, Bisaga A, Nunes EV, Brooks DJ, Levin FR. Extended-release mixed amphetamine salts and topiramate for cocaine dependence: a randomized controlled trial. Biol Psychiatry. 2012;72(11):950–6. https://doi.org/10.1016/j.biopsych.2012.05.032.
27. May, C. Transnational crime and the developing world. 2017. Retrieved from
28. May CD. How coca-cola obtains its coca. The New York Times; 1988. p. D1–5.
29. Minozzi S, Saulle R, De Crescenzo F, Amato L. Psychosocial interventions for psychostimulant misuse. Cochrane Database Syst Rev. 2016;9:CD011866. https://doi.org/10.1002/14651858.CD011866.pub2.
30. Nickley J, Pesce AJ, Krock K. A sensitive assay for urinary cocaine metabolite benzoylecgonine shows more positive results and longer half-lives than those using traditional cut-offs. Drug Test Anal. 2017;9(8):1214–6. https://doi.org/10.1002/dta.2153.
31. NIDA. Principles of drug addiction treatment: a research-based guide. 3rd ed. National Institute on Drug Abuse; 2018.
32. NIDA. Overdose Death Rates. 2020. Retrieved from https://www.drugabuse.gov/drug-topics/trends-statistics/overdose-death-rates.
33. Pani PP, Trogu E, Vacca R, Amato L, Vecchi S, Davoli M. Disulfiram for the treatment of cocaine dependence. Cochrane Database Syst Rev. 2010;1:CD007024. https://doi.org/10.1002/14651858.CD007024.pub2.
34. Pani PP, Trogu E, Vecchi S, Amato L. Antidepressants for cocaine dependence and problematic cocaine use. Cochrane Database Syst Rev. 2011;12:CD002950. https://doi.org/10.1002/14651858.CD002950.pub3.
35. Phillips KA, Epstein DH, Preston KL. Psychostimulant addiction treatment. Neuropharmacology. 2014;87:150–60. https://doi.org/10.1016/j.neuropharm.2014.04.002.
36. Pilowsky DJ, Wu LT. Screening for alcohol and drug use disorders among adults in primary care: a review. Subst Abus Rehabil. 2012;3(1):25–34. https://doi.org/10.2147/SAR.S30057.
37. Rouse B. Trends in cocaine use in the general population. NIDA Res Monogr. 1991;10:5–18.
38. SAMHSA. Key substance use and mental health indicators in the United States: results from the 2018 National Survey on Drug Use and Health. Rockville; 2019.
39. Skinner HA. The drug abuse screening test. Addict Behav. 1982;7(4):363–71. https://doi.org/10.1016/0306-4603(82)90005-3.
40. Tardelli VS, Bisaga A, Arcadepani FB, Gerra G, Levin FR, Fidalgo TM. Prescription psychostimulants for the treatment of stimulant use disorder: a systematic review and meta-analysis. Psychopharmacology. 2020;237(8):2233–55. https://doi.org/10.1007/s00213-020-05563-3.
41. Tiet QQ, Leyva YE, Moos RH, Frayne SM, Osterberg L, Smith B. Screen of drug use: diagnostic accuracy

of a new brief tool for primary care. JAMA Intern Med. 2015;175(8):1371–7. https://doi.org/10.1001/jamainternmed.2015.2438.
42. U.N. Report of the commission of enquiry on the coca Leaf. New York: Lake Success; 1950.
43. UNODC. World Drug Report. (United Nations Publication, Sales No. E.18.XI.9). 2018.
44. UNODC. Global seizures of drugs. 2019. Retrieved from https://dataunodc.un.org/drugs/global_seizures-2017
45. WHO/UNICRI Cocaine Project Briefing Kit. Geneva: World Health Organization/United Nations Interregional Crime and Justice Research Institute. 1995.

15 Opioids

Evaristo Akerele

Introduction

Approximately 271 million people, or 5.5% of the global population aged 15–64, had use drugs, while 35 million people are suffering from drug use disorders. Opioids continue to cause the most harm, accounting for two-thirds of the deaths attributed to drug use disorders. Individuals who inject drugs (11 million worldwide in 2017) endure the greatest health risks. Furthermore, over 50% live with hepatitis C, and approximately one in eight lives with HIV (*UNDOC World Drug Report 2019, Booklet* 2) [20]. More than 90% of all pharmaceutical opioids available for medical consumption were in high-income countries in 2018 comprising around 12% of the global population, while the low- and middle-income countries comprising 88% of the global population are estimated to consume less than 10% of pharmaceutical opioids. Access to pharmaceutical opioids depends on several factors including legislation, culture, health systems, and prescribing practices ([19], Booklet 1&2). There were about 34 million people who used opioids and about 19 million who used opiates. There were an estimated 27 million people who suffered from opioid use disorders in 2016. The majority of people dependent on opioids used illicitly cultivated and manufactured heroin, but an increasing proportion used prescription opioids. Overdose deaths contribute to between roughly a third and a half of all drug-related deaths, which are attributable in most cases to opioids. Opioid overdose is one of the most frequent cause of emergency room drug-related presentations [1].

Lifetime prevalence of witnessed overdose among drug users is about 70%. Although effective treatments for opioid dependence are available and could potentially prevent overdose, less than 10% of individuals who need such treatment actually receive it. The receptors to which opioids bind play a central role in susceptibility to overdose.

Opioids bind to receptors in the central and peripheral nervous systems (primarily delta, kappa, and mu), with treatment effects for pain, cough, and diarrhea. Action on these same receptors induces intense euphoria. As a result, many individuals continue to use in an effort to reproduce that first high. Most individuals misuse opioids either to reduce pain or to prevent withdrawal symptoms. However, the data suggest dispelling that opioids are not effective as long-term analgesic medications [2].

Some of the receptors matched to physiologic effects in the central nervous system are listed below (nociceptin and zeta receptors increasingly being researched):

E. Akerele (✉)
Department of Psychiatry, New Jersey Medical School, Rutgers University, Newark, NJ, USA

E. Akerele (ed.), *Substance and Non-Substance Related Addictions*,
https://doi.org/10.1007/978-3-030-84834-7_15

- Delta: analgesia, antidepressant, convulsant, physical dependence, and modulate mu-related respiratory depression.
- Kappa: analgesia, anticonvulsant, depression, hallucination, diuresis, dysphoria, miosis, neuroprotection, and sedation.
- Mu: analgesia, physical dependence, respiratory depression, miosis, euphoria, reduced GI motility, and vasodilation. Peripheral mu receptors are tissue-specific with higher concentrations in the bronchial smooth muscle and the digestive tract. This is the reason for opioids suppressing the cough reflex and causing constipation [14, 15].

Individuals experience symptoms of withdrawal either when opioids are discontinued abruptly or tapered cessation of medications. These symptoms present in acute, subacute, and chronic phases. The acute withdrawal symptoms include hot/cold flashes, nausea, vomiting, diarrhea, sweating, lacrimation, insomnia, anxiety, generalized muscle pain, tachycardia, piloerection, and dehydration.

Opioids continue to be a significant public health issue. Both overdose and withdrawal are linked to a variety of opioids, legally and illegally, that act primarily on three receptors, mu, delta, and gamma. These include heroin, fentanyl, methadone, oxycodone, and others. In the sections that follow, each one of these drugs will be addressed. The focus will be on the identification and treatment. The 2018 data suggest that approximately 128 people in the United States die daily following overdose on opioids ([7]. https://wonder.cdc.gov.).

Opioid dependence which includes *prescription pain relievers*, *heroin*, and synthetic opioids, such as *fentanyl*, is a significant public health issue that impacts socioeconomic well-being. The socioeconomic impact includes the costs of healthcare, lost productivity, addiction treatment, and criminal justice involvement. The cost of prescription drug use in the United States is approximately $78.5 million [8].

The key issue is how we arrived at this crisis. Apparently, the initial misconception in the 1990s that patients would not become addicted to prescription opioid pain relievers played a significant role. This was supported by reassurance of medical providers by pharmaceutical representatives. This enamored healthcare providers to begin prescribing opioids at greater rates. By the time it became apparent that these medications could lead to significant addiction, the diversion and misuse of these medications had become widespread [11], [16].

Gradually, opioid overdose rates began to increase. Approximately 47,000 Americans died in 2017 as a result of an opioid overdose, including prescription opioids, heroin, and illicitly manufactured fentanyl, a powerful synthetic opioid ([7]. https://wonder.cdc.gov.). An estimated 1.7 million people in the United States in 2017 met criteria for substance use disorders related to prescription opioid pain relievers, and 652,000 had heroin use disorder. Approximately 25% of individuals with chronic pain misuse their prescribed opioids [18]. Between 8 and 12% go on to develop opioid use disorder [18]. Approximately 5% of those who misuse prescription opioids transition to *heroin* [5, 3, 12].

About 80% of people who use heroin first misused prescription opioids [5] [12]. Opioid overdoses increased by 30% from July 2016 through September 2017 in 52 areas in 45 states. The Midwestern region saw opioid overdoses increase up to 70% from July 2016 through September 2017 [17].

Prescription Opioids and Heroin

Heroin is an opioid drug made from morphine, a natural substance taken from the seed pod of the various opium poppy plants grown in Southeast and Southwest Asia, Mexico, and Colombia. Heroin can be a white or brown powder, or a black sticky substance known as black tar heroin. Other common names for heroin include *big H*, *horse*, *hell dust*, and *smack*.

Heroin can be injected, sniffed, snorted, or smoked. Some individuals mix heroin with crack cocaine, a practice called speed balling. Prescription opioid pain medicines such as

OxyContin® and Vicodin® have effects similar to heroin. Research suggests that misuse of these drugs may open the door to heroin use. Data from 2011 showed that an estimated 4–6% who misuse prescription opioids switch to heroin [3, 5] and about 80% of people who used heroin first misused prescription opioids [3–6].

More recent data suggest that heroin is frequently the first opioid people use. In a study of those entering treatment for opioid use disorder, approximately one-third reported heroin as the first opioid they used regularly to get high [16]. This suggests that prescription opioid misuse is just one of the several factors leading to heroin use.

Short-Term Effects

People who use heroin report feeling a "rush" (a surge of pleasure, or euphoria). However, there are other common effects, including

- Dry mouth.
- Warm flushing of the skin.
- Heavy feeling in the arms and legs.
- Nausea and vomiting.
- Severe itching.
- Clouded mental functioning.
- Going “on the nod,” a back-and-forth state of being conscious and semiconscious.

Long-Term Effects

People who use heroin over the long term may develop:

- Insomnia.
- Collapsed veins for people who inject the drug.
- Damaged tissue inside the nose for people who sniff or snort it.
- Infection of the heart lining and valves.
- Abscesses (swollen tissue filled with pus).
- Constipation and stomach cramping.
- Liver and kidney disease.
- Lung complications, including pneumonia.
- Mental disorders such as depression and antisocial personality disorder.
- Sexual dysfunction for men.
- Irregular menstrual cycles for women.

Injection Drug Use, HIV, and Hepatitis

People who inject drugs such as heroin are at high risk of contracting the HIV and hepatitis C virus (HCV). These diseases are transmitted through contact with blood or other bodily fluids, which can occur when sharing needles or other injection drug use equipment. HCV is the most common blood-borne infection in the United States. HIV (and less often HCV) can also be contracted during unprotected sex, which drug use makes more likely.

Other Potential Effects

Heroin often contains additives, such as sugar, starch, or powdered milk, which can clog blood vessels leading to the lungs, liver, kidneys, or brain, causing permanent damage. Also, sharing drug injection equipment and having impaired judgment from drug use can increase the risk of contracting infectious diseases such as HIV and hepatitis. Heroin overdose may occur when an individual uses enough of the drug to produce a life-threatening reaction or death. Heroin overdoses have increased in recent years [4].

Overdose on heroin can result in respiratory arrest. This can reduce the quantity of oxygen reaching the brain, a condition known as *hypoxia*. Hypoxia can have short- and long-term mental effects and effects on the nervous system, including coma and permanent brain damage.

Heroin is highly addictive. People who regularly use heroin often develop a tolerance, which means that they need higher and/or more frequent doses of the drug to get the desired effects. A *substance use disorder* (SUD) is when continued use of the drug causes issues, such as health problems and failure to meet responsibilities at work, school, or home. A

SUD can range from mild to severe, the most severe form being addiction. Individuals with opioid use disorder may have severe withdrawal when they stop using abruptly. Withdrawal symptoms—which can begin as early as a few hours after the drug was last taken—include restlessness, severe muscle and bone pain, sleep problems, diarrhea and vomiting, cold flashes with goosebumps ("cold turkey"), uncontrollable leg movements ("kicking the habit"), and severe heroin cravings.

There is ongoing research on the long-term effects of opioids on the brain. Current data suggest some loss of white matter in the brain associated with the use of heroin, which is likely to affect decision-making, behavior control, and response to stress [9, 10, 13].

Key Points

- Heroin is an opioid drug made from morphine, a natural substance taken from the seed pod of various opium poppy plants.
- Heroin can be a white or brown powder, or a black sticky substance known as black tar heroin.
- Heroin can be injected, sniffed, snorted, or smoked. Mixing heroin with crack cocaine is known as *speed balling*.
- Heroin crosses the blood-brain barrier rapidly and binds to opioid receptors on cells located in many areas, especially those involved in feelings of pain and pleasure and in controlling heart rate, sleeping, and breathing.
- Individuals who use heroin report feeling a "rush" (or euphoria). Other common effects include dry mouth, heavy feelings in the arms and legs, and clouded mental functioning.
- Long-term effects may include collapsed veins, infection of the heart lining and valves, abscesses, and lung complications.
- Research suggests that misuse of prescription opioid pain medicine is a risk factor for starting heroin use.
- Heroin can lead to addiction, a form of substance use disorder. Withdrawal symptoms include severe muscle and bone pain, sleep problems, diarrhea and vomiting, and severe heroin cravings.

Treatment

Overdose Treatment

Naloxone is used to treat an opioid overdose. It works by rapidly binding to opioid receptors and blocking the effects of heroin and other opioid drugs. Sometimes more than one dose is needed for breathing to commence, hence the importance of getting to the emergency room as soon as possible. Naloxone is available as an injectable (needle) solution, a handheld auto-injector (EVZIO®), and a nasal spray (NARCAN® nasal spray). Friends, family, and others in the community can use the auto-injector and nasal spray versions of naloxone to resuscitate an individual overdosing. The increase in the number of opioid overdose deaths has resulted in an increase in public health efforts to ensure naloxone is available for at-risk persons and their families, as well as first responders and others in the community. Some states have passed laws that allow pharmacists to dispense naloxone without a prescription.

A range of treatments including medicines and behavioral therapies are effective for the treatment of opioid use disorder. Treatment approach has to be individualized. Medications are being developed to assist with the withdrawal process. The Food and Drug Administration (FDA) approved lofexidine, a non-opioid medicine designed to reduce opioid withdrawal symptoms [21, 22].

Withdrawal and Chronic Treatment

Current medications available include buprenorphine and methadone. They work by binding to the same opioid receptors in the brain as heroin, but more weakly, reducing cravings and withdrawal symptoms. Treatment with naltrexone is another option. Naltrexone blocks opioid receptors and prevents opioids from having an effect. A National Institute of Drug Abuse (NIDA) study found that once treatment is initiated, both a buprenorphine/naloxone combination and an extended-release naltrexone formulation have similar efficacy. However, since full detoxification is necessary for treatment with naloxone, initiating treatment in active users was challenging, but once detoxification was complete, the medications had similar efficacy.

Behavioral therapies for heroin addiction include cognitive behavioral therapy, contingency management, motivational therapy, network therapy, and 12-step facilitation. Cognitive behavioral therapy helps modify the patient's drug use expectations and behaviors and helps effectively manage triggers and stress. Contingency management provides motivational incentives, such as vouchers or cash rewards for positive behaviors such as drug abstinence. These behavioral treatment approaches are especially effective when used along with medicines.

Conclusion

Opioid use disorder remains a global public health issue. It significantly affects the physical, mental, and economic well-being worldwide. Approximately 271 million people globally have used opioids in the past year. 11 million are injection drug users. More than half have hepatitis C. The primary receptors that opioids interact with are delta, mu, and kappa. The main effects are analgesia, respiratory depression, euphoria, and physical dependence. Seventy percent of lifetime emergency room presentations are due to opioid overdose. There is increasing use of opioids globally. The use of prescription opioids is one modality that may lead to heroin use. Naloxone is key for the treatment of opioid overdose. Methadone and buprenorphine/naloxone are used for the chronic management of opioid use disorder. However behavioral therapies such as contingency management, network, motivational, and cognitive behavioral therapies are vital for a successful recovery from opioid addiction.

References

1. Akerele E, Olupona T. Drugs of abuse. Psychiatry Clin North Am. 2017;40(3):501–17. https://doi.org/10.1016/j.psc.2017.05.006.
2. Azadfard M, Huecker MR, Leaming JM. 2020. Opioid addiction. [updated 2020 Apr 8]. In: StatPearls [internet]. Treasure Island (FL): StatPearls publishing; 2020 Jan-. Available from: https://www.ncbi.nlm.nih.gov/books/NBK448203/.
3. Carlson RG, Nahhas RW, Martins SS, Daniulaityte R. Predictors of transition to heroin use among initially non-opioid dependent illicit pharmaceutical opioid users: a natural history study. Drug Alcohol Depend. 2016;160:127–34. https://doi.org/10.1016/j.drugalcdep.2015.12.026.
4. Centers for Disease Control and Prevention (CDC). Multiple Cause of Death, 1999–2015. CDC WONDER Online Database. https://wonder.cdc.gov/mcd-icd10.html. Accessed April 4, 2017). https://www.ncbi.nlm.nih.gov/pubmed/28582659.
5. Cicero TJ, Ellis MS, Surratt HL, Kurtz SP. The changing face of heroin use in the United States: a retrospective analysis of the past 50 years. JAMA Psychiat. 2014;71(7):821–6. https://doi.org/10.1001/jamapsychiatry.2014.366.
6. Cicero TJ, Ellis MS, Kasper ZA. Increased use of heroin as an initiating opioid of abuse. Addict Behav. 2017;74:63–6. https://doi.org/10.1016/j.addbeh.2017.05.030. Epub 2017 May 23.
7. *CDC/NCHS,* National Vital Statistics System, *Mortality. CDC WONDER, Atlanta, GA: US Department of Health and Human Services, CDC; 2018.* https://wonder.cdc.gov.
8. Florence CS, Zhou C, Luo F, Xu L. The economic burden of prescription opioid overdose, abuse, and dependence in the United States. Med Care. 2016;54(10):901–6. https://doi.org/10.1097/MLR.0000000000000625.
9. Li W, Li Q, Zhu J, et al. White matter impairment in chronic heroin dependence: a quantitative DTI study. Brain Res. 2013;1531:58–64. https://doi.org/10.1016/j.brainres.2013.07.036.
10. Liu J, Qin W, Yuan K, et al. Interaction between dysfunctional connectivity at rest and heroin cues-induced brain responses in male abstinent heroin-dependent individuals. PLoS One. 2011;6(10):e23098. https://doi.org/10.1371/journal.pone.0023098.
11. Morone NE, Weiner DK. Pain as the fifth vital sign: exposing the vital need for pain education. Clin Ther. 2013;35(11):1728–32. https://doi.org/10.1016/j.clinthera.2013.10.001.
12. Muhuri PK, Gfroerer JC, Davies MC. 2013. Associations of Nonmedical Pain Reliever Use and Initiation of Heroin Use in the United States. CBHSQ Data Rev/SAMHSA. https://www.samhsa.gov/data/sites/default/files/DR006/DR006/nonmedical-pain-reliever-use 2013.pdf#:~:text=HS%20ATA%20RI%20Associations%20of%20Nonmedical%20Pain%20Reliever,new%20formulation.%20However%2C%20the%20reformulation%20may%20have%20led.
13. Qiu Y, Jiang G, Su H, et al. Progressive white matter microstructure damage in male chronic heroin dependent individuals: a DTI and TBSS study. PLoS One. 2013;8(5):e63212. https://doi.org/10.1371/journal.pone.0063212.

14. Theriot J, Azadfard M. StatPearls [Internet]. StatPearls Publishing; Treasure Island (FL): Nov 28, 2019. Opioid Antagonists. [PubMed] Updated version:
15. Theriot J, Sabir S, Azadfard M. Opioid Antagonists. (2020) [Updated 2020 Jul 27]. In: StatPearls [Internet]. Treasure Island (FL): StatPearls Publishing; 2020 Jan-. Available from: https://www.ncbi.nlm.nih.gov/books/NBK537079/.
16. Van Zee A. The promotion and marketing of OxyContin: commercial triumph, public health tragedy. Am J Public Health. 2009;99(2):221–7. https://doi.org/10.2105/AJPH.2007.131714.
17. Vivolo-Kantor AM, Seth P, Gladden RM, et al. Vital signs: trends in emergency department visits for suspected opioid overdoses - United States, July 2016-September 2017. MMWR Morbid Mortal Weekly Rep. 2018;67(9):279–85. https://doi.org/10.15585/mmwr.mm6709e1.
18. Vowles KE, McEntee ML, Julnes PS, Frohe T, Ney JP, van der Goes DN. Rates of opioid misuse, abuse, and addiction in chronic pain: a systematic review and data synthesis. Pain. 2015;156(4):569–76. https://doi.org/10.1097/01.j.pain.0000460357.01998.f1.
19. World Drug Report 2020. https://wdr.unodc.org/wdr2020/field/WDR20_Booklet_2.pdf.
20. World Health Organization. (2020, September 16). Opioid Overdose. https://www.who.int/news-room/fact-sheets/detail/opioid-overdose.
21. Yu E, Miotto K, Akerele E, et al. A phase 3 placebo-controlled, double-blind, multi-site trial of the alpha-2-adrenergic agonist, lofexidine, for opioid withdrawal. Drug Alcohol Depend. 2008a;97(1–2):158–68. https://doi.org/10.1016/j.drugalcdep.2008.04.002.
22. Yu E, Miotto K, Akerele E, et al. Clinical pharmacokinetics of lofexidine, the alpha 2-adrenergic receptor agonist, in opiate addicts plasma using a highly sensitive liquid chromatography tandem mass spectrometric analysis. Am J Drug Alcohol Abuse. 2008b;34(5):611–6. https://doi.org/10.1080/00952990802308122.

16 Designer Drugs

Neelambika Revadigar, Ching Tary Yu,
and Isabelle Silverstone-Simard

On a Tuesday morning in 2017, 33 people were found with significant "altered mental status" in the streets of a Brooklyn neighborhood in New York City [33]. Some were found to be motionless, while some were found to be twitching on the ground reportedly consumed a bad batch of synthetic marijuana called "K2." All the victims were brought to the emergency room. Unfortunately, it was not an isolated event as mass overdose and intoxication due to designer drugs becomes more and more common. In May 2018, 56 people fell victim to K2 overdose in Brooklyn, New York. In August 2018, 99 people overdosed over just 2 days in New Haven, Connecticut [30].

These designer drugs have begun to enter mainstream toward the end of the 2000s. The goal of the manufacturers has been to evade drug laws and drug screenings by the lack of legal regulations or screening techniques on newly developed compounds. Compounded by novelty and accessibility by which users can often purchase online via the Internet or the dark web in packages labeled as "plant food" or "not for human consumption [24]." The popularity has grown considerably over the decade. Within 6 years, the number of substances being manufactured and distributed grew from less than 100 to nearly 500 in 2015 according to the United Nations Office on Drug and Crime [62, 64]. Designer drug use is most prevalent among younger adults in their 20s predominantly male, but it can affect teenagers as well as older adults upward of 40–50 years of age [9, 31, 56]. Those who are at risk include males who are single with history of conduct and behavioral issues, lower levels of education and socioeconomic status, those with family history of substance use disorders, and those with history or current poor family relationships [9, 31, 35].

Not only do these drugs are often laced with other dangerous chemical adulterants such as Krokodil, there are no standardized or safety procedures in the manufacturing process of these compounds. Theoretically, these compounds can come from raw chemical ingredients [37] through a series of chemical reactions such as reduction and dehydrocarboxylation. Given the complex chemical processes and the volatility of the chemicals involved, any mishap along the manufacturing can result in an altercation in the final molecule leading to a compound with significant different physiological effects and potentially dire consequences as seen in the victims in the mass overdose cases. These compounds are much more inherently dangerous than the traditional substances they are trying to mimic. Given the ever-growing designer drug market and the

N. Revadigar (✉) · C. T. Yu
Columbia University, New York, NY, USA
e-mail: nsr2123@cumc.columbia.edu

I. Silverstone-Simard
McGill University, Montreal, QC, Canada
e-mail: isabelle.silverstone-simard@mail.mcgill.ca

E. Akerele (ed.), *Substance and Non-Substance Related Addictions*,
https://doi.org/10.1007/978-3-030-84834-7_16

potential dire health consequences associated with these drugs, the understanding of these drugs can help with appropriate diagnoses and treatments. In this chapter, we will discuss several of the typical designer drug classes: synthetic cannabinoids, synthetic stimulants, synthetic hallucinogens, and synthetic opioids.

Synthetic Cannabinoids

Synthetic cannabinoids (SCBs) are substances with chemical properties like tetrahydrocannabinol (THC). SCBs may structurally differ from cannabinoids. SCBs are sprayed on scrapped plant material to be smoked. They are illegally sold as liquids to be inhaled via e-cigarettes and other devices, herbal supplements, or liquid incense. Sold as "K2," "Spice," and "synthetic marijuana," they are often labeled "not for human consumption" [2].

Initially, SCBs were used for cannabinoid research focusing on THC (a psychoactive and an analgesic found in the plant of cannabis) because of legal limitations on natural cannabinoids. Tritium-labeled cannabinoids such as CP-55.940 were instrumental in discovering cannabinoid receptors in the early 1990s [50]. Nabilone was the first synthetic cannabinoid used as antiemetic to tackle nausea and vomiting since 1981. Marinol or dronabinol have been used as an antiemetic since 1985 and as an appetite stimulant since 1991[14].

History of SCBs

Around the early 2000s, SCBs started being used as recreational drugs to get similar effects of cannabis because of their similar molecular structures compared to THC. As previously mentioned, abusers can easily obtain illegally manufactured compounds such as K2 or Spice in Europe and the United States. Poison control centers across the United States have reported increasing incidences of intoxications and adverse events associated with the use. Finally, the Drug Enforcement Administration (DEA) of the United States passed the Synthetic Drug Abuse Prevention Act in 2012 moving SCBs to a Schedule I drug. However, illegal laboratories have continued to work on discovering novel SCBs in order to evade detection and prosecution. By 2015, 177 types of SCBs were reported to the United Nations Office on Drugs and Crime Early Warning Advisory to be causing severe poisoning and even fatalities [13].

Classification

SCBs are classified into five major categories: classical cannabinoids, nonclassical cannabinoids, hybrid cannabinoids, aminoalkylindoles, and eicosanoids. Classical cannabinoids are analogs of THC based on a dibenzopyran ring, and many variants were discovered in the 1960s following the isolation of THC, including nabilone and dronabinol [41, 42]. Due to difficult manufacturing process, classical cannabinoids are not often seen in SCBs blends for recreational use [11]. On the other hand, aminoalkylindoles are the most common chemical structure found in SCB blends. These are less difficult to synthesize than classical and nonclassical cannabinoids.

As of today, the least difficult compounds to manufacturer are the JWHs. They were discovered by Professor John William Huffman at Clemson University in the 1990s [63]. Due to their low manufacturing cost, they are now the most widely sold and abused SCBs.

Mechanism of Action

SCBs are not direct analogs of THC. However, they do share many features with THC. They are lipid-soluble, small molecules with adequate volatility for smoking and inhalation. Common molecular features include the 5–9 full carbon side chain, which is responsible for the psychotropic activity from CB1 receptor binding. Thus, the features make them potent agonist to the cannabinoid receptor 1 (CB1) and the cannabinoid receptor 2 (CB2). These receptors are found mostly in the peripheral tissues such as the kidney, lungs, and liver, and the central nervous system, especially the basal ganglia, cerebral cortex, hippocampus, and the cerebellum where the compounds can exert most of their effects.

In contrast to THC, which is a partial CB1 receptor agonist, SCBs are full CB1 agonists with, much higher affinity for CB1 receptors than THC. As such, they are found to have greater potency and exert greater pharmacologic effects than THC.

Metabolism of SCBs

In general, the metabolisms and clearance of SCBs involve the oxidation via the cytochrome (CYP450) system [21] followed by the conjugation with a glucuronic acid via the UDP-glucuronosyltransferases (UGTs) enzymes. For example, molecules like JWH-1018, aminoalkylindoles, cyclohexylphenols, and benzylindoles are oxidized by cytochrome P450 enzymes and then conjugated by the uridine 50-diphospho (UDP)-glucuronosyltransferase enzyme presents in the liver [11]. Important CYP enzymes include CYP2D6 and CYP1A2. Studies suggest that CYP2D6 is highly expressed in the cerebral cortex, hippocampus, and cerebellum of the brain in the vicinity to CB1 receptors [43] and is involved with regulating brain concentrations of SCBs' metabolites [29]. Studies have also identified two isoforms of UDP-glucuronosyltransferase (UGT2B7 and UGT1A2) as essential roles in the glucuronidation of synthetic cannabinoid metabolites [11]. It is important to note that many metabolites of SCBs retain some pharmacological activities at the CB1 receptor [58].

Detection of SCBs

SCBs do not cross-react with marijuana's immunoassay. Thus, a urine toxicology screen is usually negative in a person suspected to have used SCBs. Recently, costly chromatographic methods for the analysis of SCBs have been reported to be useful to detect SCBs.

Adverse Effects and Treatment

SCBs are associated with higher rates of adverse effects and hospital admission compared to natural cannabis. The most common neuropsychiatric complaints associated with SCBs are agitation and irritability, hallucination, delusion, and confusion. Hypertension, tachycardia, nausea, dizziness, vertigo, and chest pain are common medical symptoms reported. Acute kidney injury is strongly associated with SCB toxicity. Treatment is mostly supportive [44] such as IV fluids, supplemental oxygen, and airway protection. Benzodiazepines can be used to treat agitation, combativeness, and muscular hyperactivity. Local poison control center should be contacted. Unfortunately, there is no available specific antidote for SCB intoxication.

Synthetic Stimulants

Among the synthetic stimulants, synthetic cathinones are among the most manufactured and abused. They fall under the family of stimulants that also encompass amphetamine, methamphetamine, and methylenedioxymethamphetamine (MDMA). Synthetic cathinones are commonly known as bath salts but also known as other street names including M-CAT and meow-meow in different countries [4, 5, 32]. There are many variants of synthetic cathinones on the market including mephedrone, methylmethcathinone (MCAT), methylenedioxypyrovalerone (MDPV), and methylone [34].

History

Cathinone is a naturally occurring beta-keto derivative of amphetamine. It can be found in khat plants in certain African and Middle Eastern countries being traditionally cultivated for their stimulant and euphoria-inducing effects [60]. The first synthetic cathinone, mephedrone, was first discovered in 1929 (13) [72]. However, it did not gain attention until in the 2000s when the compound began to be widely available on the

Internet. Based on interviews from former users, they could have easily acquired the compound online, and they preferred it for its stimulating effect on energy, mood, and sex drive [51]. Some users in Europe would specifically use these synthetic cathinones in "chemsex parties" where they would inject mephedrone intravenously and engage in risky sexual behaviors [17]. Many users described having cravings and compulsive habitual uses [70].

Mechanism of Action

In a similar fashion as the more traditional stimulant compounds such as cocaine, amphetamine, and MDMA, synthetic cathinones also facilitate extracellular release and reuptake inhibition of neurotransmitters [3–5]. Thus, like their traditional counterparts, they act by increasing the extracellular levels of serotonin, norepinephrine, and dopamine. As expected, the commonly reported effects are also similar as well. They include increased energy and feeling of social connectedness, enhanced alertness and concentration, euphoria, and sexual stimulation [65, 70].

The compounds are commonly used intranasally, but it is also known to be abused by ingestion, inhalation by smoking, or via intravenous injection. The onset of symptoms usually begins within 30 minutes of dosing with a peak within 90 minutes, lasting 2–3 hours. The effects would gradually decrease over 6–12 hours [65]. Like users of other substances, many may opt for multiple dosing to prolong the desired effects.

Metabolism of Synthetic Cathinones

Data on the metabolism of synthetic cathinones are limited but may be extrapolated from studies on naturally occurring cathinone. Cathinone undergoes first-pass hepatic demethylation to d-norpseudoephedrine via reduction of a ketone group to alcohol [48]. Both the primary compound and the metabolite can contribute to the psychoactive activity.

Detection of Synthetic Cathinones

In terms of detection in suspected cases, these synthetic stimulants may not be readily tested in a standard clinical setting. Although amphetamine immunoassays can be used to detect the more traditional psychostimulants such as MDMA based on their cross-reactivity with assay antibodies, the many newer synthetic stimulants do not possess the same level of cross-reactivity and thus are difficult to detect in most standard settings [52]. As such, these compounds are not routinely screened in a clinical setting. Detections are only conducted mainly in forensic laboratories using gas chromatography and mass spectrometry, liquid chromatography-tandem mass spectrometry, or liquid chromatography quadrupole time-of-flight/mass spectrometry [38]. Due to the prohibiting costs of these techniques, detections are generally reserved for cases involving fatalities or criminally related issues. Unfortunately, new compounds are still being developed, and the ever-growing list of de novo synthetic stimulants would further complicate the detection process in clinical settings.

Given the similar effects and pharmacologic properties between the traditional stimulants and the synthetic stimulants, drug dealers would often add synthetic cathinones into traditional stimulants such as cocaine or MDMA or substitute them all together with these synthetic cathinones [47] possibly to increase profitability. Victims would therefore unknowingly take these synthetic substitutes that are inherently more dangerous than the substances they intended to use initially [47].

Adverse Effects and Treatments

In terms of side effects and adverse effects, synthetic stimulants do manifest in similar fashions as their traditional counterparts. Most commonly, these synthetic compounds exert an increase in sympathetic tone in the body, resulting in autonomic hyperactivity such as the increase in heart rate, cardiac contractility, systolic and diastolic blood pressure, and body temperature [48]. Users might experience dysphoria, suicidal ideations, insomnia, palpitations, diaphoresis, and muscle spasms, while bruxism and mydriasis can be appreciated on physical exams [48, 70]. Furthermore, cachexia and poor physical appearance can be found in chronic users [17]. It is interesting to note that the effects of mephedrone are found to be faster and shorter in duration than MDMA [48]. Not unexpectedly, those who take the compounds intranasally or via smoke inhalation might experience epistaxis and inflamed nasal passages [15]. In 2001, it was reported that nearly 23,000 emergency room visits were related to adverse effects linked to bath salts [19].

Acute agitation is frequent among patients who experience acute toxicity on large consumption [17]. Delusions, visual, tactile, and auditory hallucinations had been documented in case reports [17, 61]. Indeed, aggressivity in the context of agitation and/or psychosis can be found among those who are acutely intoxicated [17]. Deaths from self-harm or suicide had also been documented because of the neuropsychiatric symptoms [17]. Case reports have documented the use of antipsychotics and benzodiazepines as per clinical indications for the management of psychotic, aggressive behaviors as well as delusions and hallucinations [36]. Not unexpectedly, the withdrawal symptoms are like those described for stimulant withdrawal including dysphoric mood, fatigue, dyssomnia, psychomotor agitation, and irritability [70].

Over the years, many case reports have also described the many medical complications of synthetic stimulants. Morbidities and mortalities have been well-documented. Acute reversible cardiomyopathy was found following the intravenous use of M-CAT (acute MCAT abuse, Redfern) and following smoke inhalation and intravenous use of mephedrone and MDPV [55]. Myocardial infarction, rhabdomyolysis, supraventricular tachycardia, and cardiac arrest resulting in death following MDPV intoxication were documented [22]. Fatalities related to synthetic cathinones use are not uncommon with deaths attributed to hyperthermia, hypertension, cardiac arrest, and possible serotonin syndrome [71].

Synthetic Hallucinogens

History

The most common synthetic hallucinogens include phenethylamines. These phenethylamines represent a class of chemical compounds with stimulant and psychoactive effects. They include substances such as amphetamines, methamphetamines, and MDMA [27, 69] as well as synthetic analogs commonly known as "designer drugs," gaining in popularity after the 1991 publication of *PiHKAL: A Chemical Love Story* by Alexander Shulgin and his wife Ann Shulgin [16, 53]. He was the first to describe the 2C series of phenethylamines, named after the two carbons between the amino group and benzene ring of the chemical structure [68]. Other examples of substituted substances include the 'D series of amphetamines (e.g., DOI, DOC), potent hallucinogens known as benzodifurans (e.g., Bromo-Dragonfly, 2-C-B-Fly) [12], and others such as p-methoxymethamphetamine or PMMA, sold in the drug market as a substitute for "ecstasy" (European Monitoring Centre for Drugs, & Drug Addiction,2003).

Mechanism of Action

The 2C is a series of designer drugs with a phenethylamine-based structure common to many drugs including amphetamines, cathinones, and catecholamines. Phenethylamines mainly act as stimulants, mediating the actions of dopamine, norepinephrine, and/or serotonin, or as hallucinogens, producing hallucinations via specific serotonin receptor activities [20]. The designer substitution of 2C results in increased hallucinogenic activity, which corresponds to reported effects like those of lysergic acid and psilocybin [69].

The designer hallucinogen 4-iodo-2,5-dimethoxy-N-(2-methoxybenzyl)phenethylamine (25I-NBOMe) has a methoxy group at the two and five positions on the ring and is a relative newcomer in the 2C series of phenethylamines. It gained popularity in 2011 along with several other N-benzyl phenethylamines, when a temporary Schedule I status was issued by the US Drug Enforcement Administration to these compounds, colloquially referred to as "bath salts" [19]. Initially synthesized to be used in serotonin receptor research, 25I-NBOMe has a high-affinity agonist of the serotonin 5HT2a receptor [46]. 25I-NBOMe is found both in powder and liquid forms, and its most common route of administration is oral/buccal/sublingual, as well as nasal insufflation [68]. The latter results in rapid clinical effects that peak after 20 minutes. The reported duration of action ranges from 3 to 13 hours [68].

Detection and Screening

One primary reason for designer drug use reported by individuals is the lack of detection on standard urine and serum toxicology screening. Illicit manufacturers are known to modify functional groups, substitutions frequently, and moieties to evade legal regulation [34]. Synthetic drug products may also vary in content, concentration, and chemical constituents, which add to the challenge of detection. Thus, given the lack of availability of standardized testing for designer drugs, the clinical recognition of these substances necessitates vigilance [8]. Clinicians are encouraged to directly inquire about designer drug use among young adults presenting with signs and symptoms of substance-related intoxication. Young adults are the most common demographic seeking emergency medical care for designer drug use in the United States [40]. Further, inconsistencies between observed and expected toxidrome signs and symptoms should raise suspicion of designer drug use [68].

Adverse Effects and Management

The main effects of 25I-NBOMe are visual and auditory hallucinations akin to those of compounds such as lysergic acid and psilocybin [68]. The effects of the 2C series are dose-dependent, with stimulant effects at lower doses and hallucinogenic and entactogenic effects manifesting at higher doses [23].

A wide range of psychiatric adverse effects has been reported secondary to the use of 25I-NBOMe, including delirium, paranoia, dysphoria, severe confusion, and self-harm [68]. Patients have also presented with serotonergic or sympathetic toxidromes with severe agitation, aggression, and violence. The most commonly reported adverse physiological effects are tachycardia, hypertension, and mydriasis. Hyperreflexia and clonus have also been frequently described, as well as seizures in cases that required medical attention. Severe intoxication may result in hyperthermia, pulmonary edema, and death from trauma [68].

Similar adverse effects have been found in the 'D series of phenethylamines. However, they generally have higher potency and a longer duration of effect. They are associated with more vasoconstrictive side effects which may lead to severe limb ischemia. The phenethylamines PMA, PMMA, and 4-methylthioamfetamine are the most associated with accidental deaths and higher toxicity, although there is no specific data available on deaths secondary to their use [62].

There is no specific antidote available for synthetic hallucinogens. Acute intoxication is managed with a symptom-based approach. Monitored observation is the first-line treatment of acute psychosis due to synthetic cannabinoids (SC) and 25I-NBOMe intoxication [28]. Benzodiazepines have a role in treating anxiety, agitation, and seizures [54]. Antipsychotics are used as second-line treatment for agitation, given lowered seizure threshold induced by synthetic hallucinogens [56]. Synthetic hallucinogens are not associated with severe withdrawal symptoms and do not require tapering off or replacement with a cross-tolerant drug upon abrupt cessation [67].

Synthetic Opioids

History

Among most of the synthetic opioids on the market, fentanyl has received the most attention in recent years. Fentanyl is both an analgesic and an anesthetic agent among potent opioid agonists like fentanyl, sufentanil, and alfentanil. The drug probably surfaced in the market, especially in the United States, because of side effects with existing opioid drugs like morphine [57] that can cause nausea, histamine release, bradycardia, hypertension or hypotension, and prolonged postoperative respiratory depression [39]. Around 1960, the synthesis of fentanyl brought a molecule with a higher potency among the other existing opioids, a compound that also could possess a better safety margin.

Fentanyl is among the synthetic opioid analgesics that have been used or still in use as a tranquilizer for dogs; it is also approved by the Federal Drug and Administration (FDA) to treat advanced cancer pain [1]. It can be found among compounds of several pharmaceutical formulations in the market [39]. Fentanyl is more potent than morphine (50 to 100 times). However, Dsuvia is the most potent approved opioids, and it is about ten times more potent than fentanyl [26].

Besides its clinical use, fentanyl has an illegal market value. It is also sold through illegal routes, often mixed with heroin, cocaine, or marijuana. Unlawful use of fentanyl is associated with related overdose and death in the United States [18].

Pharmacological Properties

Fentanyl selectively binds to the opioid mu-receptors in the brain by mimicking the effects of endogenous opiates. It induces a cascade of biochemical reactions by stimulating the exchange of guanosine-5′-triphosphate (GTP) for guanosine diphosphate (GDP). As a result, adenylate cyclase is inhibited, and subsequently, cAMP is decreased at intracellular level leading to a decrease in the release of substance P, gamma-aminobutyric acid (GABA), dopamine, acetylcholine, and noradrenaline. Fentanyl's metabolite is morphine. The metabolite blocks the opening of voltage-gated calcium channel, decreases Ca++ entry, and increases the outward movement of K+. The overall effect of this cascade of reaction is to hyperpolarize the cells and reduce neuronal excitability [10].

Acute and Adverse Effects

The clinical effects of fentanyl are like other opioids regardless of the route. At serum fentanyl concentrations of 0.63–1.5 ng/mL, analgesia is produced in most opioid-naïve patients [25]. At levels above 1.5 ng/mL, hypoventilation may start to manifest [25, 45]. A serum fentanyl concentration of 3.0 ng/mL may cause coma, respiratory depression, and apnea [45].

Fentanyl can cause hypotension, muscle rigidity, myoclonic movement, and localized temporal lobe electrical seizure activity [6]. As mentioned above, fentanyl overdose leads to coma and death by respiratory depression.

Detection and Screening

Fentanyl can be detected in regular urine drug screening. Other screening methods are also available such as fentanyl test strips. Studies had found that fentanyl test strips may represent a useful addition to current overdose prevention efforts when included with other evidence-based strategies to prevent opioid overdose [49].

Management

Fentanyl acute poisoning and control are not different from other opioid intoxication management. It includes support respiration with a bag-valve mask, then naloxone at 0.04 mg as an initial dose. Note that the initial pediatric dose is 0.1 mg/kg/body weight. Subsequent steps in the treatment are undertaken every 2–3 minutes based on the respiratory rate and clinical response of the intoxicated patients [7]. Up to 15 mg of naloxone can be administered.

References

1. Algren DA, Monteilh CP, Punja M, Schier JG, Belson M, Hepler BR, et al. Fentanyl-associated fatalities among illicit drug users in Wayne County, Michigan (July 2005–May 2006). J Med Toxicol. 2013;9(1):106–15.
2. Banister SD, Stuart J, Kevin RC, Edington A, Longworth M, Wilkinson SM, et al. Effects of bioisosteric fluorine in synthetic cannabinoid designer drugs JWH-018, AM-2201, UR-144, XLR-11, PB-22, 5F-PB-22, APICA, and STS-135. ACS Chem Neurosci. 2015;6(8):1445–58.
3. Baumann MH, Ayestas MA Jr, Partilla JS, Sink JR, Shulgin AT, Daley PF, et al. The designer methcathinone analogs, mephedrone and methylone, are substrates for monoamine transporters in brain tissue. Neuropsychopharmacology. 2012;37(5):1192.
4. Baumann MH, Partilla JS, Lehner KR. Psychoactive "bath salts": not so soothing. Eur J Pharmacol. 2013;698(1–3):1–5.
5. Baumann MH, Partilla JS, Lehner KR, Thorndike EB, Hoffman AF, Holy M, et al. Powerful cocaine-like actions of 3, 4-methylenedioxypyrovalerone (MDPV), a principal constituent of psychoactive 'bath salts' products. Neuropsychopharmacology. 2013;38(4):552.
6. Bowdle TA. Adverse effects of opioid agonists and agonist-antagonists in anaesthesia. Drug Saf. 1998;19(3):173–89.
7. Boyer EW. Management of opioid analgesic overdose. N Engl J Med. 2012;367(2):146–55.
8. Brewer TL, Collins M. A review of clinical manifestations in adolescent and young adults after use of synthetic cannabinoids. J Spec Pediatr Nurs. 2014;19(2):119–26.
9. Carhart-Harris RL, King LA, Nutt DJ. A web-based survey on mephedrone. Drug Alcohol Depend. 2011;118(1):19–22.
10. Chahl LA. Opioids-mechanisms of action. Aust Prescr. 1996;19(3):63–5.
11. Chimalakonda KC, Bratton SM, Le VH, Yiew KH, Dineva A, Moran CL, et al. Conjugation of synthetic cannabinoids JWH-018 and JWH-073, metabolites by human UDP-glucuronosyltransferases. Drug Metab Dispos. 2011;39(10):1967–76.
12. Collins M. Some new psychoactive substances: precursor chemicals and synthesis-driven end-products. Drug Test Anal. 2011;3(7–8):404–16.
13. Cooper ZD. Adverse effects of synthetic cannabinoids: management of acute toxicity and withdrawal. Curr Psychiatry Rep. 2016;18(5):52.
14. Crowther SM, Reynolds LA, Tansey EM. The medicalization of cannabis. London, UK: Wellcome Trust Centre for the History of Medicine; 2010. p. 4–5.
15. Dargan PI, Albert S, Wood DM. Mephedrone use and associated adverse effects in school and college/university students before the UK legislation change. QJM Int J Med. 2010;103(11):875–9.
16. Dean BV, Stellpflug SJ, Burnett AM, Engebretsen KM. 2C or not 2C: phenethylamine designer drug review. J Med Toxicol. 2013;9(2):172–8.
17. Dolengevich-Segal H, Rodríguez-Salgado B, Gómez-Arnau J, Sánchez-Mateos D. Severe psychosis, drug dependence, and hepatitis C related to slamming mephedrone. Case Rep Psychiatry. 2016;2016:8379562.
18. Drug Enforcement Administration - Department of Justice. 2015. FY 2015 Performance Budget Congressional Submission. Retrieeved from https://www.justice.gov/sites/default/files/jmd/legacy/2013/10/13/dea-justification.pdf.
19. Drug Enforcement Administration, Department of Justice. Schedules of controlled substances: temporary placement of three synthetic cathinones in Schedule I. Final Order. Federal register. 2011;76(204):65371.
20. Fantegrossi WE, Murnane KS, Reissig CJ. The behavioral pharmacology of hallucinogens. Biochem Pharmacol. 2008;75(1):17–33.
21. Fantegrossi WE, Moran JH, Radominska-Pandya A, Prather PL. Distinct pharmacology and metabolism of K2 synthetic cannabinoids compared to Δ9-THC: mechanism underlying greater toxicity? Life Sci. 2014;97(1):45–54.
22. Froberg BA, Levine M, Beuhler MC, Judge BS, Moore PW, Engebretsen KM, et al. Acute methylenedioxypyrovalerone toxicity. J Med Toxicol. 2015;11(2):185–94.
23. Garcia-Romeu A, Kersgaard B, Addy PH. Clinical applications of hallucinogens: a review. Exp Clin Psychopharmacol. 2016;24(4):229–68.
24. Gibbons, S., & Arunotayanun, W. (2013). Natural product (fungal and herbal) novel psychoactive substances. In Novel psychoactive substances. Academic Press. pp. 345–62.
25. Gourlay GK, Kowalski SR, Plummer JL, Cousins MJ, Armstrong PJ. Fentanyl blood concentration-analgesic response relationship in the treatment of postoperative pain. Anesth Analg. 1988;67(4):329–37.
26. Harrison Cook. 2018. FDA approves opioid 10 times stronger than fentanyl.Retrieved from https://www.beckershospitalreview.com/opioids/fda-approves-opioid-stronger-than-fentanyl.html.
27. Hill SL, Thomas SH. Clinical toxicology of newer recreational drugs. Clin Toxicol. 2011;49(8):705–19.
28. Hill SL, Doris T, Gurung S, Katebe S, Lomas A, Dunn M, et al. Severe clinical toxicity associated with analytically confirmed recreational use of 25I–NBOMe: case series. Clin Toxicol. 2013;51(6):487–92.
29. Holm NB, Nielsen LM, Linnet K. CYP3A4 mediates oxidative metabolism of the synthetic cannabinoid AKB-48. AAPS J. 2015;17(5):1237–45.
30. Holpuchin A. 2018. 'It's not just New Haven': mass K2 overdose symptom of national crisis. The Guardian. Retrieved from https://www.theguardian.com/society/2018/aug/17/k2-spice-synthetic-marijuana-new-haven-green-overdose.
31. Hu X, Primack BA, Barnett TE, Cook RL. College students and use of K2: an emerging drug of abuse

in young persons. Subst Abuse Treat Prevent Policy. 2011;6(1):16.
32. Iversen L, White M, Treble R. Designer psychostimulants: pharmacology and differences. Neuropharmacology. 2014;87:59–65.
33. Izaguirre A, Parascandola R, Rayman G. 2016. Thirty-three people treated in Brooklyn from possible K2 synthetic marijuana overdoses; scene compared to 'The Walking Dead'. New York daily news. Retrieved from https://www.nydailynews.com/new-york/brooklyn/multiple-people-hospitalized-k-2-overdoses-article-1.2708254.
34. Johnson LA, Johnson RL, Portier RB. Current "legal highs". J Emerg Med. 2013;44(6):1108–15.
35. Johnston LD, O'Malley PM, Bachman JG, Schulenberg JE, Miech RA. Monitoring the Future National Survey Results on Drug Use, 1975-2013. Volume 2, college students & adults ages 19–55. Institute for Social Research. 2014.
36. Khan S, Shaheen F, Sarwar H, Molina J, Mushtaq S. "Bath salts"–induced psychosis in a young woman. The primary care companion for CNS disorders. 2013;15(1).
37. Kelly, J. P. (2011). Cathinone derivatives: a review of their chemistry, pharmacology and toxicology. *Drug testing and analysis*, *3*(7-8), 439-453.\.
38. Kerrigan S, Savage M, Cavazos C, Bella P. Thermal degradation of synthetic cathinones: implications for forensic toxicology. J Anal Toxicol. 2016;40(1):1–11.
39. Kukanich B, Clark TP. The history and pharmacology of fentanyl: relevance to a novel, long-acting transdermal fentanyl solution newly approved for use in dogs. J Vet Pharmacol Ther. 2012;35:3–19.
40. Maxwell JC. Psychoactive substances—some new, some old: a scan of the situation in the US. Drug Alcohol Depend. 2014;134:71–7.
41. Mechoulam R, Feigenbaum JJ, Lander N, Segal M, Järbe TUC, Hiltunen AJ, Consroe P. Enantiomeric cannabinoids: stereospecificity of psychotropic activity. Experientia. 1988;44(9):762–4.
42. Mechoulam R, Lander N, Zahalka J. Synthesis of the individual, pharmacologically distinct, enantiomers of a tetrahydrocannabinol derivative. Tetrahedron Asymmetry. 1990;1(5):315–8.
43. Meyer RP, Gehlhaus M, Knoth R, Volk B. Expression and function of cytochrome p450 in brain drug metabolism. Curr Drug Metab. 2007;8(4):297–306.
44. Mills B, Yepes A, Nugent K. Synthetic cannabinoids. Am J Med Sci. 2015;350(1):59–62.
45. Nelson L, Schwaner R. Transdermal fentanyl: pharmacology and toxicology. J Med Toxicol. 2009;5(4):230.
46. Nichols DE, Frescas SP, Chemel BR, Rehder KS, Zhong D, Lewin AH. High specific activity tritium-labeled N-(2-methoxybenzyl)-2, 5-dimethoxy-4-iodophenethylamine (INBMeO): a high-affinity 5-HT2A receptor-selective agonist radioligand. Bioorg Med Chem. 2008;16(11):6116–23.
47. Palamar JJ, Salomone A, Vincenti M, Cleland CM. Detection of "bath salts" and other novel psychoactive substances in hair samples of ecstasy/MDMA/ "Molly" users. Drug Alcohol Depend. 2016;161:200–5.
48. Papaseit E, Pérez-Mañá C, Mateus JA, Pujadas M, Fonseca F, Torrens M, et al. Human pharmacology of mephedrone in comparison with MDMA. Neuropsychopharmacology. 2016;41(11):2704.
49. Peiper NC, Clarke SD, Vincent LB, Ciccarone D, Kral AH, Zibbell JE. Fentanyl test strips as an opioid overdose prevention strategy: findings from a syringe services program in the southeastern United States. Int J Drug Policy. 2019;63:122–8.
50. Pertwee RG. Cannabinoid pharmacology: the first 66 years. Br J Pharmacol. 2006;147(S1):S163–71.
51. Rafaeli JS. 2017. The story of Mephedrone, the party drug that boomed and went bust. Vice magazine. Retrieved from https://www.vice.com/en_us/article/9aa53a/the-story-of-mephedrone-the-party-drug-that-boomed-and-went-bust.
52. Reschly-Krasowski JM, Krasowski MD. A difficult challenge for the clinical laboratory: accessing and interpreting manufacturer cross-reactivity data for immunoassays used in urine drug testing. Acad Pathol. 2018;5:2374289518811797. https://doi.org/10.1177/2374289518811797.
53. Shulgin AT, Shulgin A. PIHKAL: a chemical love story. Berkeley: Transform Press; 1995. p. 733–9.
54. Simmons J, Cookman L, Kang C, Skinner C. Three cases of "spice" exposure. Clin Toxicol. 2011;49(5):431–3.
55. Sivagnanam K, Chaudari D, Lopez P, Sutherland ME, Ramu VK. "Bath salts" induced severe reversible cardiomyopathy. Am J Case Rep. 2013;14:288.
56. Spiller HA, Ryan ML, Weston RG, Jansen J. Clinical experience with and analytical confirmation of "bath salts" and "legal highs" (synthetic cathinones) in the United States. Clin Toxicol. 2011;49(6):499–505.
57. Stanley TH. The history and development of the fentanyl series. J Pain Symptom Manag. 1992;7(3):S3–7.
58. Su MK, Seely KA, Moran JH, Hoffman RS. Metabolism of classical cannabinoids and the synthetic cannabinoid JWH-018. Clin Pharmacol Ther. 2015;97(6):562–4.
59. Substance Abuse and Mental Health Services Administration, Center for Behavioral Health Statistics and Quality. 2011. The DAWN report: highlights of the 2011 Drug Abuse Warning Network (DAWN) Findings on Drug-Related Emergency Department Visits. Retrieved from https://www.samhsa.gov/data/sites/default/files/DAWN2k11ED/DAWN2k11ED/DAWN2k11ED.pdf.
60. Taba P, Lees AJ, Sikk K. The neuropsychiatric complications of stimulant abuse, vol. 120. Burlington: Academic Press; 2015.
61. Thornton SL, Gerona RR, Tomaszewski CA. Psychosis from a bath salt product containing flephedrone and MDPV with serum, urine, and product quantification. J Med Toxicol. 2012;8(3):310–3.

62. UN Office on Drugs and Crime. 2013. "The challenge of new psychoactive substances: a report from the Global SMART Programme" (Vienna, Austria: UNODC Laboratory and Scientific Section, March 2013), pp. 10–11. Retrieved from http://www.unodc.org/documents...
63. United Nations Office on Drugs, & Crime. 2011. 2011 World Drug Report.Retrieved from https://www.unodc.org/documents/scientific/Synthetic_Cannabinoids.pdfpdf.
64. United Nations Office on Drugs, & Crime. 2016. 2016 world drug report. United Naetions Publications. Retrieved from http://www.unodc.org/doc/wdr2016/WORLD_DRUG_REPORT_2016_web.pdf.
65. Vardakou I, Pistos C, Spiliopoulou C. Drugs for youth via internet and the example of mephedrone. Toxicol Lett. 2011;201(3):191–5.
66. Watanabe K, Itokawa Y, Yamaori S, Funahashi T, Kimura T, Kaji T, et al. Conversion of cannabidiol to Δ 9-tetrahydrocannabinol and related cannabinoids in artificial gastric juice, and their pharmacological effects in mice. Forensic Toxicol. 2007;25(1):16–21.
67. Weaver MF, Schnoll SH. Addictions: a comprehensive guidebook. In: Stimulants: amphetamines and cocaine. New York: Oxford University Press USA; 1999. p. 105–20.
68. Weaver MF, Hopper JA, Gunderson EW. Designer drugs 2015: assessment and management. Addict Sci Clin Pract. 2015;10(1):8.
69. Weaver M, Schnoll S. Hallucinogens and club drugs. In: The American Psychiatric Publishing textbook of substance abuse treatment. 4th ed. Washington, D.C.: American Psychiatric Publishing Inc; 2008. p. 191–200.
70. Winstock A, Mitcheson L, Ramsey J, Davies S, Puchnarewicz M, Marsden J. Mephedrone: use, subjective effects and health risks. Addiction. 2011;106(11):1991–6.
71. Zaami S, Giorgetti R, Pichini S, Pantano F, Marinelli E, Busardo FP. Synthetic cathinones related fatalities: an update. Eur Rev Med Pharmacol Sci. 2018;22(1):268–74.
72. Zawilska JB, Wojcieszak J. Designer cathinones—an emerging class of novel recreational drugs. Forensic Sci Int. 2013;231(1–3):42–53.

Prescription Drugs

17

Diego Garces Grosse

Introduction

Since prescription drugs can be legally obtained and are almost universally present in households, it is undeniable that the perception of their consumption is not nearly as negative as the perception of illicit drug consumption; hence, it's not uncommon that their misuse or abuse are many times overlooked [3].

Truth is, controlled medications can develop in some individuals addictive patterns equal to those of illicit drugs. This results in patients using medication differently than prescribed: using higher doses, at shorter periods, or seeking more prescriptions from different providers.

Patients who develop a misuse of prescription drugs are at higher risk to fall into illicit substance use. This is because when patients start using more medication than prescribed, it's not uncommon that they fall short of medication and will likely look out for more prescriptions. When unable to get prescriptions, patients may recur to illicit drugs and black markets in order to satisfy their cravings or keep withdrawals away.

Prescription drug abuse is a growing public health concern [3] that has been rising since the 1990s and has seen exponential growth in the past years—being now considered in epidemic levels among the United States. This growth has been noted in public health markers over the years with rising numbers from incidence and prevalence to mortality rates, having a peak in prevalence between the years 2015 and 2016 [2]. The fact that prescription drug abuse increase was noted in the three common categories (pain relievers, tranquilizers, and stimulants) resulted in efforts to control the overprescription of these types of medications and to fight the misuse of prescription drugs. These efforts to decrease the burden of prescription drug abuse have proven to be successful as can be seen in the National Survey on Drug Use and Health (NSDUH) 2018, which shows the overall decrease of prevalence in prescription drug abuse in all categories except in "tranquilizers" category. The said category showed the overall decrease of use and prescription from 2017 to 2018 but a slight increase in the abuse.

Terminology

The term prescription drug abuse, also called prescription drug misuse, encompasses a range of nonmedical patterns of prescription drug use, including, but not limited to, using a prescribed medication at higher doses or greater frequencies than prescribed or using them without a legitimate prescription. Prescription drug abuse is not a diagnosis decribed in the Fifth Edition of the Diagnostic

D. Garces Grosse (✉)
Rutgers New Jersey Medical School, Newark, NJ, USA
e-mail: dg858@njms.rutgers.edu

E. Akerele (ed.), *Substance and Non-Substance Related Addictions*,
https://doi.org/10.1007/978-3-030-84834-7_17

and Statistical Manual of Mental Disorders (DSM-5)[1]; hence, there are no criteria given to diagnose this problematic use of prescription drugs. However, since the abuse or misuse of prescription drugs usually goes along with several of the criteria for substance use disorder, prescription drug abuse can fall into different subtypes of use disorders as described in the DSM-5.

On the other hand, the National Survey on Drug Use and Health (NSDUH) 2018 [2] by the Substance Abuse and Mental Health Services Administration (SAHMSA) has a wide category referred to as "prescription psychotherapeutics" which englobes five sub-categories which are pain relivers, stimulants, tranquilizers, sedatives, and benzodiazepines. The latter three subcategories are also presented as one group, as well as independently in the NSDUH epidemiologic results.

The pain reliver subcategory encompasses several different prescription drugs, all of which are opiates, so it is safe to say that in the specific case of prescription drugs, opiates and pain relievers can be used indistinctly.

The DSM-5 presents a category which englobes sedative, hypnotic, or anxiolytic use disorders as CNS depressants. The equivalent of this category in the NSDUH would be the combination of tranquilizers, sedatives, and benzodiazepines.

Finally, the category containing stimulants is similar in both DSM-5 and NSDUH; however, the DSM-5 does not make any difference between prescribed and Illicit stimulants, whereas the NSDUH accounts for prescribed and illicit stimulants separately.

Epidemiology

The prevalence of prescription drug abuse has increased since the 1990s to a peak in 2015–2016. Aggressive efforts to counter the development of prescription drug abuse resulted in an overall decrease in prescription drug abuse reflected in the results of NSDUH in the years 2017 [13] and 2018 [2].

Grossly, the NSDUH reported that in the year 2018, 7.8% of the US population above 18 years old had a substance use disorder accounting for 19.3 million of people aged 18 or over, whereas 19.1% of the population aged 18 or over had mental illness, accounting for 47.6 million people. There is an important overlap between these two public health issues which was reported as 3.7% of the population aged 18 and older (9.2 million) as having both a substance use disorder and a mental illness.

As said before, the NSDUH showed a significant decrease in prescription drug abuse from previous years, resulting in 6.2% of the population aged 12 and older (16.9 million) as compared to 2017's 6.6% (18.1 million). The NSDUH reported that over the year 2018, 40.6% of Americans 12 years and older had any use of prescription psychotherapeutic drugs, from whose 15.2% reported nonmedical uses or misuse.

Misuse of prescription drugs is highest among young adults ages 18–25, with 12.3% reporting nonmedical use in the past year, and lowest in the ages 12–17 with 4.8% reporting past year nonmedical use of prescription medications.

It is alarming that when asked how they obtained prescription drugs for nonmedical use, greater rates responded that they got them from friends and family rather than a healthcare provider. For opioids 51.3% reported getting them from friends or family, whereas 37.6% received prescriptions from a healthcare provider. Numbers are more alarming for stimulants, whose 79.1% of users reported getting them from friends or family, while only 12.8% obtained prescriptions. The rates for tranquilizers and sedatives are not far away from that with 66.8% and 61.4% of users reporting getting them from friends or family while 20.2% and 32.5% obtaining formal prescriptions.

Within the realm of prescription drug abuse, pain medication is the one that accounts for the bigger part, which in the latest years has raised alarms due to the "opioid crisis" in the country. The numbers accounting for pain medication abuse and misuse have also shown improvement for the past few years with a decrease from 12.5 million cases of prescription pain medication misuse in 2015 to 9.9 million cases in 2018. The incidence of pain medication misuse has also decreased from 2.1 million cases per year in 2015 to 1.9 million cases per year in 2018. These decreases in both incidence and prevalence have been reflected for all age groups.

The 12-month prevalence of prescription opioid abuse disorder is approximately 3.6% among people age 12 years and older. The prevalence for people 12–17 years old is 2.8%, and the prevalence in people aged 18 years and older is 3.7%. The age group with higher prevalence is people 18–25 years old with 5.5%, and there is a decrease in prevalence with greater age, being 3.4% for the age group 26 years and older. The rate of prescription opioid abuse is higher in males than in females (3.9% vs 3.4%). Prevalence is highest in Native Americans with 5.7%, followed by non-Hispanic White with 4.4%, Hispanic with 4.0%, and African Americans with 3.5%.

The 12-month prevalence of CNS depressants is estimated to be 1.8% among 12–17-year-olds and 2.4% among adults age 18 years and older, with a prevalence for people older than 12 years of 1.9%. Rates of CNS depressant abuse are greater among adult males (2.2%) than among adult females (1.7%). The rate is greatest for the age group from 18–25 years with 6.5%, and then it decreases after 26 years with a prevalence of 1.2%. The 12-month prevalence of sedative, hypnotic, or anxiolytic use disorder varies across racial/ethnic subgroups of the US population. Prevalence is greatest among White non-Hispanics with 2.9%, followed by Hispanics with 2.2%, Native American with 1.7%, and Pacific Islanders with 1.6%, while African Americans have a rate of 1.3%.

The estimated 12-month prevalence of prescription stimulant abuse in the United States is 1.5% among 12–17-year-olds and 1.9% among individuals 18 years and older, with a global prevalence of people 12 years and older of 1.9%. Rates are considerably higher in males (2.1%) than females (1.6%) for all age groups and especially noticeable in age group 18–25 years old with rates of male and female being 6.8% and 6.2%. For ethnic groups, White non-Hispanics have the highest prevalence with 2.2%, followed by Asians with 1.6% and Hispanic with 1.4%. The prevalence of prescription stimulant abuse increases with higher education levels as seen in rates of people who did not complete high school of 0.7%, finished high school 1.4%, some college 2.9%, and then decreases for college graduates with 2.2%.

Prescription Opioid Abuse

Prescription opioid abuse refers to the use of opioid substances that are used for no legitimate medical purpose or, in the presence of a medical condition that requires opioid treatment, greatly in excess of the amount needed for that medical condition. For example, an individual prescribed with opioid analgesics for pain using higher doses than required to control pain. People who develop prescription opioid abuse usually start with prescriptions for valid medical uses, most commonly pain control [3]. Patients who develop prescription opioid abuse tend to exaggerate symptoms to obtain prescriptions or seek prescriptions from several physicians. Healthcare professionals who abuse prescription opioids can often obtain them by prescribing for themselves or by diverting pharmacy supplies. Prescription opioid abuse can begin at any age, but problems associated with opioid use are most commonly first observed in the late teens or early 20s as seen in the NSDUH results [2]. It has also been noted that receiving prescription for opioids during adolescence increases the risk of future opioid misuse. Once opioid use disorder develops, it usually continues over a period of many years, even though brief periods of abstinence are frequent. In treated populations, relapse following abstinence is common [1].

Complications following prescription opioid abuse are not uncommon. Given that the use of opioids is associated with decreased mucous membrane secretions, it can cause dry nose and mouth. The slowing of GI tract motility may lead to constipation. Opioids can also cause decreased visual acuity due to pupillary constriction. Sexual functioning can also be affected; males often experience erectile dysfunction during intoxication or chronic use, while females may have disturbances of reproductive function and irregular menses. Infants born to mothers with opioid use disorder can have low birth weights which do not generally carry consequences, and they may also experience withdrawal syndrome, requiring medical treatment [1, 5].

Prescription CNS Depressants Abuse

This class of substances includes all prescription sleeping medications and almost all prescription antianxiety medications. Non-benzodiazepine antianxiety agents, like buspirone, are not included in this section because they have not been associated with significant misuse.

CNS depressant abuse usually starts at younger ages as shown in the NSDUH, and almost 80% of people abusing these types of substances obtain them from friends or family. While some people who get this category of drugs for medical purposes develop a use disorder, some who misuse them will not develop a use disorder. Most commonly, substances with shorter half-lives or faster onset of action are used for intoxication purposes, although longer-acting dugs may also be used.

The frequent use of CNS depressants can lead to significant levels of tolerance and withdrawals. Withdrawals and tolerance can also be seen in individuals without a use disorder, but who have used these drugs for long periods at prescribed and therapeutic doses and stop abruptly. In such cases, additional criteria are required to diagnose a substance use disorder, and it is necessary to determine if the drugs are being appropriately prescribed and used.

The usual pattern of CNS depressants abuse starts with individuals in their teens or 20s, who escalate their occasional use of the drug to the point that they meet criteria for diagnosis of substance use disorder. This pattern is more likely in individuals with other substance use disorders, who may use CNS depressants to overcome side effects from other substances such as stimulants or to decrease withdrawal symptoms or increase "the high" when using opioids or alcohol. Earlier onset of use has been associated with higher risk for developing use disorders.

The less frequently observed pattern starts with an individual who is prescribed the medication, most commonly for the treatment of anxiety or insomnia. Because the use of some of these medications can result in the rapid development of tolerance, a gradual increase of dose and frequency of administration is commonly seen. Patients will likely justify this increase based on original symptoms; however, drug-seeking behaviors become more prominent. Some patients will exaggerate symptoms; some may even recur to multiple physicians to obtain more prescriptions [1, 3, 4]. Given that these patients can develop high levels of tolerance and need higher doses, withdrawals, including seizures, could occur if not appropriately tapered down.

Acute intoxication with CNS depressants often results in disinhibition, like with alcohol, which can cause interpersonal difficulties in different instances of the individual's life, sometimes resulting in aggression. Cognitive impairment is very common during acute intoxication as well, which often results in interference in educational and professional performance. Because of impairment in motor coordination during intoxication, automobile accidents are a serious and common outcome [1, 3]. Physical examination often reveals a decrease in most aspects of autonomic nervous system functioning, which is evidenced by decreased heart and respiratory rates as well as decreased blood pressure.

Effects in memory, cognition, and motor coordination tend to increase as the individual ages because of pharmacodynamic and pharmacokinetic age-related changes. Also, individuals with dementia are more likely to develop intoxication at lower doses. In other cases, chronic intoxication could resemble a progressive dementia. In elderly individuals, the use of any sedative medication can increase the risk for falls.

Chronic intoxication or repeated use, especially at high doses, can result in substance-induced mood disorders that can resemble a severe depression, although temporary, that could even lead to suicide attempts or completed suicide.

Most of the drugs in the category of CNS depressants can be identified qualitatively in urine and quantitatively in blood tests. Longer-acting substance such as diazepam or flurazepam usually remain positive in urine for up to 1 week [1].

Prescription Stimulant Abuse

This category includes the different types of substances which can be divided into amphetamine or amphetamine-type and stimulants that are structurally different but have similar effects. Stimulants are usually prescribed for ADHD, obesity, and narcolepsy. The common medications prescribed are either methylphenidate or amphetamine salts. The NSDUH 2018 reported that 79.1% users of prescription stimulants obtain them through friends or family. People who abuse these drugs without a prescription usually start using them for weight control or for improvement in school, work, or athletics, and because of this, prescribed stimulants are easily diverted into the illegal market [2].

Intoxication usually results in individuals feeling a "rush" or euphoria, and they may present with rambling speech. At higher doses ideas of reference and paranoia might be present as well as aggressive behavior and auditory or most commonly, tactile hallucinations. Other effects on the body are notable for increased heart rate and blood pressure and dilation of airways. Decreased appetite is also usually present, the reason for which individuals may misuse stimulants for weight loss. Overdoses can also happen with prescription stimulants which may result in several different presentations ranging from restlessness, tremors, overactive reflexes, confusion to arrhythmias, heart attack, seizures, or coma [16].

Stimulant abuse can develop in as short as 1 week in individuals who use amphetamine-type stimulants, although the onset is not always this rapid. Repeated use will result in the development of tolerance and decrease of pleasurable effects and the risk of withdrawals, which include hypersomnia, increased appetite, and dysphoria. Withdrawal symptoms can cause and enhance cravings. Withdrawal states can also be associated with depressive episodes which can be intense and can resemble a major depressive disorder. These depressive states usually resolve within 1 week. Suicidal ideations or behavior can occur during these depressive episodes [1]. Withdrawals present with physiological changes which are opposite to those of intoxication, with increased appetite and somnolence, and can even present with bradycardia.

Differences with Nonprescription Drug Abuse

Several differences can be noted in the patterns of use and misuse of prescription and illicit drugs, being the most notorious the legal availability of the former. Because of their legality, the perception of prescription drugs is more benign, despite having the same potential for abuse.

There have also been reported differences in the use of prescription versus illicit drugs of the same class. For example, cravings appear to be milder in patients who abuse prescription opioids as compared to heroin users. Because of this, it is suspected that response to treatment might be different between those groups. A study by Stein et al. found that heroin and prescription opioid users report different concerns. For example, heroin users express more concern of infectious diseases, whereas prescription opioid users tend to report more concern about alcohol use [17].

Johnston et al. found that college students are more likely to use prescription stimulants as compared to college-age young adults not enrolled in higher education, which is not consistent with other stimulants such as cocaine [18]. This trend is consistent with the prevalence of prescription stimulants use in the NSDUH 2018 results.

Comorbidity

Multiple studies have shown association between prescription drug misuse and problematic use of other substances such as tobacco, alcohol, and illicit drugs among the US population in all age groups [1–3]. Other substances are often taken to reduce withdrawal symptoms or to enhance the effects of the drug of choice [3].

Opioid users are at greater risk to develop mild to moderate depression to the point of meeting criteria for major depressive disorder, which can be an opioid-induced mood disorder or an exacerbation of a primary depressive disorder [1, 4]. Periods of depression are common during chronic intoxication.

Commonly, the nonmedical use of CNS depressants is associated with alcohol use disorder, tobacco use disorder, and/or illicit drug use. There appears to be an overlap between CNS depressants use and antisocial personality disorder, depressive, bipolar, and anxiety disorders.

Stimulant abuse is also often associated with other substance use disorders, especially those involving substances with sedative properties, which are often taken to reduce insomnia, nervousness, and other unpleasant side effects. Stimulant use disorder may be associated with posttraumatic stress disorder, antisocial personality disorder, attention-deficit/hyperactivity disorder, and gambling disorder. The use of stimulants is associated with decreased appetite and weight loss, sometimes, to the point of malnutrition.

Treatment

Research has consistently shown that substance use disorders can be treated effectively. For treatment to be effective, it must consider the type of drug being abused along with the patient's needs [13]. To achieve this, treatment can be designed using different strategies, which include detoxification, counseling, and medications. Withdrawals of abused drugs must also be taken in consideration because of their risk of increased morbidity and mortality. Most individuals will require more than one course of treatment before achieving full recovery.

There are two main categories of treatment for substance use disorder; these being behavioral treatments and medication [11]. Common behavioral treatments are cognitive behavior therapy, as well as individual, family, or group therapy. Behavioral treatments help patients to change unhealthy patterns of behavior and thought as well as teach them coping mechanisms and strategies to manage cravings.

Addiction to prescription opiates can be treated with medications which include buprenorphine, methadone, and naltrexone. These drugs can prevent or relieve withdrawal symptoms and cravings (methadone and buprenorphine) or prevent other opioids from affecting the brain (naltrexone), both of which will result in decreasing relapses. Withdrawal from opioids can also be treated with non-opioid medications such as clonidine or lofexidine and adjuvants for symptom management. Medications for opioid use are often administered in combination with behavioral treatments [13].

The treatment for CNS depressants, such as tranquilizers, sedatives, and hypnotics, should start with medically supervised detoxification with down-taper since withdrawals from this type of drugs can be severe and potentially life-threatening [13, 14]. The process of supervised detoxification is usually done in an inpatient basis, whereas counseling can be followed as inpatient or outpatient. There is currently no medical treatment for CNS depressants abuse; however, cognitive behavioral therapy has shown success in treatment by modifying the patient's thinking, expectations, and behaviors while increasing coping skills with life stressors.

The treatment for prescription stimulants abuse is based on behavioral therapies that are effective for treating cocaine and methamphetamine addiction following detoxification via drug tapering and withdrawal prevention and management [11]. There are currently no FDA-approved medications for the treatment of stimulant use disorders. The National Institute for

Drug Abuse (NIDA) is supporting research on this topic [13]. Contingency management has been also used for prescription stimulant abuse, which consists of motivational incentives such as providing vouchers or small cash rewards for positive behaviors such as staying drug free [16].

Oftentimes misuse of prescription drugs occurs along with use of other substances such as alcohol, tobacco, or opioids. In such cases, the treatment approach should address the multiple addictions [13].

Risk Factors

Like with other substance use disorders, the risk for prescription drug abuse is increased for individuals who present already any other type of substance use disorder [2, 3]. The lack of knowledge about the prescriptions and their potential for abuse has also been identified as a risk factor [3, 8]. Genetic factors and family history of substance abuse have also been identified as risk factors [1]. Impulsivity and novelty seeking have been associated with an increased risk for prescription drug abuse, although these may also be genetically predisposed.

Co-occurrent mental illness is also a significant risk factor, as seen in the 2018 NSDUH, where they reported that out of the 7.6% of the population over 18 years of age with substance use disorders, near half (3.4% of that population) presented with both mental illness and substance use disorders [2].

Environments with easy access to prescription drugs and peer pressure play an important role especially in teenagers and young adults who obtain prescription drugs from friends or family in the greater part [2]. Easy access at home, such as unlocked cabinets, might result in the risk for the preservation of prescription drug abuse.

It is also important to acknowledge the impact of overprescription as a risk factor, especially related to prescription opioids for pain management in the past few years, which is now decreasing due to tremendous efforts by governments to control the opiates crisis [2].

Prevention

Efforts to decrease prescription drug abuse have proved worthy with a reduction in prevalence from 6.8% Americans in 2017 to 6.2% in 2018. Prevention is a crucial step to decrease the burden of prescription drug abuse, and it can be approached by both physicians and patients.

Physicians should always ask about drugs and help patients to identify any potential misuse. Also, when prescribing medications, physicians should inform patients about the abuse potential and try to keep the treatment as short as possible in order to reduce the risk of tolerance along with planning a tap-down protocol in order to avoid patients going into withdrawals, which is commonly why people start seeking medications elsewhere. Prescribers should take note of any rapid increase in amount of medication needed and of any unscheduled refill requests.

Prescription drug medication programs (PDMPs) are electronic databases to which providers can access to track prescription and dispensing of prescription drugs. These programs can be used to prevent and identify prescription drug abuse by checking frequency of refills as well as the number of different prescribers. The use of PDMPs has been associated in some states with lower rates of opioid prescribing and overdose [7].

Other measures that can be considered by physicians are the use of informed consent forms, treatment agreements, risk documentation tools, and guided management based on treatment goals [9, 10, 14]. By using universal precautions, and being aware of aberrant behaviors, physicians may feel more confident in identifying and addressing problematic behaviors.

When dealing with prescription opioids for pain management, the prescriber should monitor the "four As" which are analgesia, activities of daily living, adverse reactions, and aberrant behaviors [9, 10]. Aberrant behaviors usually include refusal to do random urine tests, like selling their medication or buying from nonmedical sources, complaining of multiple episodes of "lost" or "stolen" scripts, recurring to multiple physicians and pharmacies, and nonadherence to other recommendations.

Not only prescribers are responsible for preventing prescription drug abuse, but patients, as users of the medication, should also be counseled to identify aberrant patterns of use and to inform their doctor if they notice any concerning behavior or pattern [3]. To ensure this, patients should be advised to only take medications as prescribed and to be aware of the potential risk of abuse. Patients should be advised to keep track of their treatments and to make sure that they are taking the correct medication at the correct dosage and frequency.

Appropriate disposal should also be advised, so to prevent making unused drugs available to third parties. Appropriate storage and away from children's reach should also be advised. Patients should also be advised not to save any unused medication and to avoid using someone else's medication and to avoid sharing their prescribed medications with others [14].

References

1. American Psychiatric Association. Substance-related and addictive disorders. In: Diagnostic and statistical manual of mental disorders. 5th ed. Arlington: American Psychiatric Publishing; 2013.
2. Substance Abuse and Mental Health Services Administration Results from the 2018 national survey on drug use and health: detailed tables. Retrieved from https://www.samhsa.gov/data/report/2018-nsduh-detailed-tables.
3. McHugh RK, Nielsen S, Weiss RD. Prescription drug abuse: from epidemiology to public policy. J Subst Abus Treat. 2015;48(1):1–7. https://doi.org/10.1016/j.jsat.2014.08.004.
4. Votaw VR, Geyer R, Rieselbach MM, McHugh RK. The epidemiology of benzodiazepine misuse: a systematic review. Drug Alcohol Depend. 2019;200:95–114. https://doi.org/10.1016/j.drugalcdep.2019.02.033. Epub 2019 May 7. PMID: 31121495
5. Monheit B, Pietrzak D, Hocking S. Prescription drug abuse—a timely update. Aust Fam Physician. 2016;45:862–6.
7. Pardo B. Do more robust prescription drug monitoring programs reduce prescription opioid overdose? Addiction. 2017;112:1773–83.
8. Brady KT, McCauley JL, Back SE. Prescription opioid misuse, abuse, and treatment in the United States: an update. Am J Psychiatry. 2016;173:18–26.
9. Antman KH, Berman HA, Flotte TR, Flier J, Dimitri DM, Bharel M. Developing core competencies for the prevention and management of prescription drug misuse: a medical education collaboration in Massachusetts. Acad Med. 2016;91:1348–51.
10. Manubay J, Muchow C, Sullivan M. Prescription drug abuse: epidemiology, regulatory issues, chronic pain management with narcotic analgesics. Prim Care. 2011;38:71–90.
11. Jones JD, Mogali S, Comer SD. Polydrug abuse: a review of opioid and benzodiazepine combination use. Drug Alcohol Depend. 2012;125(1–2):8–18. https://doi.org/10.1016/j.drugalcdep.2012.07.004.
13. National Institute on Drug Abuse. Principles of drug addiction treatment: a research-based guide. 3rd ed. Rockville: National Institute on Drug Abuse, National Institutes of Health; 2018.
14. National Institute on Drug Abuse. Misuse of prescription drugs. 2018. https://www.drugabuse.gov/publications/misuse-prescription-drugs/overview.
15. NIDA. Trends & statistics. 24 Apr 2017. Retrieved from https://www.drugabuse.gov/related-topics/trends-statistics on 20 Sept 2019.
16. National Institute on Drug Abuse. Prescription stimulants. 2018. https://www.drugabuse.gov/publications/drugfacts/prescription-stimulants.
17. Stein M, et al. Comparing the life concerns of prescription opioid and heroin users. J Subst Abus Treat. 2015;48(1):43–8.
18. Johnston LD, O'Malley PM, Backman JG, Schulenberg JE. Monitoring the future national survey results on drug use, 1975–2012: volume 2, college students and adults ages 19–50. Ann Arbor: Institute for Social Research, The University of Michigan; 2013.

Part V

Special Issues in Substance Use

18 Drug Policy

Olaniyi Olayinka

Introduction

Illicit drug use constitutes a major public health concern given its significant negative impact on users, families, and society. Illicit drugs are substances that have addictive potential and generally regarded by the international community as having no medical use [1]. Globally, approximately 1 in 20 people aged 15–64 years reported using at least 1 illicit drug in 2016 [2]. Morbidity and mortality related to drugs are a global health burden with over 167,000 drug-related deaths reported in 2015. Globally, opioids are implicated in over 70% of drug-related deaths and as such have been one of the main targets of international and national drug policies [1]. The illegal production, distribution, and use of cannabis, opioids, cocaine, and amphetamine-type stimulants continue to dominate the global drug market, with sociopolitical and public health ramifications [1, 3]. Hence, it is crucial to develop effective, evidence-based policies targeted to major illicit drugs.

While various drug policies exist, most are based on political ideologies, beliefs, and national priority rather than evidence-based practice. For example, the professional background and political affiliation of policy makers may influence to what extent punitive international drug laws are enforced in a country [4–6]. Over the years, a range of national drug policies have emerged ranging from draconian to liberal. In addition to policies that criminalize the production, distribution, and use of illicit drugs, recent policies attempt to (1) prevent the initiation of drug use, (2) reduce drug use and its ill effects by improving access to harm reduction programs as well as mental health services and substance use treatment programs, and (3) create effective drug law enforcement strategies (e.g., establishing drug courts and monitoring system for prescribers of controlled substances).

International Drug Control

Establishing a balanced, global drug policy is a herculean task, given the varied national, political, and economic interests of governments as well as nongovernmental institutions. The stakes are high, however, if individuals, families, communities, and society are not protected from the scourge of illicit drugs. Since its formation in 1945, countries have turned to the United Nations (UN) (through the Economic and Social Council [ECOSOC], a main UN organization) to coordinate global efforts targeted to mitigate the local and transnational effects of drugs. Subsequently, international drug policies have been consolidated

O. Olayinka (✉)
Department of Psychiatry and Behavioral Sciences, Interfaith Medical Center, Brooklyn, NY, USA

E. Akerele (ed.), *Substance and Non-Substance Related Addictions*,
https://doi.org/10.1007/978-3-030-84834-7_18

into three UN treaties, namely, the Single Convention on Narcotic Drugs of 1961 as amended by the 1972 Protocol, the Convention on Psychotropic Substances of 1971, and the United Nations Convention Against Illicit Traffic in Narcotic Drugs and Psychotropic Substances of 1988 [7].

The Commission on Narcotic Drugs was established by ECOSOC in 1946 to supervise and advise on all matters related to global drug control in the context of the international treaties. Membership of the Commission is globally representative with each ECOSOC-elected member serving a 4-year term (11 members each representing Africa and Asia, 10 from Latin America and the Caribbean, 6 from Eastern Europe, and 14 members from the remaining member states).

The Commission, with the World Health Organization (WHO) and the International Narcotics Control Board (INCB), work to place psychotropic drugs or precursor substances under international control. For example, the Commission recently agreed with the WHO's recommendation to place carfentanil, a synthetic opioid far more potent than fentanyl, in Schedules I and IV of the 1961/1971 conventions. Additionally, the Commission governs the United Nations Office on Drugs and Crime by approving and financing its budget and field operations related to global drug control. Overall, the success of international drug control depends on the collective effort of governments to implement and enforce control measures.

Single Convention on Narcotic Drugs of 1961 as Amended by the 1972 Protocol

In 1961, the first international convention on drugs was birthed, namely, the Single Convention on Narcotic Drugs of 1961, which was later amended and jointly adopted by over 90 United Nations member states representing all geographic regions of the world. In 1972, amendments were made to the 1961 Convention which included emphasis on a "coordinated and universal" approach to drug control (Resolution II) and a reminder of the bidirectional, causal relationship between drug-related behaviors of individuals and their social environment (Resolution III). The increased risk of drug abuse in socially disadvantaged populations is well-recognized and continues to be recommended to public health decision-makers for incorporation into current drug policies at all levels [8, 9].

Convention on Psychotropic Substances of 1971

As newer mind-altering drugs (other than cannabis, cocaine, and opioids) emerged, and their abuse potential became apparent, the international community would develop a protocol for controlling psychotropic drugs that is broad in scope. The Convention on Psychotropic Substances of 1971 was the product of this effort. The evidence base for adjudging a substance as requiring international control falls within the purview of the WHO as mandated under the Conventions. Specifically, the WHO conducts a comprehensive evaluation of narcotic and psychotropic substances to determine which of the Convention's drug schedules to place them. The WHO's recommendation is then forwarded to the UN Commission on Narcotic Drugs (CND) that decides, in a final and administrative step, whether to schedule a drug [10]. As of the time of writing of this chapter, 184 Parties have adopted the provisions of the 1971 Convention on Psychotropic Substances including Afghanistan, China, Colombia, Ethiopia, Netherlands, Mexico, and the United States among others [11].

Aspects of the 1971 drug treaty that are worth mentioning include Article 5 and Articles 20–22 [7]. The Convention is categorical about Parties limiting the use of Schedule I drugs—including cocaine, cannabis, heroin, fentanyl, and methadone—to "medical and scientific purposes" (Article 5). Articles 20–22 mandate Parties to seek legal recourse against drug abusers and traffickers, which may include serving jail/prison time. Some public health experts and policy makers argue that this tough legal stance—the so-called "war on drugs" strategy—lacks evidence base in reducing drug trafficking and abuse [12, 13]. In fact, there are studies suggesting that illicit drug markets/traffickers are able to adapt to strict regulations, helping them to thrive in the long run [14].

The legalization of the recreational use of cannabis a Schedule I substance is one that has drawn attention locally and globally. Despite being the subject of contentious debate, two Parties to the 1971 Convention, namely, Uruguay (2013) and Canada (2018), have legalized the cultivation, sales, possession, and use of cannabis at the national level [15]. Uruguay's decision to legalize cannabis in 2013, reportedly, was motivated by its president's aim to reduce the negative health and social effects of drugs [16]. While legalizing cannabis may benefit local and national economies (e.g., a source of tax revenue), reduce drug-related crimes, and prevent unnecessary criminalization of drug addicts, evidence regarding the physical and mental health benefits of cannabis use remains equivocal. There is evidence of negative effects of cannabis use (either from acute intoxication or chronic use) on the health of individuals [17, 18]. These include impairment of motor and cognitive functioning as well as an increased risk of psychotic illness following early cannabis exposure [17, 18]. Accidental childhood exposure has also been cited as a major public health concern by those who oppose the legalization of marijuana [18]. Of note, he 2018 Cannabis Act of Canada shares similar sentiments as that of Uruguay's which includes diverting the profit from cannabis sales from criminals to other legal outlets [13]. Canada also has clear statements on its goal to prevent youths from accessing cannabis and ensure the public's safety by reforming its impaired driving laws [19].

United Nations Convention Against Illicit Traffic in Narcotic Drugs and Psychotropic Substances of 1988

Drug trafficking is a multibillion-dollar trade and a major target of national and transnational policies. The 1988 Convention aimed to address upstream issues related to the production, distribution, and trade of controlled substances by organized criminal entities. Under this Convention, proceeds from drug trafficking are subject to seizure, and individuals behind illicit drug trade can be extradited among countries. The spillover effect of the 1988 Convention is the criminalization of drug possession, an ineffective drug control strategy that has done little to stem the ever-increasing rate of drug abuse in society.

International Schedules of Narcotic Drugs

The goal of the Schedules is to limit the generation, trade, distribution, and use of substances with abuse potentials to medical and scientific uses. Since the harmful and abuse potentials of each narcotic drug and psychotropic substance vary (e.g., morphine is more potent and addictive than codeine due to its greater mu receptor binding), the degree of control of these substances would also vary, but not in a chronological order (e.g., very strict control of Schedules I and IV drugs, compared with Schedules II and III, is advised under the 1961/1971 Conventions). Popular naturally occurring and synthetic drugs that have been scheduled include cannabis/cannabis resin, coca leaf, cocaine, hydromorphone, methadone, morphine, and opium (Schedule I); codeine (Schedule II), preparations of codeine and buprenorphine (Schedule III, which have the least strict control); and cannabis/cannabis resin (Schedule IV). Interestingly, few substances are placed in two different Schedules. Cannabis/cannabis resin is an example. Being placed in Schedule IV reflects the notion that cannabis and cannabis resin have a high risk of addiction and with negative public health effects that outweigh their therapeutic benefits [20]. Of note, the recreational use of cannabis has been legalized in Uruguay (the first country to do so in 2013), ten states, and the District of Columbia in the United States (California being the first state in 1996), and more recently Canada (2018).

Adopting the recommendation of the international drug control treaties has its merit. For example, nations without the resources to develop drug policies from ground up have something to work with. Additionally, operating under common drug control treaties provide an opportunity for countries that serve as major transit routes for drugs (e.g., heroin and cocaine) to effectively coordinate effort to combat global drug epidemics. This is particularly important with respect to the opioid epidemic where an intricate global network of production and distribution of heroin contributes to opioid-related overdose and deaths worldwide. The role prescription pattern of opioids plays in recent opioid epidemics in countries like the United States and Canada has also been well-documented. That is why public health strategies designed to monitor the prescription pattern of certain medications and offer treatment for persons with substance use, among other programs, are considered a critical piece of national drug policies [21, 22].

Although the international drug scheduling system is widely referenced globally, slight variations exist in some countries. The US Drug Enforcement Administration classifies drugs, substances, and precursor chemicals into five categories, based on their abuse potentials. Drugs considered to have the highest abuse potential are placed in Schedule I, while those with the least abuse potential are placed in Schedule V. Unlike the international system, cocaine is a Schedule II drug under the US drug scheduling scheme. The United Kingdom runs a drug scheduling system that is somewhat similar to that of the United States.

Overall, the goal of and basis for creating various drug control strategies remain fairly the same globally. These include limiting the use of addictive substances to medical and scientific uses while offering avenues to rehabilitate individuals who have a substance use disorder.

Conclusion

International drug policies appear to play a critical role in controlling global drug trafficking. However, challenges remain as unlawful drug trade continue to thrive, as they become more organized and sophisticated in their adaptation to national and international drug policies. Additionally, the current pandemic of opioid-related overdose and deaths have added to the global burden of illicit drug use. Despite the aforementioned, the fight against illicit drugs (and prescription drugs misuse) can only be won by the collaborative effort of the international community.

References

1. Degenhardt L, Hall W. Extent of illicit drug use and dependence, and their contribution to the global burden of disease. Lancet. 2012;379(9810):55–70.
2. United Nations Office on Drugs and Crime. World Drug Report 2018. 2018. Available from: https://www.unodc.org/wdr2018/prelaunch/WDR18_Booklet_1_EXSUM.pdf.
3. Crowley R, Kirschner N, Dunn AS, Bornstein SS. Health and public policy to facilitate effective prevention and treatment of substance use disorders involving illicit and prescription drugs: an American College of Physicians position paper. Ann Intern Med. 2017;166(10):733–6.
4. Ammerman S, Ryan S, Adelman WP, Abuse CS. The impact of marijuana policies on youth: clinical, research, and legal update. Pediatrics. 2015;peds:2014–4147.
5. MacGregor S, Singleton N, Trautmann F. Towards good governance in drug policy: evidence, stakeholders and politics. Int J Drug Policy. 2014;25(5):931–4.
6. Sweileh WM, Zyoud SH, Al-Jabi SW, Sawalha AF. Substance use disorders in Arab countries: research activity and bibliometric analysis. Subst Abuse Treat Prev Policy. 2014;9:33.
7. United Nations. The international drug control conventions. Vienna 2013. Available from: http://www.unodc.org/documents/commissions/CND/Int_Drug_Control_Conventions/Ebook/The_International_Drug_Control_Conventions_E.pdf.
8. Cooper HL, Linton S, Kelley ME, Ross Z, Wolfe ME, Chen Y-T, et al. Racialized risk environments in a large sample of people who inject drugs in the United States. Int J Drug Policy. 2016;27:43–55.
9. Pauly B. Harm reduction through a social justice lens. Int J Drug Policy. 2008;19(1):4–10.
10. World Health Organization. Guidance on the WHO review of psychoactive substances for international control. 2010. Available from: http://www.who.int/medicines/areas/quality_safety/GLS_WHORev_PsychoactSubst_IntC_2010.pdf.

11. United Nations. United Nations treaty collection. 2018. Available from: https://treaties.un.org/pages/viewdetails.aspx?src=treaty&mtdsg_no=vi-16&chapter=6&lang=en.
12. Beletsky L, Davis CS. Today's fentanyl crisis: Prohibition's Iron Law, revisited. Int J Drug Policy. 2017;46:156–9.
13. Cooper HL. War on drugs policing and police brutality. Subst Use Misuse. 2015;50(8–9):1188–94.
14. Astorga L, Shirk DA. Drug trafficking organizations and counter-drug strategies in the US-Mexican context. 2010.
15. BBC News. Canada becomes second country to legalise recreational cannabis. 2018. Available from: https://www.bbc.com/news/world-us-canada-45806255.
16. Hetzer H, Walsh J. Pioneering cannabis regulation in Uruguay. NACLA Rep Am. 2014;47(2):33–5.
17. Volkow ND, Baler RD, Compton WM, Weiss SR. Adverse health effects of marijuana use. N Engl J Med. 2014;370(23):2219–27.
18. Wilkinson ST, Yarnell S, Radhakrishnan R, Ball SA, D'Souza DC. Marijuana legalization: impact on physicians and public health. Annu Rev Med. 2016;67:453–66.
19. Watson TM, Erickson PG. Cannabis legalization in Canada: how might 'strict' regulation impact youth? Taylor & Francis; 2018.
20. World Health Organization. Cannabis and cannabis resin. 2014. Available from: http://www.who.int/medicines/areas/quality_safety/8_2_Cannabis.pdf.
21. Kolodny A, Courtwright DT, Hwang CS, Kreiner P, Eadie JL, Clark TW, et al. The prescription opioid and heroin crisis: a public health approach to an epidemic of addiction. Annu Rev Public Health. 2015;36:559–74.
22. Volkow ND, Frieden TR, Hyde PS, Cha SS. Medication-assisted therapies—tackling the opioid-overdose epidemic. N Engl J Med. 2014;370(22):2063–6.

Global Drug Use

19

Evaristo Akerele

Introduction

Non medical use of marijuana increased during the pandemic. Cocaine manufacture was initial disrupted but returned to normal in the USA the was an increase in opioid overdose deaths. (World drug report 2021 booklet 1. http://www.unodc.org/res/wdr2021/field/WDR21_Booklet_1.pdf). Due to movement restrictions, some producers could potentially seek out new modalities to manufacture drugs.

As a result of the economic crisis of 2008, some users began seeking out cheaper synthetic substances and patterns of use shifted toward injecting drugs.

Potentially the largest immediate impact on drug trafficking can be expected in countries where large quantities are smuggled through commercial airlines. Rising unemployment and the lack of opportunities will make it more likely that poor and disadvantaged people engage in harmful patterns of drug use, suffer drug use disorders, and turn to illicit activities linked to drugs.

Approximately 269 million people used drugs worldwide in 2018, which is 30% more than in 2009, while over 35 million people suffer from drug use disorders, according to the World Drug Report [13]. Restrictions due to the pandemic have resulted shortages of drugs on the street, increased prices, and reduced purity.

The rising unemployment and reduced opportunities caused by the pandemic are also likely to disproportionately affect the poorest countries, making them more vulnerable to drug use and also to drug trafficking and cultivation to boost income.

Due to COVID-19, traffickers may have to find new routes and methods, and trafficking activities via the dark net and shipments by mail may increase, despite the international postal supply chain being disrupted. The pandemic has also led to opioid shortages, which in turn may result in people seeking out other available substances such as alcohol, benzodiazepines, or mixing with synthetic drugs. Interception operations and international cooperation may also become less of a priority, making it easier for traffickers to operate.

Cannabis was the most used substance worldwide in 2018, with an estimated 192 million people using it worldwide. Opioids, however, remain the most harmful, as over the past decade, the total number of deaths due to opioid use disorders went up to 71%, with a 92% increase among women compared with 63% among men.

Drug use increased far more rapidly among developing countries over the 2000–2018 period than in developed countries. Adolescents and young adults account for the largest share of those using drugs, while young people are also

E. Akerele (✉)
Department of Psychiatry, New Jersey Medical School, Rutgers University, Newark, NJ, USA

E. Akerele (ed.), *Substance and Non-Substance Related Addictions*,
https://doi.org/10.1007/978-3-030-84834-7_19

the most vulnerable to the effects of drugs because they use the most and their brains are still developing.

Cannabis Trends

While the impact of laws that have legalized cannabis in some jurisdictions is still hard to assess, it is noteworthy that the frequent use of cannabis has increased in all of these jurisdictions after legalization. In some of these jurisdictions, more potent cannabis products are also more common in the market.

Cannabis also remains the main drug that brings people into contact with the criminal justice system, accounting for more than half of drug law offence cases, based on data from 69 countries covering the period between 2014 and 2018.

More than 90% of all pharmaceutical opioids available for medical consumption were in high-income countries in 2018 comprising around 12% of the global population, while the low- and middle-income countries comprising 88% of the global population are estimated to consume less than 10% of pharmaceutical opioids. Access to pharmaceutical opioids depend on several factors including legislation, culture, health systems, and prescribing practices.

Poverty, limited education, and social marginalization remain the major factors increasing the risk of drug use disorders, and vulnerable and marginalized groups may also face barriers to getting treatment services due to discrimination and stigma (WDR 2020 Executive Summary). In the following sections, the challenges with the primary drugs of abuse will be addressed.

Cocaine

Cocaine production and seizures reach record highs. Cocaine production reaches a record level amid transition in Colombia. The estimated global illicit manufacture of cocaine reached an all-time high of 1976 tons (estimated as 100% pure) in 2017, an increase of 25% on the previous year. This was mainly driven by increases in cocaine manufacture in Colombia, which produced an estimated 70% of the world's cocaine. Colombia experienced a 17% expansion in the area under coca bush cultivation in 2017, and a 31% rise in the amount of cocaine produced, mainly due to a marked rise in the productive areas under coca bush cultivation. The Colombian Government's 2016 peace deal with the Revolutionary Armed Forces of Colombia (FARC) has helped to drastically reduce cocaine production in the central areas of the country, where farmers in areas previously controlled by the FARC have abandoned cultivation. But in other areas previously controlled by the FARC, criminal groups have moved in to continue and expand coca bush cultivation. A third dynamic in Colombia saw entirely new areas given over to coca bush cultivation during 2016, reflected in the production data for 2017. These areas are often far away from major cities, making it difficult for the central authorities to provide incentives to farmers to stop cultivation. Also, a reduction in eradication efforts might have fostered the idea that cultivation was relatively risk-free. Record seizures help to keep cocaine supply in check. The global quantity of cocaine seized in 2017 increased to 1275 tons – the largest quantity ever reported, and an increase on the previous year of 13%. While cocaine seizures have risen by 74% over the past decade, production has risen by 50%. Overall, the data suggest that the amount of cocaine available for consumption has increased at a slower rate than has manufacture. This suggests that at the global level, law enforcement efforts and international cooperation have likely become more effective with the interception of a larger share of cocaine products than in the past. The bulk of cocaine seizures are in the Americas, which accounted for almost 90% of the global total in 2017. Interception close to the source of manufacture is significant; Colombia alone intercepted 38% of the global total in 2017.

Cocaine use is on the rise in North America and Western and Central Europe. An estimated 18.1 million people used cocaine in the past year, with the highest rates reported in North America (2.1%) and Oceania (1.6%). North America had seen a decline in cocaine use between 2006 and

2012, but there are now signs of an increase, as there are in Western and Central Europe, Oceania, and some South American countries. In parts of Asia and West Africa, increasing amounts of cocaine have been reported to be seized, which suggests that cocaine use could potentially increase, especially among affluent, urban dwellers in subregions where use had previously been low. Cocaine trafficking has expanded into a global phenomenon since the 1980s. Some 143 countries across all regions reported cocaine seizures over the period 2013–2017, up from 99 countries over the period 1983–1987. Most of the cocaine trafficked from the Andean countries of South America is destined for the main consumer markets in North America and Western and Central Europe. Seizures in North America have more than doubled in recent years, from 94 tons in 2013 to 238 tons in 2017. The second most important cocaine trafficking flow worldwide is from the Andean countries to Western Europe. The quantity of cocaine seized in Western and Central Europe has also more than doubled in the past 5 years, from 65 tons in 2013 to 141 tons in 2017 [10, 11].

Health Consequences of Cocaine

Cocaine damages many other organs in the body. It reduces blood flow in the gastrointestinal tract, which can lead to tears and ulcerations [8]. Many chronic cocaine users lose their appetite and experience significant weight loss and malnourishment. Cocaine has significant and well-recognized toxic effects on the heart and cardiovascular system [5, 6, 8]. Chest pain that feels like a heart attack is common and sends many cocaine users to the emergency room [6, 8]. Cocaine use is linked with increased risk of stroke [5], as well as inflammation of the heart muscle, deterioration of the ability of the heart to contract, and aortic ruptures [6].

Cocaine users increasingly seek treatment in Europe, most often for polydrug use. The number of people seeking treatment for the first time for cocaine use disorders has increased over the past 2 years in the European Union countries. Three-quarters of those who accessed specialized drug treatment services for the first time were reported in just three countries: Italy, Spain, and the United Kingdom. Among all cocaine users entering drug treatment in the European Union, one-third were seeking treatment only for cocaine use disorders. The rest also reported the use of secondary substances, especially alcohol and cannabis. Many of the "crack" cocaine users entering treatment reported using heroin as a secondary drug.

Marijuana

Marijuana is derived from the plant *Cannabis sativa*. The major psychoactive constituent in cannabis is Δ-9-tetrahydrocannabinol (THC). Compounds which are structurally similar to THC are referred to as cannabinoids. The term marijuana usually refers to cannabis leaves or other crude plant material. Cannabis plants contain 70 unique compounds, collectively known as phytocannabinoids [7], the main psychoactive substance being THC, which provides the psychoactive effects of cannabis. The unpollinated female plants are called hashish. The cultivation of unpollinated female cannabis plants (sinsemilla) has resulted in increased potency. This selective breeding yields higher THC levels but has also resulted in the selection of varieties containing lower levels of CBD [3]. Cannabis oil (hashish oil) is a concentrate of cannabinoids obtained by solvent extraction of the crude plant material or of the resin.

There are a number of marijuana products. These include but are not limited to concentrates, shake, and edibles.

"Concentrates" are made from the cannabis plant processing ensures they contain only the most desired compounds (primarily cannabinoids and terpenes). "Shake" refers to small pieces of cannabis flower that have broken off the larger buds. "Trim" refers to leftover leaves that are trimmed from the cannabis flower. Shake and trim provide reasonable levels of THC for extraction. Both are sold directly to the consumer, usually in the form of pre-rolled joints. "Cannabis-infused products" or "edibles" may include a range of products such as cookies, brownies, and cakes, as well as cannabis-infused drinks and capsules. The ingredients may include cannabis tincture, butter, or oil.

Cannabis is the most widely abused illicit drug globally. Half of all drug seizures worldwide are cannabis seizures. Approximately 188 million people, 2.5% of the world population, consume cannabis [12]. This is at least ten times as much as the consumption of cocaine (0.2%) and opiates, also 0.2% [15].

The majority cannabis seizures occur in the Americas. Approximately 38% of the global total in 2017 were from South America and 21% from North America. This represents a change from previous years when North America had the most seizures. Apparently, the seizures of cannabis in North America are on the decline; down by 77% from the level in 2010. Simultaneously the decline in seizures in North America has been accompanied by a rise in the nonmedical use of cannabis in a context in which measures legalizing the nonmedical use of cannabis were implemented in some jurisdictions. Despite the aim of preventing criminals from generating profits from the illicit trade in cannabis, residual illicit cannabis markets continue to exist in many of the states that have legalized the nonmedical use of the drug. This is especially evident in Colorado and the State of Washington, which were among the first jurisdictions to allow such measures, in 2012. In California, the initial attempts to license the sale of cannabis in 2018 resulted in prices that were higher than in the illicit market and thus failed to entice users away from the illicit market. The intensity of cannabis use has been increasing in the context of cannabis legalization. While more people are using cannabis in North America than they were a decade earlier, the increase has been more pronounced in the regular (nonmedical) use of the drug. For instance, in the United States, the number of past year users of cannabis rose by some 60% between 2007 and 2017, while the number of daily or nearly daily users of cannabis more than doubled over the period. This group of regular users accounts for the largest share of the cannabis consumed. Cannabis products have diversified and increased in potency since legalization. In Colorado, while the potency (tetrahydrocannabinol (THC) level) of cannabis flower has remained lower than that of cannabis concentrates (20% versus 69%, in 2017), the potency of both product types increased by about 20% over the period 2014–2017. The market for cannabis concentrates has also evolved rapidly, with a wide range of products now available, each with varying levels of THC, although the proportion of tested cannabis concentrates that contain over 75% THC has increased fivefold in recent years. There is also an increase in Colorado in the demand for non-flower products such as oil-filled vaporizer cartridges, wax/shatter concentrates, and infused edibles [12].

Nonmedical use of marijuana is legal in Canada, Uruguay (Law No. 19.172), and 11 states in the United States ((34) In the United States, cannabis is federally prohibited as a substance in Schedule I of the Controlled Substances Act. (35) Home cultivation is not allowed in the State of Washington. The number of plants allowed in each state varies. (36) National Conference of State Legislatures, "Marijuana overview", 14 December 2018). All have laws to restrict access of children to marijuana [15].

Marijuana may impair cognitive development including associative processes such as recall of previously learned items. Psychomotor performance in performance in a wide variety of tasks, such as motor coordination, divided attention, and operative tasks of many types; human performance on complex machinery can be impaired for as long as 24 hours after smoking as little as 20 mg of THC in cannabis; there is an increased risk of motor vehicle accidents among persons who drive under the influence of cannabis. This includes the organization and integration of complex information involving various mechanisms of attention and memory processes. Prolonged use may lead to greater impairment, which may not recover with cessation of use and which could affect daily life functions.

The data suggest that marijuana use can cause functional impairment in cognitive abilities but that the degree and/or duration of the impairment depends on the age of onset of use, quantity, and duration [9, 10].

Among nearly 4000 young adults in the Coronary Artery Risk Development in Young Adults study tracked over a 25-year period until mid-adulthood, cumulative lifetime exposure to marijuana was associated with lower scores on a test of verbal memory but did not affect other cognitive abilities such as processing speed or executive function. The effect was sizeable and significant even after eliminating those involved with current use and after adjusting for confounding factors such as demographic factors, other drug and alcohol use, and other psychiatric conditions such as depression [2].

Marijuana may exacerbate of psychosis in individuals with schizophrenia. However, the data suggest that some antipsychotics reduce marijuana craving in individuals with schizophrenia [1]. Epithelial injury of the trachea and major bronchi is caused by long-term cannabis smoking. Airway injury, lung inflammation, and impaired pulmonary defense against infection often results from persistent cannabis consumption over prolonged periods. Heavy cannabis consumption is associated with a higher prevalence of symptoms of bronchitis. Cannabis used during pregnancy is associated with impairment in fetal development leading to a reduction in birth weight.

Opioids

"Opioids" is a generic term that refers both to opiates and their synthetic analogues [14]. Opiates are naturally occurring alkaloids found in the opium poppy, such as morphine, codeine, and thebaine, as well as their semisynthetic derivatives, such as heroin, hydrocodone, oxycodone, and buprenorphine. (All opiates are controlled under the Single Convention on Narcotic Drugs of 1961, except for buprenorphine, which is controlled under Schedule III of the Convention on Psychotropic Substances of 1971.) The term "opioids" also includes synthetic opioids, which are structurally diverse substances. Most pharmaceutical opioids are controlled under the Single Convention on Narcotic Drugs of 1961 with the exception of some, such as buprenorphine, which are controlled under the Convention on Psychotropic Substances of 1971. Tramadol is an example of a pharmaceutical opioid that is currently not controlled under the drug conventions.

In some countries, heroin is used in a medical context as part of heroin-assisted treatment directed at people for whom other opioid treatment options have previously failed. Such treatments can help those people to remain in treatment, limit their use of street drugs, reduce their illegal activities, and possibly reduce their likelihood of overdose and mortality. In such heroin-assisted programs, heroin is administered, preferably in a clinical setting as unadulterated, subsidized, or even cost-free [4].

North America has seen a rising number of overdose deaths resulting from the use of opioids. More than 47,000 opioid overdose deaths were recorded in the United States in 2017, an increase of 13% from the previous year. Those deaths were largely attributed to synthetic opioids such as fentanyl and its analogues, which were involved in nearly 50% more deaths than in 2016. In Canada, nearly 4000 opioid-related deaths were reported in 2017, a 33% increase from the 3000 overdose deaths reported in 2016. Fentanyl or fentanyl analogues were involved in 69% of those deaths in 2017, compared with 50% in 2016. Trafficking of fentanyl and its analogues rises and expands outside North America. North America is the principal market for fentanyl, but seizure data suggest that trafficking has expanded worldwide. While just 4 countries reported fentanyl seizures to UNODC in 2013, 12 countries did so in 2016 and 16 countries in 2017. Europe hosts a small but growing market for fentanyl. Seizures or use have been reported in most European countries. In Western and Central Europe, seizures have risen from 1 kg in 2013 to 5 kg in 2016 and 17 kg in 2017. The substances are often sold on the Internet, sometimes as "legal" replacements for controlled opioids. Tramadol: The other opioid crisis in low- and middle-income countries West and Central and North Africa are currently experiencing a crisis of another synthetic opioid, tramadol, which has been used as a painkiller for decades. Limited information on the supply of tramadol for nonmedical use points to tramadol being (illicitly) manufactured in South Asia and trafficked to African countries and parts of the Middle East. Global seizures of tramadol rose from less than 10 kg in 2010 to almost 9 tons in 2013 and reached a record high of 125 tons in 2017. New data from Nigeria suggest the problem is greater than previously thought. The national drug use survey conducted in 2017 shows that 4.7% of the population aged 15–64 reported the nonmedical use of prescription opioids in the previous year, with tramadol being by far the most common opioid misused. With the rapidly growing number of synthetic opioid, new psychoactive substances (NPS) emerge on the market. The number of new psychoactive substances that are synthetic opioids, mostly fentanyl analogues, reported on the market has been rising at an unprecedented rate. It rose from just 1 substance in 2009 to 15 in 2015 and 46 in 2017, while the overall number of NPS present on the market stabilized at around 500 substances per year over the period 2015–2017. Synthetic opioids have become the second most important substance group, after stimulants, in terms of NPS reported for the first time. The group accounted for 29% of the newly identified NPS in 2017. Heroin is still reaching the market despite declining opium production and rising seizures. The drought in Afghanistan causes decline in the cultivation and production of opium in 2018. Afghanistan was again the country responsible for the vast majority of the world's illicit opium poppy cultivation and opium production in 2018. The 263,000 ha under cultivation in Afghanistan in 2018 dwarfs cultivation in nearest rivals, Myanmar (37,300 ha in 2018) and Mexico (30,600 ha in 2016/2017). Overall, the global area cultivated fell by some 17% in 2018 to 346,000 ha, largely as a result of a drought in Afghanistan. Also, opium prices in Afghanistan fell rapidly between 2016 and 2018, probably because of overproduction in previous years, making the crop less lucrative for farmers. However, the area under cultivation today is more than 60% larger than it was a decade ago, and the estimated cultivation area in Afghanistan in 2018 is the second largest estimate ever. The global production of opium was even more affected than was cultivation by the drought in Afghanistan, which produced 82% of the world's opium in 2018. After an upward trend over the last two decades, the global production fell by 25% from 2017 to 2018, to some 7790 tons. Despite that drop, the amount of opium produced was the third largest amount since UNODC started to systematically monitor opium production in the 1990s. Opiate seizures increase to record levels. Quantities of opiates seized globally again reached an all-time high in 2017. Some 693 tons of opium were seized, which was 5% more than in the previous year. In addition, 103 tons of heroin were intercepted, 13% more than in 2016, and 87 tons of morphine, a 33% rise. Expressing these seizures in common heroin equivalents, heroin seizures exceed those of morphine and opium. Some 86% of all opiates seized in 2017 were intercepted in Asia, the region that accounts for more than 90% of global illicit opium production. Global interceptions of heroin have increased at a faster pace than production, suggesting a likely increase in the efficiency of law enforcement efforts and international cooperation. The greatest burden of disease is seen in East and South-East Asia, North America, and South Asia, reflecting the large numbers of opioid users and people who inject drugs (PWID) in those subregions.

Health Consequence

More than 11 million people worldwide inject drugs. People who inject drugs (PWID) experience multiple negative health consequences. They are at an increased risk of fatal overdose and are disproportionately affected by blood-borne infectious diseases such as HIV and hepatitis C. The number of people who inject drugs worldwide stood at 11.3 million in 2017. A small number of countries account for a considerable proportion of the global number of PWID. Some 43% of all PWID reside in just three countries: China, the Russian Federation, and the United States.

Patterns of HIV infection among people who inject drugs have wide regional variations. Roughly one in eight people who inject drugs lives with HIV, amounting to 1.4 million people. The UNAIDS estimates that injecting drug users are 22 times more likely than the general population to be infected with HIV. The prevalence of HIV among PWID is the highest by far in South-West Asia and in Eastern and South Eastern Europe, with rates that are 2.3 and 1.8 times the global average, respectively. Those two subregions also have higher than average proportions of injecting drug users. Action to tackle hepatitis C epidemic among people who inject drugs has been slow. Hepatitis C is highly prevalent among PWID, with almost one-half of PWID, or some 5.6 million people, living with hepatitis C. Highly effective treatment for hepatitis C has recently become available in the form of direct-acting antivirals, potentially transforming the management and outlook for PWID living with hepatitis C. However, despite the opportunity afforded by these new medications in addressing the high burden of hepatitis C among PWID, progress in scaling up prevention and treatment services among PWID has been slow. Deaths and years of "healthy" life lost attributed to the use of drugs remain unacceptably high. Some 585,000 people are estimated to have died as a result of drug use in 2017. More than half of those deaths were the result of untreated hepatitis C, leading to liver cancer and cirrhosis; almost one-third were attributed to drug use disorders. Most (two-thirds) of the deaths attributed to drug use disorders were related to opioid use. Some 42 million years of "healthy" life were lost (premature deaths and years lived with disability) as a result of drug use. They were also mostly attributed to drug use disorders, especially from the use of opioids.

Conclusion

Cocaine has no therapeutic use. There is currently no pharmacological treatment for cocaine. Marijuana has some therapeutic utility and increasing legal for recreational use. Long-term effects on both economy and health remain to be determined. Opioids have therapeutic utility and probably the most frequent cause of death in drug users. Global efforts ought to focus on the prevention of drug abuse especially the abuse of opioids. The modality in which drugs are use also has a significant impact on the likelihood of adverse health effects. Coca leaves have been used in Latin America in countries like Peru to this day for tea and other apparently innocuous purposes. Peyote has neen used by Native Americans prior to the advent of colinization. Marijuana and its components have some therapeutic use. The legalization of marijuana for recreational use is increasing rapidly. There is a need for the education of both prscribers and users of opioids. Furthermore the global opioid crisis requires the implementation of novel modalities that will enhance prevention of opioid overdose. Prescription opioids are useful when prescribed nd used appropriately. Most important, substance use disorder is a global health challenge that requires global solutions. These include, rapid identification of individuals at risk, access to treatment and regulation to limit availablity of opioids.

References

1. Akerele E, Levin FR. Comparison of olanzapine to risperidone in substance-abusing individuals with schizophrenia. Am J Addict. 2007;16(4):260–8. https://doi.org/10.1080/10550490701389658.
2. Auer R, Vittinghoff E, Yaffe K, et al. Association between lifetime marijuana use and cognitive function in middle age: the coronary artery risk development in young adults (CARDIA) study. JAMA Intern Med. 2016;176(3):352–61. https://doi.org/10.1001/jamainternmed.2015.7841.
3. European Monitoring Centre for Drugs and Drug Addiction. Cannabis production and markets in Europe (EMCDDA Insights Series No 12). 2012. https://www.emcdda.europa.eu/attachements.cfm/att_166248_EN_web_INSIGHTS_CANNABIS.pdf.
4. Ferri M, Davoli M, Perucci CA. Heroin maintenance for chronic heroin-dependent individuals. Cochrane Database Syst Rev. 2011;(12):CD003410. https://doi.org/10.1002/14651858.CD003410.pub4.
5. Fonseca AC, Ferro JM. Drug abuse and stroke. Curr Neurol Neurosci Rep. 2013;13(2):325. https://doi.org/10.1007/s11910-012-0325-0.
6. Maraj S, Figueredo VM, Lynn MD. Cocaine and the heart. Clin Cardiol. 2010;33(5):264–9. https://doi.org/10.1002/clc.20746.

7. Meyer JS, Quenzer LF, editors. Psychopharmacology: drugs, the brain, and behaviour. 3rd ed. Sunderland: Sinauer Associates; 2019.
8. Riezzo I, Fiore C, De Carlo D, Pascale N, Neri M, Turillazzi E, Fineschi V. Side effects of cocaine abuse: multiorgan toxicity and pathological consequences. Curr Med Chem. 2012;19(33):5624–46. https://doi.org/10.2174/092986712803988893.
9. Volkow ND, Swanson JM, Evins AE, DeLisi LE, Meier MH, Gonzalez R, Bloomfield MAP, Curran HV, Baler R. Effects of cannabis use on human behavior, including cognition, motivation, and psychosis: a review. JAMA Psychiat. 2016;73(3):292–7. https://doi.org/10.1001/jamapsychiatry.2015.3278.
10. United Nations. World Drug Report 1, Executive summary. United Nations publication, Sales No. E.19.XI.8. 2019a. https://wdr.unodc.org/wdr2019/prelaunch/WDR19_Booklet_1_EXECUTIVE_SUMMARY.pdf
11. United Nations. World Drug Report 4, Stimulants. United Nations publication, Sales No. E.19.XI.8. 2019b. https://wdr.unodc.org/wdr2019/prelaunch/WDR19_Booklet_4_STIMULANTS.pdf
12. United Nations. World Drug Report 5, Cannabis and hallucinogens. United Nations publication, Sales No. E.19.XI.8. 2019c. https://wdr.unodc.org/wdr2019/prelaunch/WDR19_Booklet_5_CANNABIS_HALLUCINOGENS.pdf
13. World Drug Report 2020. https://www.unodc.org/unodc/press/releases/2020/June/media-advisory%2D%2D-global-launch-of-the-2020-world-drug-report.html
14. WHO. Lexicon of alcohol and drug terms. Geneva: WHO; 2014.
15. World Health Organization. 14 Sept 2020. Cannabis. https://www.who.int/substance_abuse/facts/cannabis/en/.

Drug Abuse and Education

20

Biren Patel, Mohammad Naqvi, and Nidal Moukaddam

Introduction

In this chapter, we will discuss how addiction is taught in medical curricula. Addictive disorders are very common in the population than any clinician will come in contact with, yet the skills to properly identify, diagnose, and manage addictive disorders are not taught frequently enough or with sufficient depth. According to the Healthcare Cost and Utilization Project (HCUP) Statistical Briefs, derived from the Nationwide Inpatient Sample and base figures from the US Census Bureau, in 2014, the findings from HCUP indicate that "among approximately 30 million annual adult inpatient stays for physical health conditions or mental and/or substance use disorders (M/SUDs), the co-occurrence of these two types of conditions increased from 38.4 percent of stays in 2010 to 45.0 percent of stays in 2014" [1].

In the next sections, we will examine the background history of medical learners' exposure to addiction training. This can occur in various stages during a medical learner's training, such as medical school, residency, fellowship training, and as a physician in practice [2]. We will first begin with the history of modern medical education.

Background

Medical learner's education first began in the United States in 1765 with the establishment of the first medical school in Pennsylvania [3]. At that time courses involved chemistry, botany, pharmacology, anatomy, surgery, and midwifery. Over the years, medical schools in the United States would continue to modify their curriculum according to practices set forward by regional medical societies. Each regional medical society would be independent from another, and this could lead to discrepancies in their curriculum. To address the disparity between medical colleges and their regionally based education, 40 medical societies from 28 institutions met in 1847 and established the American Medical Association (AMA) [4]. The establishment of the AMA set uniform standards for the curriculum for medical schools. The medical school

B. Patel
Behavioral Health, Kelsey-Seybold Clinics, Houston, TX, USA
e-mail: biren.patel@kelsey-seybold.com

M. Naqvi
Department of Investigational Cancer Therapeutics, The University of Texas MD Anderson Cancer Center, Houston, TX, USA
e-mail: mfnaqvi@mdanderson.org

N. Moukaddam (✉)
Menninger Department of Psychiatry & Behavioral Sciences, Baylor College of Medicine, Houston, TX, USA
e-mail: nidalm@bcm.edu

E. Akerele (ed.), *Substance and Non-Substance Related Addictions*,
https://doi.org/10.1007/978-3-030-84834-7_20

curriculum was re-evaluated during the early twentieth century and made more rigorous after examination by Abraham Flexner. He was an educator who in 1910 published a guide deemed the Flexner Report [5]. He recommended that the best learning came from doing and that clinical teaching should be conducted at the dispensary as well as the hospital wards. His report impacted the basis of medical education for the twentieth century, as medical school would continue to emphasize a curriculum of basic sciences followed by equally important clinical rotations.

During the middle to late twentieth century, medical learners would continue to engage in a similar curriculum during their medical education. A search of the literature for alcoholism and medical education revealed few articles from the 1950s to the 1960s. One explanation for this is that it was not a required part of the curriculum until much later [6]. Another explanation can be alcohol and substance use disorders were not given enough attention by the medical community. This began to change in the early 1970s, as it was noted medical learners had limited experience and opportunities to learn about how to treat patients with alcohol and substance use disorders [7]. The American Medical Association (AMA) and National Institute on Alcohol Abuse and Alcoholism (NIAAA) examined medical learners' education and developed reports that cited the need for the importance of addiction training for medical learners. As substance addictions began to become more evident, the federal United States government initiated the Career Teacher Program in 1971. This program was established to develop faculty specifically for substance addictions and to implement curriculum changes. It was implemented at 59 medical schools and marked the first-time addiction training which was added in the United States in the medical learners' education. In 1979, the AMA recognized the importance of addiction training for all medical learners and published the Guidelines for Physician Involvement in the Care of Substance Abusing Patients [6].

As a response to the continued importance of teaching about substance use, an additional Career Teacher Program was implemented in 1988 at 13 medical schools. This time the program also included increasing the faculty that are specialized in addictions from three to five at every medical school. The AMA also recognized the importance of training medical learners in addiction with the passage of H295.922, which stated that alcohol and other drug abuse education needed to be an integral part of medical education [6]. Medical schools began adding substance abuse education into their curriculums as well during this time. By 1992, 93% of the US medical schools had at least one curriculum unit in substance abuse [7]. The medical schools continued adding courses in substance abuse during the 2000s, and by 2005–2006, all but 1 out of 125 medical schools offered either a required or an elective course in substance abuse [6]. The medical education process started to include addiction curriculums in response to the increasing importance of addiction as a field. We will now begin discussing how medical learners increase their knowledge about addictive disorders.

Medical Learner's Curriculum

Medical learners embark on their journey of gaining knowledge to become a physician during their graduate studies. Medical learners in the United States initially complete coursework focusing on basic sciences for the first 18–24 months depending on the medical school curriculum. This coursework is then followed by exposure to clinical rotations for the last 2 years. Medical learners can be exposed to addiction training at various times during their education. We will begin discussing challenges faced by medical learners including medical learners' own prior experience with substance use disorders, biases toward patients with substance use disorders, opportunities for medical learners, and methods in which substance abuse education can be improved.

Some challenges for medical learners can be the medical learner's own personal experience with substance use disorders. Medical learners can be juxtaposed between learning about the treatment of patients with substance use disorders as well as currently having symptoms of their own. A 2015 survey of 855 medical learners from 49 medical schools across the United States revealed a variety of substance use, with the most common being alcohol, marijuana, and tobacco use [8]. In this survey, approximately 85.2% of medical learners used alcohol in the past month, with 33.8% (n = 290) having consumed five or more drinks in one sitting. Approximately 26.2% of medical learners had consumed marijuana, and 17.3% had consumed tobacco within the past month. Having a medical learner with concurrent substance use could present a challenge to both identifying substance use disorders and for the learner to receive help. Despite being in training within the medical field, only 30% of the medical learners surveyed were aware of substance use prevention programs within their own institutions. Several medical learners in the survey also experienced negative consequences due to their substance use, including 22.3% of learners experiencing memory loss, 13.2% missing class, and 10.3% having driven a car while under the influence. This could present a challenge to medical learners as the current use of substances could impact their ability to learn about various substance use disorders. Another challenge can be a lack of knowledge about available programs which could affect their ability to learn about the effective treatments for substance use disorders.

Another challenge often encountered by medical learners can be the biases encountered when treating patients with substance use disorders. A survey in 1989 of 386 medical students at a single medical school in the United States revealed several findings on the views of medical students on substance users [9]. Fourth-year learners were more likely than third-year learners to see addiction as a character weakness and that treatment was ineffective. Another finding was that those medical learners that felt confidence in their ability to screen for substance use disorders were also more likely to felt responsible for treating the patient's substance use disorder. Medical learners' views on substance use disorders could impact their confidence and subsequent referring of the patient for additional treatment. A learner's personal view of addiction as a disease is just a few of the many challenges that can arise when treating substance use disorders.

Internationally, studies from around the world have cited similar concerns about medical learners' exposure to substance use disorder treatment and the views medical learners have about substance users. A survey of 671 students including both first-year and fourth-year medical learners was conducted in the United Kingdom in 2000 [10]. This survey revealed that 34% of first-year medical learners felt that drug users were less deserving of treatment than patients with other medical conditions. This view of substance abuse disorder in a negative light did decline by the fourth year, as only 28% of medical learners in their fourth year believed patients were undeserving of care. This study revealed that bias can still exist within medical learners in terms of how they perceive substance use disorders and the care that the medical learner perceives the patient should receive. Having a negative view of addiction and the care that a patient can receive can create a bias within a medical learner.

Another challenge that medical learners face could be the limited opportunity to interact with patients with substance use disorders. Different clinical rotations occur during the third and fourth years in the US medical school training, and medical learners experience a variety of rotations across varying disciplines at this time. A survey was conducted in 1992 of program directors across the nation regarding how many had substance abuse curriculum unit in their rotations for third-year medical learners. The program directors that were reported having one curriculum unit of substance abuse training in their clerkships was as follows: 95% in psychiatry, 87% in family medicine, 59% in pediatrics, 46% in internal medicine, 46% in emergency medicine, and 45% in obstetrics gynecology [7]. Substance abuse training was not equally present in all of the core clerkship rotations. As a result, limited exposure depending on the clerkship could limit a medical learner's exposure to both the recognition and treatment of substance use disorders.

There is a way that medical learners can increase their exposure to the field of substance abuse treatment with an interesting opportunity in the United States. Medical learners can apply for the Summer Institute for Medical Student (SIMS) program. The SIMS program encompasses a 1-week program at the Betty Ford Center in California, where a medical learner can participate as an active participant in a residential treatment facility [11]. Medical learners are given the opportunity to engage in group psychotherapy with patients. One participant who completed the program reported having an increased understanding of the neurobiology of addictive diseases. Increasing medical learners' exposure to residential treatment settings is one way to increase future clinicians' knowledge of substance abuse treatment.

Medical learners can also face a challenge in their comfort level with educating patients about their substance use disorders. One intervention that has been evaluated to increase medical learners' confidence in screening for substance use disorder is to increase their exposure to standardized patients. These screenings would also have to be able to be observed by clerkship preceptors. A study in 2015 of 1065 third-year medical learners in the United States was conducted with medical learners from 10 different medical schools. The study inquired about learners' comfort level with counseling patients on tobacco cessation [12]. The medical learners were asked their confidence in tobacco cessation counseling for patients using the 5A model of asking about smoking history. The 5A model encompasses advising to quit smoking, assessing willingness to quit, assisting with developing a quit plan, and arranging follow-up contact related to smoking. The medical learners were surveyed using a Likert scale of how likely they were to continue to refer patients for treatment of tobacco dependence. The study found that those medical learners who had greater tobacco treatment self-efficacy scores would have a greater frequency of 5A use. Those medical learners with intentions to use 5A behaviors were also significantly associated with 5A use frequency. Another important finding was that reported greater 5A instruction ($B = 0.06$ (0.03); $p < 0.05$) as well as observation of tobacco treatment skills ($B = 0.35$ (0.02); $p < 0.001$) were found to be significant predictors for greater 5A behaviors in medical learners. This emphasizes the importance of education regarding substance use disorders for medical learners as well as an opportunity for their skills to be assessed. Medical learners who are provided with the opportunity to practice their skills often improve their ability to assess and provide treatment for patients.

Internationally, studies have been conducted around the world regarding medical learners and their preparation to treat substance use disorders. A survey of 556 third-year medical learners in Sao Paulo in 2017 was conducted to assess medical learners' views on various topics including tobacco use and counseling patients as treatment for nicotine use [13]. The study found that 62.95% of the learners surveyed believed that smoking health professionals were less likely to advise smoking patients to quit smoking. Interestingly in the survey, 5.23% of learners surveyed were current cigarette smokers, and 43.82% had experimentation of waterpipe tobacco smoking. This study revealed that even among the medical community of future clinicians, there can be bias regarding counseling patients to quit using tobacco products.

After a medical learner successfully completes their medical degree, they begin a postgraduate training which is also known as residency in the United States.

Resident's Exposure to Addiction

The medical learner begins a residency program which varies in length based on specialty. All programs require an intern year during their first year of training, and then the learner is known as a resident during the subsequent years. The resident can experience exposure to substance use disorders at various times during their residency, with several receiving education through a formal curriculum at didactics as well as by learning from experience with patients that they will be treating.

Residents can also face similar challenges similar to medical learners. Residents can display bias when treating patients with substance use disorders, as well as have limited exposure to substance use curriculums based on their specialty. Residents can also face the challenge of having less expertise in treating patients with medications to prevent and treat substance use disorders. We will then examine who among the residents can improve on their skills, such as by engaging in objective structured clinical exams.

Residents can have bias similar to medical learners in terms of the resident's view of treating patients with substance use disorders. A study conducted in 2002 of 95 internal medicine residents and 49 faculty clinicians at a single residency program in Boston consisted of surveying clinicians after they treated patients with a variety of disorders [14]. The survey found that residents had significantly less satisfaction when treating patients with alcohol problems, substance use, or depression compared to when the residents treated patients with hypertension. The survey found similar results in faculty clinicians as they reported lower satisfaction for treating patients with alcohol or substance use compared to patients with hypertension. This study revealed that residents as well as faculty clinicians can have more satisfaction when treating patients with a "traditional" medical disorder such as hypertension compared to when they are treating alcohol or substance use.

Residents can also have limited exposure to patients with substance use disorders based on the specialty that they choose. In 1997, a survey of residency directors across the United States was conducted, and 1183 of the 1832 residency directors responded to the survey [15]. These residency directors were chosen in six fields including emergency medicine, family medicine, internal medicine, obstetrics-gynecology, pediatrics, psychiatry, and osteopathic medicine. Of the programs surveyed, only the following programs had a required curriculum in substance abuse education for residents: 95% in psychiatry, 75% in family medicine, 55% in emergency medicine, 51% in internal medicine, 41% in osteopathic medicine, 40% in obstetrics-gynecology, and 32% in pediatrics. This survey revealed the discrepancy between residency programs and the percentage of programs that had a required substance use education component.

Within the United States, residency programs are evaluated by a governing organization of the Accreditation Council of Graduate Medical Education (ACGME). Beginning in 2001, the field of psychiatry began to include a 1-month full-time equivalent rotation in their psychiatric residency programs [16]. The growing importance of substance use disorders in the curriculum and training of residents has only increased as the field of addictions becomes more prevalent and diverse.

Currently in the United States, there are concerns for an opioid epidemic which can be affected by a clinician's inability to recognize signs and symptoms of opioid abuse. Residents can often have difficulty in treating disorders for which they are not accustomed to treating [17]. One example can be seen within internal medicine residency, as residents within internal medicine often treat patients who present with chronic pain. These residents may not receive adequate education in prescribing opioids safely, and the impact of education while in residency is continuously assessed and evaluated. A study in 2017 examined 91 internal medicine residents at a single residency program in the United States [17]. These residents completed a training program of a 4.5-hour educational didactic while in their second or third year of training. The training included dimensions including defining chronic pain, defining opioid use disorder, roles of opioids in treating chronic pain, developing and practicing of skills, utilizing managerial strategies, and explaining their clinical reasoning. This survey included a four-point Likert scale which assessed if residents agreed or disagreed with statements regarding the treatment of patients with chronic pain. After completing the didactic sessions, the residents were able to work with faculty clinicians who treated patients with chronic pain; after completing the training, the internal medicine residents were more likely to feel comfortable managing patients with chronic pain. The surveyed residents also reported increased confidence in their ability to recognize patients with chronic pain who developed an opioid use disorder. Another positive outcome from the didactics was that the residents also reported more confidence in their increased knowledge of resources that are available for chronic pain and opioid use disorders.

It is important that residents continue to receive education regarding substance use disorders. Several methods have been employed, such as increasing the availability of faculty, initiating a brief didactic session, and implementing an objective-structured clinical exam (OSCE). An OSCE entails having a standardized patient and observing resident interviews by faculty supervisors. A study of 265 third year family medicine and internal medicine residents at a medical school in New York was conducted using OSCEs [18]. These exams were used to evaluate residents' ability to communicate, assess, and manage various conditions in standardized patients. One of the cases included heroin use disorder, and the faculty would observe the resident during their interview. The study found that residents' skills were significantly better in communication than the assessment or management portion of heroin abuse. The residents' inexperience with assessing and managing heroin abuse was noted on 59–81% of the standardized patients. Another important finding from this survey was that 35% of the residents that were surveyed had no prior exposure to a similar case during their training. This could impact a resident's ability to successfully treat a patient with heroin use disorder, as this study revealed inexperience, impacting the ability to assess and recommend management.

Fellows' Exposure to Addiction

Once a resident completes their postgraduate residency training, they are given the opportunity to continue their training in a fellowship training program or to enter the workforce as an independent practitioner. For those medical learners who completed residency and decide on pursuing additional addiction training, fellowships are available to further increase one's knowledge and comfort with treating patients with addictions.

In the United States, addiction fellowships are offered by the American Board of Preventive Medicine (ABPM) and by the American Board of Psychiatry and Neurology (APBN). The field of addiction medicine was first recognized as a self-designated specialty in 1990 [19]. The addiction medicine fellowship is a 12- to 24-month fellowship which can be accomplished after completing a residency in internal medicine, family medicine, or psychiatry. The American Society of Addiction Medicine (ASAM) supervised certification in Addiction Medicine from 1984–2008, after which time the American Board of Addiction Medicine (ABAM) administers the supervision of the certification. In March of 2016, the American Board of Medical Specialties recognized addiction medicine as a subspecialty under the American Board of Preventative Medicine.

Another specialty certification for addiction training is the field of addiction psychiatry. This fellowship is 12 to 24 months in duration and completed after a general psychiatry residency is completed. Addiction psychiatry certification first began in 1993 [20]. As of 2017, there are currently only 1959 board-certified addiction psychiatrists who maintain an active certification in the United States [21]. These fellowships have been established to further increase the knowledge and expertise of physicians to aid the treatment within the growing field of addictive disorders. These fellowships encompass 1 to 2 years of training in a variety of sites including inpatient and outpatient settings, as well as the completion of a board examination at the end of training.

Internationally, several other countries have adopted similar addiction training programs to help further train specialized physicians. Australia has established the Chapter of Addiction Medicine in 2001 through the Royal Australasian College of Physicians [22]. This training program involves 3 years of basic general medical training after internship followed by 3 years of discipline-specific supervised training. In the Netherlands, a 2-year curriculum has been established in the field of addiction medicine, which is open to all medical clinicians and not just psychiatrists [23].

Practicing Physician's Ability to Continue Education in Addiction

The medical field is a unique one in that the knowledge that is learned is never finalized. The medical field has evolving principles and new findings that will continue to change the landscape of how medicine is practiced. Independent practitioners who have completed training are required to complete continuing medical education, or CME, in the United States to maintain board certification [24]. These CME credits are given for a variety of educational opportunities, including online assessments, attending conferences, and attending lectures. Practicing physicians can also continue to further their knowledge in the treatment of addictions by attending a conference sponsored by the American Academy of Addiction Psychiatry, the American Psychiatric Association, or the American Society of Addiction Medicine.

Another innovation that has occurred is the ability for clinicians to be able to prescribe medication for medication-assisted treatment. Treatment for alcohol and nicotine use disorder does not require additional training or certifications. In 2000, the passage of the Drug Addiction Treatment Act allowed physicians to prescribe more outpatient treatments [20]. This includes buprenorphine, a medication that is used for opioid use disorder. Physicians in the United States can complete an 8-hour CME course with the AAAP, APA, or ASAM in order to be granted a waiver in order to prescribe buprenorphine. This waiver is another example of the benefit of clinicians continuing on their path of gaining knowledge about the ever-changing field of substance use disorders.

Potential Improvements in the Establishment of Medical Education

Even with the establishment of addiction medicine curriculum and improved exposure to addictive disorders assessment/treatments, there exists a discrepancy with clinicians and their ability to treat patients with substance use disorders. What can continue to account for this difference? One explanation can be clinicians having a negative view of addiction as a whole and the bias that can arise from having this view. We will begin with the discussion of how addiction has been viewed historically.

The field of addiction medicine has had several different models to help conceptualize the understanding of the disorder. Five basic models that are used to describe chemical dependency include the moral, learning, disease, self-medication, and the social model [25]. The oldest model that has been used is the moral model, and this includes the view of substance use as the result of moral weakness and a lack of willpower. A variant of the moral model is the spiritual model, which stresses a patient's substance use disorder is due to a misalignment with God and the universe. The spiritual model has been used by several 12-step groups such as Alcoholics Anonymous. One challenge from the moral model is that the clinician can develop an antagonist, judgmental relationship with the patient. The moral model can lead to countertransference, in which the clinician can place their views and judgments toward a patient in recovery [25]. Clinicians may have to replace the model that is held by the clinician, as it is best to meet the patient at the model that they are in. The disease model is one that can often be utilized to help explain for addiction as a disease. The disease model is based on genetic and other biological factors and does not focus on the lack of willpower or the lack of self-control. If clinicians could explain these models among themselves but also with patients, there could be less stigma being perceived by the patient. There is also a gap in the current literature regarding the moral model and outcomes among medical learners. Future areas for improvement could include increasing the awareness of the moral model among medical learners and potential biases that can arise.

Another potential improvement in the field of addiction medicine can be earlier intervention and exposure to substance abuse curriculum. A systematic review of 29 articles was conducted regarding addiction medicine curricula around the globe [26]. A finding that was present in nine articles in this study was that there was almost no undergraduate teaching in addiction medicine. This highlighted a need to teach about the potential signs and symptoms of substance use disorders prior to a medical learner beginning medical school. Earlier exposure and knowledge could help medical learners establish an interest in treating patients who suffer from addictive disorders.

Another area for potential improvement could be finding the best method to teach medical learners about addiction medicine. While in medical school, learners are often taught by professors in their first 2 years and by clinical faculty during their third and fourth year rotations. One analysis examined tobacco use dependence education around the world in a variety of medical schools. A 2008 global survey revealed that in 37 of 48 countries (78%), a formal didactic existed regarding tobacco cessation education [27]. In these 37 countries, the median course length was 16 hours, and a variety of methods were used to complete the didactics. These included lectures (98%), small groups sessions (94%), observed practice with clients (70%), one-on-one teaching (48%), and online training (25%). Medical learners can experience these methods to learn about substance use disorders during several rotations during their third year, although this occurs most often within their psychiatric clerkship [28]. It is important for medical learners to establish a solid foundation regarding substance use disorders, their treatments, and to view the addiction as a life-altering disorder that the patient is seeking aid for.

Residents often obtain their education through formal didactics and exposure to various cases. Psychiatry (95%) and family medicine residencies (75%) were the most likely to have a curriculum regarding substance abuse education [15]. A study conducted in 1999 revealed approximately 50% of other postgraduate residency programs had no substance abuse curriculum at all [28]. Residents are a key component to the treatment of substance use disorders as they have the ability to treat patients as well as provide medical learner education. Residents at several programs in the United States have undergone a training known as screening, brief intervention, and referral to treatment (SBIRT) [29]. This brief intervention includes routine screening for alcohol/drug use, performing a brief intervention for patients whose patterns of use can pose potential risks to health (i.e., advice to cut back or counseling to increase motivation for change), and referring to specialized addiction treatment programs for patients with severe substance use disorders. SBIRT has been shown to improve resident's knowledge/satisfaction [30] and confidence in treating patients with substance use disorders [31]. A study was conducted among all training programs, and SBIRT was able to be implemented across all fields of graduate medical education [32]. Resident education is a transitional role from medical learners to faculty, and this time can provide an opportunity for different interventions to be learned [33]. Residents also have the ability to practice certain aspects of treatment that they will carry forward with them when they complete training. One important aspect is keeping compassion, as patients with addictions can be easily overlooked by clinicians in terms of compassion. A lack of compassion can lead to a greater chance of not treating the patient adequately and to less likely to refer patients to the proper resources. It is most important to be cognizant of resident clinicians, as they are still able to change their practice habits easily. The compassion clinicians have with patients with addictive disorders can be limited, and this was evident in several faculty physicians.

Faculty clinicians in the field of medicine often have little education in the field of substance use disorders. There is a need for education in certain aspects of faculty clinicians, including both how addictive disorders are viewed and how the treatments are viewed. A survey of 149 internal medicine clinicians at a single institution in Boston was conducted in 2014 [34]. This survey consisted of both hospitalists and primary care clinicians who are assessed for their views with treating patients with substance disorders as well as views on substance use. Of the faculty surveyed, more than one-third of hospitalists felt that patients with addiction were making a choice and that substance use disorders were different than other chronic diseases. Another finding was that 12% of the hospitalists and 6% of primary care clinicians surveyed viewed that someone who had used drugs had committed a crime and deserved a punishment. The view a clinician has in terms of conceptualizing a disease can impact the stigma regarding the disease, and patients could be less likely to obtain care for a disorder if they perceive being stigmatized. This study revealed not only how faculty clinicians perceived substance use disorders but also how faculty viewed their treatment. The view the faculty have on treatments can impact the likelihood to refer a patient to treatment. In this study, 14% of the internists viewed opioid agonist treatment as replacing one addiction with another. This finding in a fairly recent survey was concerning as there have been decades of evidence showing the benefits of treating opioid use disorder with medication. A systemic change in the way substance use disorders are seen would have to be completed by faculty clinicians as they are often the guidance for future residents, students, and medical education.

Improvement can begin at increasing awareness at the undergraduate level, as well as changing the way clinicians see and treat addictive disorders. Teaching medical learners the five-model system earlier in their careers could also help to increase their awareness of which model the clinician is using. Lastly, improving the way addiction is viewed by the medical community can be beneficial for reducing a clinician's countertransference as well as increasing the clinician's willingness to treat a patient. Current medical learners are the most important group that can be targeted to change the way addiction is viewed and treated in the future.

References

1. Owens PL, et al. Co-occurrence of physical health conditions and mental health and substance use conditions among adult inpatient stays, 2010 versus 2014: statistical brief #240, Healthcare cost and utilization project (HCUP) statistical briefs. Rockville: Agency for Healthcare Research and Quality (US); 2006.
2. American Association of Medical Colleges. www.aamc.org. Accessed 17 Oct 2018.
3. Fee E. The first American medical school: the formative years. Lancet. 2015;385:1940–1.
4. Doctor of Medicine profession. https://medlineplus.gov/ency/article/001936.htm. Accessed 17 Oct 2018.
5. Ebert RH. Flexner's model and the future of medical education. Acad Med. 1992;67:737–42.
6. Hawk C, Hyland J, Rupert R, Colonvega M, Hall S. Report 11 of the council on medical education (A-07). AMA-ASSN. 2006;14:3.
7. Fleming M, Karry K, Davis A, Kropp S, Kahn R, Rivo M. Medical education about substance abuse changes in curriculum and faculty between 1976 and 1992. Acad Med. 1994;69:362–9.
8. Ayala EE, Roseman D, Winseman JS, Mason HRC. Prevalence, perceptions, and consequences of substance use in medical students. Med Educ Online. 2017;22:1392824.
9. Geller G, Levine DM, Mamon JA, Moore RD, Bone LR, Stokes EJ. Knowledge, attitudes, and reported practices of medical students and house staff regarding the diagnosis and treatment of alcoholism. JAMA J Am Med Assoc. 1989;261:3115–20.
10. Landy J, Hynes J, Checinski K, Crome IB. Knowledge of and attitudes to substance misuse in undergraduate British medical students. Drugs Educ Prev Policy. 2005;12:137–48.
11. Palma N. A medical student's education in addiction. Acad Psychiatry. 2015;39:342–3.
12. Hayes RB, Geller AC, Crawford SL, et al. Medical school curriculum characteristics associated with intentions and frequency of tobacco dependence treatment among 3rd year U.S. medical students. Prev Med (Baltim). 2015;72:56–63.
13. Martins SR, Paceli RB, Bussacos MA, Fernandes FLA, Prado GF, Lombardi EMS, Terra-Filho M, Santos UP. Effective tobacco control measures: agreement among medical students. J Bras Pneumol. 2017;43:202–7.
14. Saitz R, Friedmann PD, Sullivan LM, Winter MR, Lloyd-Travaglini C, Moskowitz MA, Samet JH. Professional satisfaction experienced when caring for substance-abusing patients: faculty and resident physician perspectives. J Gen Intern Med. 2002;17:373–6.
15. Isaacson JH, Fleming M, Kraus M, Kahn R, Mundt M. A national survey of training in substance use disorders in residency programs. J Stud Alcohol. 2000;61:912–5.
16. ACGME. ACGME program requirements for graduate medical education in psychiatry. Med Educ. 2017:1–13.
17. Ruff AL, Alford DP, Butler R, Isaacson JH. Training internal medicine residents to manage chronic pain and prescription opioid misuse. Subst Abus. 2017;38:200–4.

18. Parish SJ, Stein MR, Hahn SR, Goldberg U, Arnsten J. NIH public access. Subst Abus. 2013;34:1–10.
19. Billington M. EMRA fellowship guide. https://www.emra.org/books/fellowship-guide-book/addiction-medicine/. Accessed 23 Oct 2018.
20. Polydorou S, Gunderson EW, Levin FR. Training physicians to treat substance use disorders. Curr Psychiatry Rep. 2008;10:399–404.
21. Tongaat Hulett (2017) ABPN annual report. https://doi.org/10.1017/CBO9781107415324.004.
22. Haber PS, Murnion BP. Training in addiction medicine in Australia. Subst Abus. 2011;32:115–9.
23. De Jong C, Luycks L, Delicat J-W. The master in addiction medicine program in the Netherlands. Subst Abus. 2011;32:108–14.
24. ABPN. Maintenance of certification program enhancements. APBN. 2018. https://doi.org/10.3122/jabfm.19.2.211.
25. Brower KJ, Blow FC, Beresford TP. Treatment implications of chemical dependency models: an integrative approach. J Subst Abus Treat. 1989;6:147–57.
26. Ayu AP, Schellekens AFA, Iskandar S, Pinxten L, De Jong CAJ. Effectiveness and organization of addiction medicine training across the globe. Eur Addict Res. 2015;21:223–39.
27. Rigotti NA, Bitton A, Richards AE, Reyen M, Wassum K, Raw M. An international survey of training programs for treating tobacco dependence. Addiction. 2009;104:288–96.
28. Fleming MF, Manwell LB, Kraus M, Isaacson JH, Kahn R, Stauffacher EA. Who teaches residents about the prevention and treatment of substance use disorders? A national survey. J Fam Pract. 1999;48:725–9.
29. Pringle JL, Kowalchuk A, Meyers JA, Seale JP. Equipping residents to address alcohol and drug abuse: the national SBIRT residency training project. J Grad Med Educ. 2012;4:58–63.
30. Clemence AJ, Balkoski VI, Schaefer BM, et al. Multispecialty screening, brief intervention, and referral to treatment (SBIRT) training in an academic medical center: resident training experience across specialties. Subst Abus. 2016;37:356–63.
31. Whittle AE, Buckelew SM, Satterfield JM, Lum PJ, O'Sullivan P. Addressing adolescent substance use: teaching screening, brief intervention, and referral to treatment (SBIRT) and motivational interviewing (MI) to residents. Subst Abus. 2015;36:325–31.
32. O'Sullivan PS, Yuan P, Satre DD, Wamsley M, Satterfield J. A sequential implementation model for workforce development: a case study of medical residency training for substance use concerns. Teach Learn Med. 2018;30:84–94.
33. Ryan S, Pantalon MV, Camenga D, Martel S, D'Onofrio G. Evaluation of a pediatric resident skills-based screening, brief intervention and referral to treatment (SBIRT) curriculum for substance use. J Adolesc Health. 2018;63:327–34.
34. Wakeman SE, Pham-Kanter G, Donelan K. Attitudes, practices, and preparedness to care for patients with substance use disorder: results from a survey of general internists. Subst Abus. 2016;37:635–41.

Drug Abuse and Pain

21

Anil A. Thomas

Pain conditions and substance use disorder are dynamic conditions. Pain conditions are debilitating and also complex to manage. It can fluctuate in intensity based on physical, psychological, and social circumstances and also over time. Similarly, substance use disorders (SUD) can be debilitating and complex to manage. It can fluctuate from remission to relapse over time, and it can be influenced by physical, psychological, and social circumstances. These factors have both objective and subjective aspects to the patients, thus making assessing and effectively managing extremely challenging. People suffering from addiction are susceptible to chronic pain, and pain increases vulnerability to addiction [21]. To further complicate the treatment, caregivers may face pragmatic, ethical, and legal issues when managing patients with pain and SUD, as treatment of one condition can support or conflict with the treatment of the other [2]. However, as clinicians, we are best positioned to balance the treatment of pain against the risk of serious adverse outcomes, including addiction, unintentional overdose, and ultimately death.

Pain can be acute, acute intermittent, or chronic and these are not mutually exclusive. Pain is referred to as the "fifth vital sign" and has been broadly defined as "whatever the experiencing person says it is, existing whenever the person says it does," implying that it may involve more than a physical sensation (Ed Salsitz). Pain and the responses to pain can be shaped by culture, temperament, psychological state, memory, cognition, beliefs and expectations, co-occurring health conditions, gender, age, and other biopsychosocial factors [4]. Pain is both a sensory and an emotional experience and thus subjective in nature [4]. Most chronic pain is due to central sensitization and less due to peripheral nociception, and the diagnostic findings guiding decision-making is a patient report, thus increasing the risk of undertreating an actual pain syndrome or inappropriately supporting an addiction (Asam 98).

With injury nociceptors are excited, the stimulus travels to the dorsal horn of the spinal cord and subsequently travels to the brain along multiple pathways in the spinal cord. They terminate in the somatosensory cortex, where the pain is evaluated; the limbic system, where emotional reactions are mediated; the autonomic centers, where breathing, heart rate, and perspiration are mediated; and other parts of the brain where behavior to the stimulus is mediated [5]. Impulses to nearby terminals of the same nerve can lead to diffuse pain and the release of inflammatory substances, which are a protective response to tissue injury [5]. Nociceptive response also triggers pain-inhibiting responses, and this involves endorphins, enkephalins, gamma-amino butyric

A. A. Thomas (✉)
Department of Psychiatry, NYU Grossman School of Medicine, New York, NY, USA
e-mail: anil.thomas@nyulangone.org

E. Akerele (ed.), *Substance and Non-Substance Related Addictions*,
https://doi.org/10.1007/978-3-030-84834-7_21

acid, norepinephrine, serotonins, oxytocin, and relaxin [5].

Acute or chronic pain affect more than 30% of Americans [1, 6, 9]. Among older persons, the prevalence of chronic pain is higher [1, 6]. Given the prevalence of pain and its disabling effects, opioid analgesics are the most commonly prescribed class of medications in the USA [1, 11]; the highest rates of opioid prescriptions being in rural counties; the highest rates are among Whites and American Indians or Alaska Natives. Opioid analgesics relieve many types of acute pain and improve function; the benefits of opioids when prescribed for chronic pain are more debatable.

Addiction or substance use disorder by definition is a chronic, neurobiological disease with genetic (family history, child-rearing practices), developmental (early exposure especially during the vulnerable adolescent periods), psychological (mood disorder, attention-deficit hyperactivity disorders, anxiety disorders), social (poor social/familial supports at vulnerable times), and environmental (easy access of drugs and a permissive attitudes) influences factoring in its manifestation. It is overall characterized as impaired control over drug use, continued use despite harm, and cravings. The *Diagnostic and Statistical Manual of Mental Disorder V* (*DSM-V*) of mental disorder further defines it (Fig. 21.1).

Substance use disorders are complex, multistage diseases that are characterized by dysregulations in three neurocircuits: basal ganglia, binge/intoxication stage; extended amygdala, withdrawal/negative effect stage; and prefrontal cortex, preoccupation/anticipation stage. The rewarding effects of the substance emerge after neurons in the ventral tegmental area of the limbic system release the neurotransmitter dopamine into the nucleus accumbens. Other areas of the broader brain reward circuit exert influences including the amygdala, emotional valence; the hippocampus, memory; and the prefrontal cortex

Criteria for Substance Use Disorders
1. Taking the substance in larger amounts or for longer than you're meant to.
2. Wanting to cut down or stop using the substance but not managing to.
3. Spending a lot of time getting, using, or recovering from use of the substance.
4. Cravings and urges to use the substance.
5. Not managing to do what you should at work, home, or school because of substance use.
6. Continuing to use, even when it causes problems in relationships.
7. Giving up important social, occupational, or recreational activities because of substance use.
8. Using substances again and again, even when it puts you in danger.
9. Continuing to use, even when you know you have a physical or psychological problem that could have been caused or made worse by the substance.
10. Needing more of the substance to get the effect you want (tolerance).
11. Development of withdrawal symptoms, which can be relieved by taking more of the substance.

Fig. 21.1 APA DSM criteria

including the anterior cingulate and the orbital frontal cortex, executive function, and salience. The reward circuits within the brain are intensely interconnected, and thus multiple other areas, i.e., the insula and the cerebellum, add to the complexity of the addiction. Impaired signaling of dopamine and glutamate in the prefrontal regions of the brain weakens their ability to resist strong urges or to follow through on decisions to stop taking the substance [19].

Physical dependence is the physiological adaptation in the brain to taking an opioid regularly, defined broadly by the development of withdrawal signs and symptoms when the opioid is withdrawn. Physical dependence occurs within days of dosing with opioids, it varies among patients due to the individual metabolic variance and is a normal and expected response to continued opioid use. Physical dependence does not necessarily mean addiction. The risk factors for opioid-related aberrant behavior include family history of substance abuse: alcohol, illegal drugs, prescription drugs which carry greater risk; personal history of substance abuse; age range of 16–45 years; history of preadolescent sexual abuse especially in women; psychological disease including attention deficit disorder (ADD) and depression. An individual will not meet the *Diagnostic and Statistical Manual of Mental Disorder* (*DSM*) *V* criteria for substance use disorder if the individual only has physical dependence and tolerance with no aberrant behavioral patterns (Ed Salsitz).

Addiction and chronic pain share several risk factors including posttraumatic stress disorder, early childhood trauma, and adult trauma (Asam 98).

Pseudo-addiction is a behavior that mimics addictive behavior; however, this is the result of inadequate pain management rather than an addiction; the addictive behavior is extinguished when the pain is adequately controlled. Differentiating pseudo-addiction and addiction can be challenging and is usually done retrospectively (Asam 98).

Epidemiology data imply that persons with SUDs are at higher risk of developing chronic pain conditions; the converse also holds true [8]. The diagnosis of pain can also be complicated by SUDs as the patient may or may not appreciate the SUD. Similarly, pain complicates the diagnosis of SUD, and here again the patient might not recognize that a SUD has developed [8]. To further complicate the therapeutic relationship, patients may maximize pain complaints and minimize relief from alternative methods of therapies; the patient may believe they are entitled to pain relief; the caregiver may risk undertreating actual pain with the thought of not supporting a substance use disorder (Asam 98).

Over the last few decades, there has been a significant increase in the prescribing of opioids, resulting in a concomitant increase in prescription opioid-associated overdose deaths, emergency department visits, and admission to drug treatment centers. The CDC reports approximately 16,000 overdose deaths related to prescription opioids annually, and total poisoning deaths now outnumber motor vehicle accident deaths. (Ed Salsitz). Opioid and many more opioid prescription overdose deaths occur in men than women.

With proper diagnosis comes effective treatment. The goal of opioid therapy should be to improve and or stabilize pain intensity, improve function, and improve the quality of life. The Center for Disease Control and Prevention (CDC) Guideline for Prescribing Opioids for Chronic Pain [20] published in 2016 promotes non-opioid medications and non-pharmacological intervention as preferred when managing patients with chronic noncancer pain. They make 12 recommendations about opioid prescribing; non-opioid pharmacological therapy and non-pharmacological therapy are the preferred treatment for chronic pain; opioid should be used only when benefits for pain and functionality outweigh risks; before initiating opioid therapy the clinician establish realistic treatment goals; before initiating and periodically thereafter, discuss with the patient how the opioids will be discontinued if realistic benefits do not outweigh risks; immediate-release opioids instead of extended-release/long-acting (ER/LA) opioids should be prescribed for chronic pain therapy; opioid should be prescribed at the lowest-effective dosage; opioid should be prescribed at no greater quantity than needed; careful reassessment of benefits and risk when considering dosage increase; avoid concurrent opioids and benzodiazepine therapy; evaluate benefits and harms of continued opioid therapy every 3 months including reviewing the prescription monitoring program data; urine drug testing conducted before initiating and periodically thereafter to assess prescribed medications and other controlled substance; for patients with opioid use disorder, they should be offered evidence-based treatments including medication-assisted treatment (MAT) with buprenorphine or methadone [20]. The guidelines also indicate the lack of evidence in the efficacy of long-term opioid treatment.

General principles for safe opioid prescribing include a full and detailed history and physical examination with assessment of the risk versus the benefits of opioid treatment; obtain a written agreement or "contract" with established goals; stratify risk, monitoring, and treatment; check the prescription monitoring data (PMP) with each prescription; baseline urine drug test and thereafter do urine drug test and pill count as indicated; taper and discontinue if goals are not met; caution if dose is high; do not use concomitant sedatives hypnotics; and finally document all encounters in detail.

Shared comorbidities of chronic pain and addiction such as anxiety and depression, human suffering, financial problems, functional disability, cognitive disturbances, sleep disturbances, family and social problems, and secondary physical problems are commonly encountered and must be addressed concomitantly.

Conclusion

The treatment of acute pain with opioids is a common gateway for long-term opioid use. Opioid analgesic efficacy often declines with continuous use because of adaptation of dependence. Opioid use for chronic pain is open ended and usually requires higher doses than what is needed for acute pain or end-of-life pain. Chronic pain and addiction should be approached as chronic disease involving the reward, limbic, cortical, and associated areas of the brain and the peripheral nervous system, thus requiring a multi-model approach to treatment to improve outcomes and prevent debilitation and possibly death. Guidelines, principles, and criteria have been developed to help in optimizing results in patients with pain and drug abuse.

Bibliography

1. American Psychiatric Association. Diagnostic and statistical manual of mental disorders. Arlington: American Psychiatric Association; 2013.
2. Ballantyne J, Massachusetts General Hospital. The Massachusetts General Hospital handbook of pain management. 3rd ed. Philadelphia: Lippincott Williams & Wilkins; 2006.
3. Brookoff D. In: McCarberg B, Passik SD, editors. Chronic pain as a disease: the pathophysiology of disordered pain. Philadelphia: American College of Physicians; 2005.
4. Cheatle M, Comer D, Wunsch M, Skoufalos A, Reddy Y. Treating pain in addicted patients: recommendations from an expert panel. Popul Health Manag. 2014;17:79–89.
5. Dowell D, Haegerich TM, Chou R. CDC guideline for prescribing opioids for chronic pain--United States, 2016. JAMA. 2016;315:1624–45.
6. Flanagan O. The shame of addiction. Front Psych. 2013;4:1–11.
7. Herron AJ, Brennan T, American Society of Addiction Medicine. The ASAM essentials of addiction medicine. 3rd ed. Philadelphia: Wolters Kluwer Health/Lippincott Williams & Wilkins; 2020.
8. Koob GF, Volkow ND. Neurocircuitry of addiction. Neuropsychopharmacology. 2010;35:217–38.
9. Koob GF, Volkow ND. Neurobiology of addiction: a neurocircuitry analysis. Lancet Psychiatry. 2016;3:760–73.
10. Martin C, Comer D, Wunsch M, Skoufalos A, Reddy Y. Pain in addicted patients: recommendations from an expert panel. Popul. Health Manag. 2014;17(2):79–89.
11. Miller SC, Fiellin DA, Rosenthal RN, Saitz R, American Society of Addiction Medicine. The ASAM principles of addiction medicine. 6th ed. Philadelphia: Wolters Kluwer; 2019.
12. Odegaard S, Peller A, Shaffer HJ. Addiction as syndrome in paradigm. Fall. 2005;2005. pp. 12,13,22.
13. Prater CD, Zylstra RG, Miller KE. Successful pain management for the recovering addicted patient. Prim care companion. J Clin Psychiatry. 2002;4:125–31.

14. Quinan J, Cox F. Acute pain management in patients with drug dependence syndrome. Pain Rep. On Line. 2017:1–7.
15. Salsitz EA. Chronic pain, chronic opioid addiction: a complex Nexus. J Med Toxicol. 2016;12:54–7.
16. (US) SAAMHSA. Chronic pain in adults with or in recovery from substance use disorder. (TIP) CFSATTIP, 5 TN, editors. USA.
17. Tompkins DA, Hobelmann JG, Compton P. Providing chronic pain management in the "fifth vital sign" era: historical and treatment perspectives on a modern-day medical dilemma. Drug Alcohol Depend. 2017;173(Suppl 1):S11–21.
18. Volkow ND, Koob G. Brain disease model of addiction: why is it so controversial? Lancet Psychiatry. 2015;2:677–9.
19. Volkow ND, Koob GF, McLellan AT. Neurobiologic advances from the brain disease model of addiction. N Engl J Med. 2016;374:363–71.
20. Volkow ND, McLellan AT. Opioid abuse in chronic pain--misconceptions and mitigation strategies. N Engl J Med. 2016;374:1253–63.
21. Volkow ND, Michaelides M, Baler R. The neuroscience of drug reward and addiction. Physiol Rev. 2019;99:2115–40.

Index

E. Akerele (ed.), *Substance and Non-Substance Related Addictions*,
https://doi.org/10.1007/978-3-030-84834-7

MIX
Papier aus verantwortungsvollen Quellen
Paper from responsible sources
FSC® C105338

If you have any concerns about our products,
you can contact us on
ProductSafety@springernature.com

In case Publisher is established outside the EU,
the EU authorized representative is:
Springer Nature Customer Service Center GmbH
Europaplatz 3, 69115 Heidelberg, Germany

Printed by Libri Plureos GmbH
in Hamburg, Germany